NEUROANATOMY
A Conceptual Approach

C. Romero-Sierra, M.D., D.Sc.

Professor
Department of Anatomy
Queen's University
Kingston, Ontario
Canada

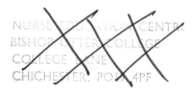
Churchill Livingstone
New York, Edinburgh, London, Melbourne
1986

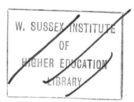

Library of Congress Cataloging-in-Publication Data

Romero-Sierra, C.
  Neuroanatomy: a conceptual approach.

  Bibliography: p.
  Includes index.
  1. Neuroanatomy. I. Title. [DNLM: 1. Nervous
System—anatomy & histology. WL 101 R763n]
QM451.R66   1986   611'.81   85-28060
ISBN 0-443-08361-4

Distributed in the United Kingdom by Churchill Livingstone, Robert Stevenson
House, 1-3 Baxter's Place, Leith Walk, Edinburgh EH1 3AF, and by associated
companies, branches, and representatives throughout the world.

Acquisitions Editor: *Gene C. Kearn*
Production Designer: *Charlie Lebeda*
Production Supervisor: *Joe Sita*
Cover Design: *Paul Moran*

Printed in the United States of America

First published in 1986

NEUROANATOMY

A Conceptual Approach

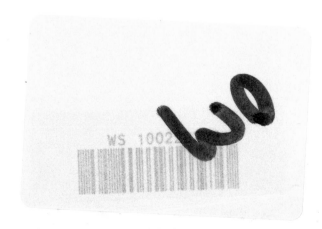

Dedicated to
Kerstin Bergström
and to past, present, and future
students, teachers, and writers of anatomy

Foreword

Some 3,000 years ago, Solomon, King of Israel, wrote: "Of the making of books there is no end." Further, we know that in recent years tens of thousands of books on medical sciences appear annually. Some of these are on the topic of neuroanatomy, and generally they are quite good. Against this realistic background, I began reading Dr. Romero-Sierra's new book as a courtesy.

Soon, I was truly amazed and delighted. Here is a truly original and highly useful book for students of neuroanatomy. Suddenly and with little or no fanfare, it leaps into the arena, and immediately it will become the champion.

What accounts for the great success this text is sure to enjoy? Perhaps one could cite the author's enormous experience and wide education—Dr. Romero-Sierra has doctorates in science, medicine, and psychiatry and has worked with distinguished mentors including Bror Rexed and Sten Skoglund in Uppsala, Sweden, and N.A. Buchwald at the Brain Research Institute at the University of California, Los Angeles. For two decades, he has taught neuroanatomy to medical students, graduate students, and other health professionals while carrying on a superb program of research projects.

All that is true, but it simply does not explain why he, and not another distinguished neuroscientist, has produced the best textbook of neuroanatomy. The book must speak for itself, and it does so brilliantly. No current textbook of neuroanatomy comes close to this one in its profound concern for the learning process of students. While many other books also have profuse illustrations, few of them are so tailored as to explain to the student the real significance of the matter being described in the text. The integration between the text and the great many specially drawn figures is unrivalled.

This book is written by a brilliant teacher with a true conceptual approach which appears to have been guided by an inspiration: the student's appreciation and learning from words and pictures form the object of the exercise. It does not rely on just "laying out the facts, take it or leave it," which many other authors seem to adopt. Nor does Dr. Romero-Sierra lay out the facts by gimmicks (a widely used approach); he explains the facts patiently and carefully. The student's learning process is the author's constant concern, and as a consequence, the result is brilliant.

This is a great textbook of neuroanatomy and I am thrilled to have had the good fortune of writing this foreword.

John V. Basmajian M.D., F.A.C.A., F.R.C.P.(C)
Professor of Anatomy and Medicine
McMaster University
Hamilton, Canada
President, American Association of Anatomists, 1985–86

Preface

The progress made in the neurosciences in the last few years is impressive. Neuroanatomy is part of an exciting domain of study and our time is witnessing a discipline which is developing before our very eyes. Awesome technological advances are making it possible to investigate increasingly finer neuroanatomical details. Yet we seem to have just begun to learn about what is perceived to be nature's most sophisticated life-form: the human brain.

Neuroanatomy: A Conceptual Approach is written for medical and other health science students as an introduction to neuroanatomy. The nervous system is composed of complex entities intricately interrelated and functioning as an integrated system. In approaching the study of the nervous system, students are well advised to learn about the simple concepts of the nervous system components first and the integrated structures and functions later, and I have used this approach in the organization of the text.

The book is divided into five sections, beginning with the evolutionary development of the nervous system and a description of the basic cellular components. Next the basic anatomical structures are described followed by a review of the various nervous system tracts. The fourth section classifies the structures by function and emphasis is given to the performance of the system as units at all levels of the nervous system. Lastly, the integration of the nervous system is considered, with chapters covering the central nervous system as a visceral unit, the cerebral cortex as an analytical integrating entity, the vascular supply of the system, and the role of neurotransmitters.

Examples of malfunction and their relation to structural lesions are presented throughout the text only when they serve to reinforce the understanding of basic concepts.

Given the individual and distinct scope of the curriculum in each university program, different teachers choose to stress different topics within a course in neuroanatomy. This book hopes to "cover the bases" by providing a basic text suitable for any university course that teaches neuroanatomy.

Visualization is indispensable in the study of neuroanatomy, and more than 500 drawings illustrate the text. In order not to overwhelm the students, the labels to the figures, with few exceptions, have been limited to structures described in the text.

The references given at the end of each chapter provide other sources related to the topic of the chapter in part or as a whole. Moreover, at the end of the book are two lists of references, one regarding recommended textbooks of neuroanatomy and related topics and the other regarding atlases.

My more than 20 years of dedication to the teaching of neuroanatomy underlie this text. Throughout the years my students have helped improve the manuscript with their criticisms and suggestions. I want especially to thank the now practicing physicians, Drs.

Susan A. Halter, Peter Lane, and Jerry Tan, as well as Dr. Marc R. Marien and Miss Edi Alvarez. My colleagues Drs. Richard I. Barnett, Roland J. Boegman, Henry B. Dinsdale, David C. House, David M. Robertson, and Anders Sima have made valuable suggestions after reading the draft, and I wish to express to them my deep gratitude.

To the illustrators, Miss Joan Bennett, Mrs. Susan Clow, Mr. Ralph Idema, Mrs. Marie Lehman, Mrs. Shelley Lupu-Krehm, Mr. Stan Morton, and Mr. Henry Verstappen, who patiently labored to align the illustrations with the demands of the text, I am sincerely thankful.

At Queen's University the staff of the Visual Aids Centre and the Departments of Medical Photography and Medical Arts worked diligently to contribute to this book, and I would like to acknowledge my appreciation for their able assistance.

Finally I wish to thank the staff of Churchill Livingstone, especially Gene Kearn, Donna Balopole, and Charlie Lebeda, for all their assistance in the production of this book.

C. Romero-Sierra, M.D., D.Sc.

Acknowledgments

I wish to acknowledge the following authors and publishers for their courtesy:

Almquist and Wiksell, Stockholm
Eccles TC (1966): Functional organization of the
cerebellum in relation to its role in motor control.
In Granit R, Ed: Muscular Afferents and Motor
Control, First Nobel Symposium. (Figure 15-14A)

Blakiston Company, Philadelphia
Krieg WJS (1942): Functional Neuroanatomy. (Figure 18-10B)

WH Freeman and Company, San Francisco
Bullock TH, Orkand R, Grinnell A (1977):
Introduction to Nervous Systems. (Figure 4-11)

Hafner Publishing Company, New York
Wolf-Heidegger G (1962): Atlas of Systematic (Figures 5-12
Human Anatomy. and 5-14)

Harper & Row, Publishers, Philadelphia
Barr M, Kiernan JA (1983): The Human Nervous (Figures 6-23,
System: An Anatomical Viewpoint. Fourth Edition. 6-24, and 6-25)

Little, Brown and Company, Boston
Daube JR, Sandok BA (1978): Medical Neurosciences:
An Approach to Anatomy, Pathology, and Physiology (Figures 21-1
by Systems and Levels. and 22-1)

McGraw-Hill Book Company, New York
House EL, Pansky B (1967): A Functional Approach
to Neuroanatomy. (Figure 5-16)

Mohr JP, Fisher CM, Adams RD (1980): Cerebrovascular
diseases. In Iselbacher KJ, Adams RD, Braunwald E,
et al, Eds: Harrison's Principles of Internal
Medicine. Ninth Edition. (Figure 22-22)

Oxford University Press, New York
Brodal A (1981): Neuroanatomical Anatomy in (Figures 5-18
Relation to Clinical Medicine. Third Edition. and 17-5)

WB Saunders Company, Philadelphia
Bloom W, Fawcett D (1975): A Textbook of
Histology. Tenth Edition. (Courtesy of D. Kent   (Figures 4-9
Morest.)   and 4-14)

Curtis BA, Jacobson S, Marcus EM (1972): An   (Figures 11-2
Introduction to the Neurosciences.   and 11-3)

Fulton JF (1955): A Textbook of Physiology.   (Figure 16-4)

McDowell FH (1979): Cerebrovascular diseases.
In Beeson PB, McDermott W, Eds: Textbook of
Medicine. Fifteenth Edition.   (Figure 22-23)

Williams PL, Warwick R (1975): Functional   (Figures 5-15
Neuroanatomy of Man.   and 9-13B)

Springer-Verlag, New York
Heimer L (1983): The Human Brain and Spinal Cord: (Figures 15-14B,
Functional Neuroanatomy and Dissection Guide.   15-15 and 16-1)

Urban & Schwarzenberg, Baltimore
Sobotta J (1978): Atlas of Human Anatomy.   (Figure 5-11)

Williams & Wilkins, Baltimore
Carpenter MB (1976): Human Neuroanatomy. Seventh
Edition.   (Figure 9-16)

Contents

V. Integration

I

Introduction

1

Phylogeny

Life

Primitive unicellular organisms like the **amoeba** (Fig. 1-1) do not have a nervous system. Nevertheless, they manage two basic vital functions: to accept or to avoid stimuli from the environment. The structure of the amoeba is simple, and it involves itself in unelaborate interactions with its environment. It accepts a pleasant stimulus, e.g., food which it engulfs, and shuns an unpleasant one, e.g., a toxin, which it tries to avoid. It is entirely dependent on its environment and dies if removed from its medium.

The **vorticella** (Fig. 1-2) has a fibrous stem that enables it to contract, for instance, when it is in danger. In order to obtain nutrients, it uses its cilia to move a continuous stream of water across its oral aperture. These are examples of organisms that can live only in particular environments with which they can interact. In fact, this can be expressed as a universal law of the plant and animal kingdoms: **Life** is the active interplay between organisms and their environment. This concept is central in neuroanatomy, because the nervous system develops for this very reason, i.e., it feeds upon and fosters the interaction between the organism and its environment.

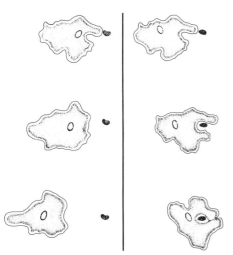

Fig. 1-1. Amoeba rejecting a stimulus (left) and accepting one (right).

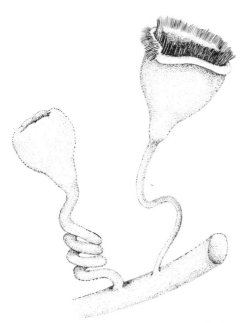

Fig. 1-2. Two vorticellae, one extended and one contracted.

Cell Specialization

The **specialization** of cells for specific functions within an organism is advantageous for the organism. It increases its economy and efficiency. This specialization regarding structure and function of cells is far from being completely under-

stood, and much is to be gained in this area from continued investigation.

Higher in the phylogenetic scale in coelenterates like the **hydra** (Fig. 1-3), the organisms develop a set of cells, primitive neurons, which are specialized in receiving stimuli and transmitting them to other cells. Structurally, primitive neurons have a cell body and processes that are spread throughout the organism, forming a network (primitive nervous system). This cell specialization is a further improvement in the evolution of the organism and results in an improved capacity to sense, accept, and avoid stimuli offered by the environment.

Neurons and Neural Network

The nervous system consists of cells that are called **neurons.** These, more so than any other type of cell, vary enormously in size and shape.

The neuronal cell consists of a **body** and **processes.** These processes are arranged to permit the cell to receive, conduct, and

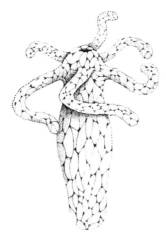

Fig. 1-3. Neural network of hydra.

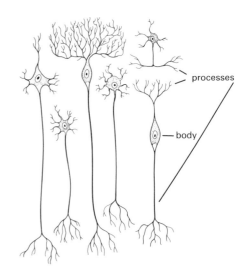

Fig. 1-4. Some shapes of neurons.

transmit stimuli to another cell or cells (Fig. 1-4).

Although the **neural network** of a hydra is an evolutionary improvement over a simpler form of life, it still has limitations. A major one is that it lacks an auxiliary system of cells to facilitate the conduction and transmission of stimuli. The network itself is rudimentary; in fact, it offers resistance to the passage of a signal initiated by the stimulus, thereby decreasing its intensity as it travels farther away from the source.

Another limitation of the neural network is that the signals become diffused through the network, and the ability of the organism to pinpoint the source of the stimulus is lacking in precision.

Glial Cells

In higher organisms, the neurons gain efficiency through special **glial** (Gr. *glia* glue) **cells** (Fig. 1-5). These surround the neurons, adhering to their surfaces and helping to resolve the problem of resistance to the passage of excitation. The neurons and glial cells establish a structural and functional symbiotic union of mutual benefit as long as both kinds of cells remain healthy.

There are different sizes and shapes of glial cells. Those of the human nervous system outnumber the neurons 10 to 1 and constitute two-thirds of its volume, while the neurons account for the remaining third.

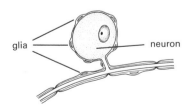

Fig. 1-5. Glial cells covering a neuron.

Centralization

When nature improves on the neural network of the hydra in higher organisms like the **earthworm** (Fig. 1-6), again the laws of economy are applied. In the earthworm, many neuronal cell bodies are placed in the center of the organism, thus saving the paths of the connecting processes.

Figure 1-6A represents an organism in which four points of the body surface are interconnected. Each point represents a nerve cell that may communicate with the other three. In Figure 1-6B the neurons are placed in the center of the organism. Each nerve cell still manages the same number of connections and the same volume of information as before, but a large amount of connecting material or wiring has been saved.

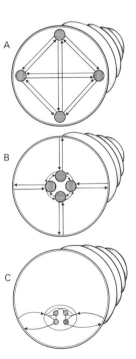

Fig. 1-6. Centralization. (A) Peripheral network; (B) central network; (C) schematic representation of the nervous system of the earthworm.

This change in the basic design of the nervous system is very significant and reflected in the name—the **central nervous system**—where its structural elements, the neurons, are concentrated close to each other. This process of **centralization** vastly improves the economy and efficiency in the operation of the nervous system. The geometrical circumstances that produce economy of wiring have already been mentioned. Efficiency is gained, because in this system impulses reach their destination quicker, as the neurons are closer to one another. Thus time is saved and risk of errors or damage to the neuronal structures is reduced. Nature is neither luxuriously generous nor mean, but economical; because where and when an organism is not economical, life for it ends.

Centralization of the nervous system occurs in worms and all other animals higher on the phylogenetic scale.

Afferents (Sensory), Efferents (Motor): Loops

Some peripheral neurons specialize in conducting the detected stimuli in the form of impulses from the periphery toward the center of the organism. These are called **afferent neurons** (L. *afferere* to

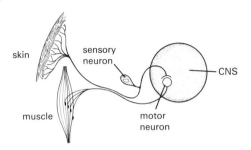

Fig. 1-7. Sensorimotor loop, also called pathway or circuit.

carry toward) and also **sensory neurons,** because they sense stimuli in the environment (Fig. 1-7).

Other neurons that have their cell bodies in the central nervous system specialize in conducting impulses transmitted to them in the central nervous system toward the periphery to reach a muscle or a gland. These are called **efferent neurons** (L. *efferere* to carry away). They are also called **motor neurons,** as the majority creates movement by causing muscle cells to contract.

The nervous system of earthworms, and even more deservedly that of higher animals, can be considered as a set of **circuits** or **loops.** One of these circuits is made up of a sensory neuron and a motor neuron. The connection between these neurons for the transmission of a neural impulse is called a **synapse** (Gr. *synapsis* contact) (Fig. 1-8).

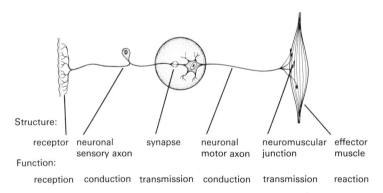

Structure:					
receptor	neuronal sensory axon	synapse	neuronal motor axon	neuromuscular junction	effector muscle
Function:					
reception	conduction	transmission	conduction	transmission	reaction

Fig. 1-8. Components of a two-neuron circuit.

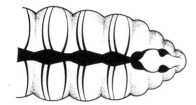

Fig. 1-9. Segmental body and neural pattern of earthworm.

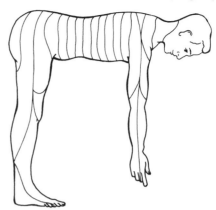

Fig. 1-10. Segmental innervation of the human body.

Segmentation

The schematic diagram of the body of an earthworm and certain aspects of its nervous system illustrates that (1) the earthworm is built up of **body segments,** (2) each body segment contains a **nervous system segment** of its own, and (3) each nervous system segment has circuits as described above (sensory—synapse—motor).

If the surface of one segment is stimulated, the sensory neurons of this segment transmit a signal through synapses to motor neurons of the same segment; in turn, the motor neurons produce a response in that segment. The repetitive organization of this segmental pattern in all higher animals is called **segmentation,** which hence is the organization of the human nervous system, i.e., a segmental cord (Figs. 1-9 and 1-10).

The simple concept of segmentation is very important in medicine, e.g., in the exploration of the nervous system and the diagnosis of its diseases. Since there is a close correlation between a segment of the body and its nerve supply, it is possible to localize a lesion of a specific segment of the nervous system simply by observing abnormalities of the corresponding body segment. If one knows the normal response to the stimulation of the surface of each segment, one can find which area of the nervous system is damaged by detecting an abnormal response. For example, if we touch the eye of a normal person with a wisp of cotton, the subject will blink; fail-ure to blink in response to such a stimulus may indicate a lesion in the neural circuit of the eye.

Interneurons and Intercircuit Message Paths

The neural segments are dependent on each other in order to function in a coordinated manner. Therefore, neural connections are established between the segments by means of **interneurons** and **intersegmental paths.**

In Figure 1-11 we recognize the sensory neuron (SN), the synapse (SY), and the motor neuron (MN). An interneuron (I) of this segment receives information from the sensory neuron of the same segment and then transmits this message to other neurons of adjacent segments.

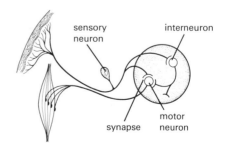

Fig. 1-11. Three neurons and pathways.

This does not mean, however, that all segments react to the same stimulus in the same way. For instance, not all muscles in these circuits contract equally. One and the same stimulus may inhibit the contraction of certain muscles while causing other muscles to contract. This is due to the nature of synaptic contact; some synapses enhance and others inhibit the excitability of the neuron. Thus the interneuron acts as a gate, either permitting or preventing passage of an impulse.

The interneuron can also perform in a more complex way. It may act as an amplifier (excitatory) by enhancing or as an attenuator (inhibitory) by putting a damper on an incoming signal, or it may act as a polarity reversal switch, transforming a positive signal into a negative one or vice versa.

Visceral and Somatic Nervous Systems

The **visceral nervous system** is that part of the nervous system that innervates the viscera, blood vessels, and glands. It can be subdivided into **visceral sensory, visceral intercalary,** and **visceral motor** systems (Fig. 1-12).

The **somatic** (Gr. *soma* body) **nervous system** is that part of the nervous system that innervates the body, e.g., skin, skeletal muscles, but not the viscera, blood vessels, or glands. It can also be subdivided into **somatic sensory, somatic intercalary,** and **somatic motor systems** (Fig. 1-12).

Glands and, even to a larger extent, blood vessels are found throughout the whole body, in skin (glands and vessels) and skeletal muscles (vessels). These two subsystems of the nervous system, i.e., the somatic and the visceral, spread through the body, each with its own function but in harmony with the other. For instance, the somatic nervous system is concerned with the tactile sense of the skin, whereas the visceral nervous system is involved with the supply of blood to the skin or the secretion of sweat.

Integration— Encephalization

Nature succeeds with greater perfection in terms of economy and efficiency in elongated animals by giving them a favored direction of displacement. Thus the buccal end of an organism consistently comes into contact first with the environment. Naturally, there is great advantage in developing sensors here, as well as centralizing the decision-making apparatus fed by these sensors.

In higher animals, the eyes, nose, and ears are placed near the mouth to permit quick transfer of information from one sense organ to another through nervous tissue inside the head to check and recheck each bit of information. This mass of nervous tissue needs to receive information from all the segments of the body in order to "know" how the body is positioned, and it has to send down command signals to the body to move it as needed in a coordinated manner. The more connections there are established between the nervous tissue concerned with the sense organs of the head and the segmental cord, the more the nervous tissue in the head develops. Billions of interneurons are developed to coordinate all the information in an effort

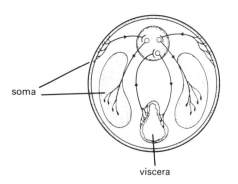

Fig. 1-12. Somatic and visceral sensorimotor loops.

to act as an integrating force in the operation of the nervous system as a unit.

The most highly developed part of the nervous system is the **encephalon** (Fig. 1-13) (Gr. *enkephalos* **brain**), the dynamic process of which is called **encephalization.** It consists of the accumulation of cells concerned with inter- and multisegmental relations to centralize, coordinate, and integrate the activities of all the segments.

The Human Nervous System and its Main Divisions

The human nervous system is divided into the **peripheral nervous system (PNS)** and the **central nervous system (CNS).**

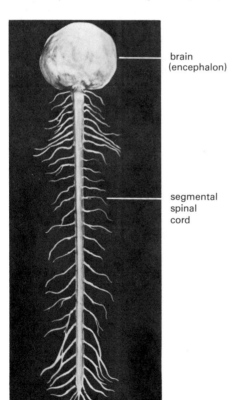

Fig. 1-13. Human nervous system.

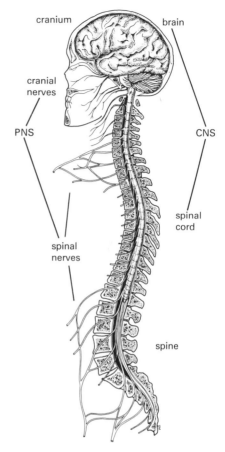

Fig. 1-14. Nervous system components.

The peripheral nervous system is that part of the nervous tissue which extends to and from the central nervous system and its bony enclosures. It appears as threads, called **nerves,** to and from the central nervous system and extends to the periphery of the body. The nerves connected with the brain and passing through the cranium are the **cranial nerves,** and those connected with the spinal cord are the **spinal nerves.** The nerves leave the skull or the spinal canal through special orifices called **foramina** (L. *foramen* opening, hole).

The structure of the central nervous system is enclosed in bone. The part that is contained in the **cranium** is called **brain** or **encephalon,** and the part contained in the **vertebral column,** or **spine,** is called **spinal**

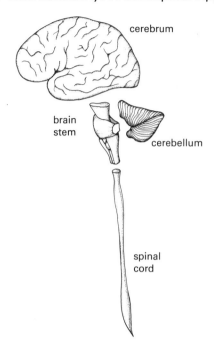

Fig. 1-15. Divisions of the CNS.

Table 1-1. The Main Structures and Functional Areas of the Human Nervous System

CNS

Cerebrum
  Feelings, thoughts, highest control of all functions
Brain stem
  Basic vital functions, e.g., respiration rate, heart beat, sleep; sensory and motor components of the head and their control
Cerebellum
  Equilibrium, posture, locomotion
Spinal cord
  Sensory and motor components of the body and their control

PNS

Cranial nerves
  Conductors toward or away from the brain
Spinal nerves
  Conductors toward or away from the spinal cord

Thus the main structures and functional areas of the human nervous system are as shown in Table 1-1.

Planes of Orientation— Topographical Terms

The position of a person standing with arms hanging, palms facing anteriorly, and the head looking straight forward (Fig. 1-16) is called the **anatomical position.** In this position, the **horizontal, frontal (coronal),** and **sagittal** planes of orientation can be drawn. The frontal and sagittal planes are longitudinal, vertical planes that are perpendicular to the horizontal planes. The sagittal plane along the midline is usually referred to as **median** or **midsagittal,** whereas planes parallel to it are called **parasagittal** planes. The intersection of the midfrontal and midsagittal planes defines the midline.

The following adjectives describe the

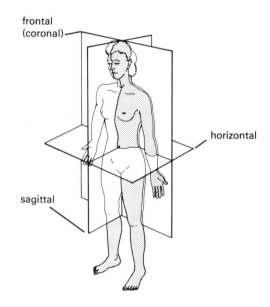

Fig. 1-16. Planes of orientation in anatomical position.

cord, because of its shape and position (Fig. 1-14). The brain can be subdivided into **forebrain,** or **cerebrum, brain stem,** and **cerebellum** (L. dim. *cerebrum* little brain) (Fig. 1-15).

relative position of a structure in the human nervous system:

medial—close to or toward the midsagittal plane
lateral—away from the midsagittal plane, i.e., to the sides
posterior—in the back, behind the mid-frontal plane
anterior—in the front, in front of the mid-frontal plane
superior—high, up, above
inferior—low, down, below

Due to the differences in position between man in a vertical position on his two legs and animals in a horizontal position on four legs, there is sometimes understandable confusion in the terminology regarding orientation in cases where terms which have originated in veterinary or comparative anatomy have spilled over into the terminology of human anatomy and vice versa. For instance, anterior in human anatomy means "in the chest or belly" and also "in the face" (Fig. 1-17). The same word means "in the head or face" in the dog.

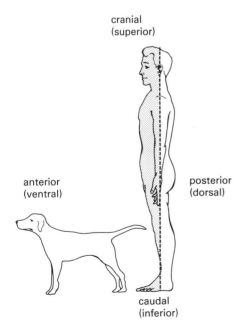

cranial
(superior)

anterior
(ventral)

posterior
(dorsal)

caudal
(inferior)

Fig. 1-17. Topographical terminology.

Other terms that may be unclear depending on the context are

caudal—on the tail, toward the tail
dorsal—on the back
ventral—on the belly

Proper correlation of these terms in human anatomy is as follows:

caudal—inferior, in an inferior position (direction)
dorsal—posterior, behind
ventral—anterior, in front

Other terms to denote position in human anatomy are

rostral—in the face
ipsilateral—on the same side
contralateral—on the opposite side
bilateral—on both sides

To indicate direction there are terms like **afferent**—conducting toward; **efferent**—conducting away from.
The suffix -ad, which also indicates direction, is sometimes used: caudal or **caudad**—toward the tail; cephalic or **cephalad**—toward the head.
Other terms regarding orientation are

stereotaxis—pertaining to or characterized by precise positioning in space
stereotaxy—procedure for localizing and inserting instruments into a precise area of the brain without exposing it
stereology—the three-dimensional definition of a feature in space
topography—the mapping of the structural features of a region

This terminology will be further explained in Chapter 2.

Arterial Vascular Supply to the Brain

Fifty trillion cells form the adult human body. The brain is made up of one trillion cells. It weighs 1.4 kg and constitutes 2

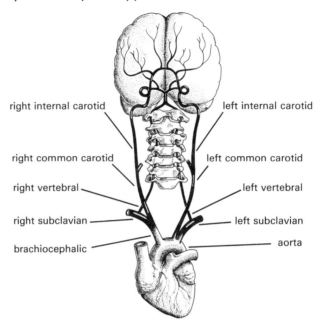

Fig. 1-18. Arterial trees to the brain.

percent of the body's total weight. This 2 percent receives 20 percent of the blood pumped from the heart to the body; it requires 20 percent of all the oxygen supplied to the body and 20 percent of the calories supplied to the body as glucose. Improper diet, faulty respiration, or impaired blood circulation to the brain may cause emotional instability. Vascular insufficiency to the brain may result in unconsciousness in 5 to 10 seconds and irreversible damage after 3 to 8 minutes.

Accurate knowledge of the vascular supply to the nervous system is important, because many disturbances of nervous system functions arise as a consequence of impaired circulation.

The cerebral circulation depends first and foremost on adequate pumping action of the heart. It is important to recognize that any obstruction in any of the extracranial branches of the blood supply to the brain can result in circulatory insufficiency to the brain. The symptoms of such a disorder will be evident in the brain long before they appear in other tissues supplied by the arteries.

The four main arteries supplying the brain (Fig. 1-18) are

1. the **right internal carotid artery** (branch of the **right common carotid artery,** in turn a branch of the **brachiocephalic artery**);
2. the **left internal carotid artery** (branch of the **left common carotid,** a branch of the **aorta**);
3. the **right vertebral artery** (a branch of the **right subclavian artery**); and
4. the **left vertebral artery** (a branch of the **left subclavian artery**).

Neural Pathways

A **neural pathway** is a chain of neural cells (two or more) linked together to convey a signal from one part of the body to another.

The sensorimotor segmental loops are

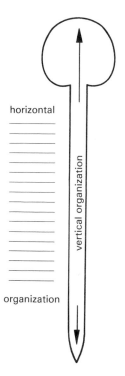

horizontal

vertical organization

organization

Fig. 1-19. Segmental and ascending-descending loops.

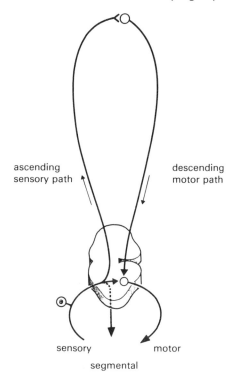

ascending
sensory path

descending
motor path

sensory

motor

segmental

Fig. 1-20. Organizational arrangements of neural pathways.

called **horizontal pathways.** They conduct the input from the exterior and the output to the exterior.

The **ascending sensory paths** and the **descending motor paths** within the CNS are called **vertical pathways** that along their course connect different regions of the central nervous system (Fig. 1-19).

Sound anatomical knowledge of the horizontal and vertical organizations of the human nervous system and their coupling is fundamental for diagnosis in clinical neurology.

1. one branch (the horizontal) for the segment it enters;
2. one descending branch (the descending vertical) to establish contact with segments below; and
3. one ascending branch (the ascending vertical) to establish contact with segments above and to link together with the vertical motor (descending) pathways (Fig. 1-20).

The horizontal motor processes exiting the spinal cord and the brain stem constitute the final motor path.

Spinal Cord: Input-Output Signals and Their Paths

The sensory processes entering the spinal cord give off three branches, i.e.,

Classification of the Nervous System

To ease the task of understanding the nervous system, one can make use of various classifications, e.g., (1) the central nervous system and (2) the peripheral nervous system. Another classification is (1) the somatic nervous system and (2) the visceral nervous system. Yet another classification identifies only portions of the nervous system, for example, in terms like *thermoregulatory system, nociceptive system,* and **auditory system.**

In the study of these systems, one must take into careful consideration the segmental (horizontal) and vertical components.

Historical Perspective of Neurosciences

In any developing scientific field a historical perspective of related acquired knowledge is of great importance not only for a proper evaluation of what is considered known but also for what is still to be explored. The history of the neurosciences is readily available in the literature, and in this text only some general annotations to the historical perspective are made here:

In the last fifty years no other scientific field has grown faster than the neurosciences.

The number of scientists active in this field is now larger than in any other.

This area is the most complex and fascinating one, attracting the interest, efforts, and expertise of scientists from all disciplines.

The rate of discoveries made in this sphere of work keeps increasing.

Every neuroscientist is aware of our still profound and fundamental ignorance of the subject matter.

The task ahead to explore fully this territory is awesome, and society's need for this knowledge is imperative.

There is room for any one at every level of knowledge and expertise to contribute in this field. If 20 percent of the efforts generated by mankind were concentrated on studying how man actually functions in the fine-tuning of his complexities, we would be establishing a parallel to what nature does by providing 20 percent of the body's oxygen supply to the brain.

Suggested Readings

Basmajian JV: Primary Anatomy. Eighth Edition. Williams and Wilkins, Baltimore, pp. 297–347, 1982.

Bogoch S, Ed.: The Future of the Brain Sciences, Plenum Press, New York, 1969.

Bullock TH, Orkand R, Grinnell A: Introduction to Nervous Systems, WH Freeman and Co., San Francisco, 1977.

Cotman CW, McGaugh JL: Behavioral Neuroscience: An Introduction, Academic Press, New York, pp. 1–2, 1980.

Heym C, Forssmann WG, Eds.: Techniques in Neuroanatomical Research, Springer-Verlag, Heidelberg, 1980.

Jacobson M: Developmental Neurobiology, Developmental Biology Series, Holt, Rinehart and Winston, Inc., New York, 1970.

McLoughlin JC: Archosauria, A New Look at the Old Dinosaur, Viking Press, New York, 1979.

Ranson SW, Clark SL: The Anatomy of the Nervous System, WB Saunders, Philadelphia, pp. 1–19, 1964.

Sarnat HB, Netsky MG: Evolution of the Nervous System. Second Edition. Oxford University Press, New York, 1981.

Shepherd GM: Neurobiology, Oxford University Press, New York, pp. 3–45, 1983.

Sidman RL, Sidman M: Neuroanatomy, a Programmed Text, Vol. 1, Little, Brown and Co., Boston, 1965.

Williams PL, Warwick R: Functional Neuroanatomy of Man, WB Saunders, Philadelphia, pp. 746–765, 1975.

2

Ontogeny

Ontogeny is the development of an organism from its beginning to its maturity, i.e., from the fertilized cell to the adult form.

When following the development of the human (**human ontogeny**), within the first embryonic week one observes the formation of three layers: the **ectoderm, mesoderm,** and **endoderm** (Fig. 2-1).

A thickening of the dorsal ectoderm, called the **neural plate,** appears in the sixteenth embryonic day. It invaginates and forms the **neural groove.** By the twenty-first day it starts to form the **neural tube** as well as the **neural crests,** which are **neuroectodermal cells** left dorsolaterally in clusters along the outside of the tube (Fig. 2-1).

The tubular structure is the beginning of the central nervous system. The neural tube grows in length and width. Its cephalic portion grows the most and in such a manner that the tube develops three **primary vesicles** (Fig. 2-2A):

1. The uppermost cephalic vesicle is called the **prosencephalon** or **forebrain.**
2. The middle vesicle is called the **mesencephalon** or **midbrain.**
3. The lower vesicle is called the **rhombencephalon** or **hindbrain.**

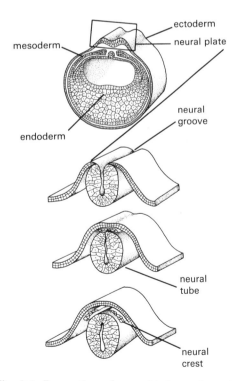

Fig. 2-1. Formation of neural tube and crests.

15

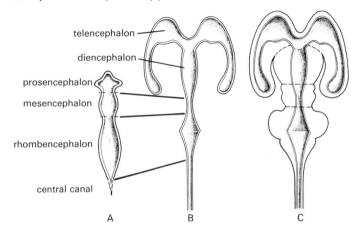

Fig. 2-2. Brain vesicles.

More caudally, the remaining portion of the neural tube with its cavity, the so-called **central canal,** does not change to any large extent.

During the fifth embryonic week, **secondary vesicles** form. The prosencephalon develops two vesicles on each side of its rostral end, thus changing the shape of the structure and motivating an expansion of the related nomenclature (Fig. 2-2B and C). The two lateral vesicles, left and right, together called the **telencephalon** (Gr. *telos* end), grow more than the other vesicles.

The middle portion is called the **diencephalon** (Gr. *dia* through) or **interbrain.**

For the understanding of these vesicles and their terminology it is important to first study the cavities of them as a system, i.e., the **vesicular ventricular system,** and,

subsequently, the walls of these cavities in their final adult stage as generators of nervous tissue.

Ventricular System

The cavities of the telencephalon are the **right** and **left lateral ventricles.** These ventricles are roughly C-shaped and consist of a body, an **atrium** (L. hall), and projections, which are called the **anterior, posterior,** and **inferior horns** (Fig. 2-3).

The cavity of the diencephalon is called the **third ventricle.** This is a narrow slit-like ventricle situated in the midline (Fig. 2-4).

Each lateral ventricle communicates

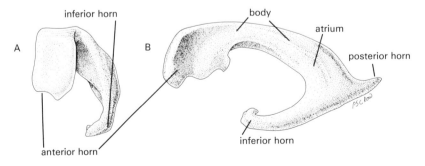

Fig. 2-3. Left lateral ventricle. (A) Frontal view; (B) lateral view.

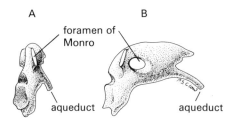

Fig. 2-4. Third ventricle. (A) Frontal view; (B) lateral view.

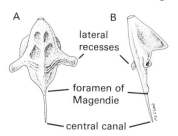

Fig. 2-5. Fourth ventricle. (A) Frontal view; (B) lateral view.

with the third ventricle through the **interventricular foramen** (L. hole, opening; pl. **foramina**) **of Monro** (Fig. 2-4).

The cavity of the mesencephalon is narrow and appears as a canal or **aqueduct** (Fig. 2-4). It is variously called **aqueduct of the mesencephalon, aqueduct of Sylvius, aqueduct of the midbrain, cerebral aqueduct,** or simply aqueduct.

The cavity of the rhombencephalon is called the **fourth ventricle.** It appears rhomboid-shaped from an anterior view and as a distorted pyramid from a lateral view. It has two recesses, the **right** and **left lateral recesses,** with openings called the **foramina of Luschka.** In the midline posteromedially it has another opening called the **foramen of Magendie** or **median aperture of the fourth ventricle** (Fig. 2-5).

The aqueduct permits communication between the third and fourth ventricles (Fig. 2-6).

The fourth ventricle continues inferiorly with the central canal (Fig. 2-6).

The fourth ventricle is the only ventricle with openings to the surface of the brain (Fig. 2-6A and B). These openings are the lateral foraminal and the foramen of Magendie.

Note: To understand why these vesicles were numbered third and fourth, one must be aware that in older times the lateral ventricles were known as the first and second ventricles. Hence the four brain ventricles were then numbered as follows: first ventricle—right lateral; second ventricle—left lateral; third ventricle; fourth ventricle; the fifth secondary vesicle remains as the aqueduct.

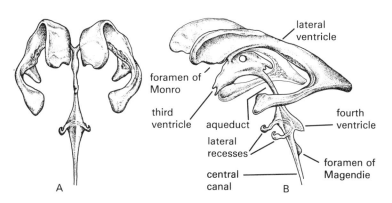

Fig. 2-6. Ventricular system. (A) Frontal view; (B) lateral view.

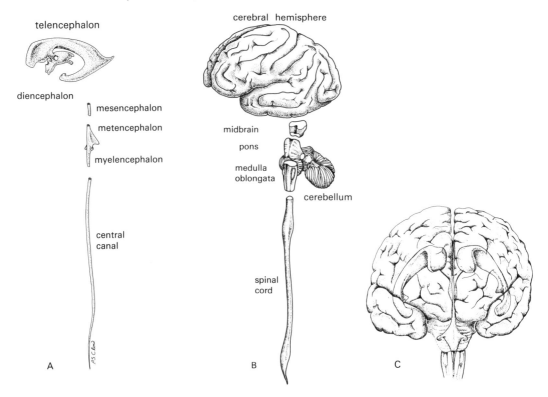

Fig. 2-7. (A) Brain ventricles; (B) derivations of ventricular walls; (C) position of brain ventricles within brain, a frontal view.

Main Regions of the Central Nervous System

The wall of the central canal gives rise to the **spinal cord** (Fig. 2-7).

The wall of the fourth ventricle, or rhombencephalon, gives origin in its caudal portion to the **myelencephalon** (Gr. *myelos* marrow), or **medulla** (L. marrow) **oblongata.** The rostral part of the rhombencephalon is the origin of the **metencephalon,** which in turn becomes the **pons** (L. bridge) and the **cerebellum.**

The wall of the aqueduct, or mesencephalon, gives origin to the midbrain.

The walls of the lateral ventricles, or telencephalon, develop the **cerebral hemispheres.**

The walls of the third ventricle, or diencephalon, grow, although the region retains its original name, diencephalon. It is hidden by the cerebral hemispheres.

Nomenclature— Developmental Terms and Synonyms

The study of neuroanatomy offers a plethora of terms, whose definitions often are conflicting. To circumvent this problem it may be tempting to weed out some of the terms in an introductory textbook. This, however, is an unsound strategy, since in consequence the student will not ready herself or himself to grasp the contents of other neuroanatomy texts, where

Table 2-1. Divisions of the Central Nervous System

Telencephalon Endbrain **Cerebral hemispheres** **Diencephalon** Interbrain	}	Prosencephalon Forebrain **Cerebrum**	}	
Mesencephalon **Midbrain**	}			**Brain** Encephalon }
Metencephalon Afterbrain **Pons** **Cerebellum** }	Rhombencephalon Hindbrain }	**Brain stem** }		} **CNS**
Myelencephalon **Medulla oblongata** }			**Spinal cord** Medulla spinalis }	

A vertical line indicates synonyms.

the terminology includes additional names and synonyms. It is better to make the student aware of as much of the existing nomenclature as possible, while at the same time attempting to provide guidance regarding the maze of synonyms and classification systems with special reference to developmental aspects.

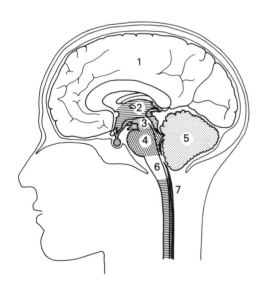

Fig. 2-8. Divisions of CNS. 1. Cerebral hemisphere; 2. diencephalon; 3. midbrain; 4. pons; 5. cerebellum; 6. medulla oblongata; 7. spinal cord.

A glossary with aforementioned terms is presented in Table 2-1. The most commonly used names related to developed brain are bolded. They are the prevalent terms in problems of clinical medicine (Fig. 2-8).

Derivatives of Neuroectodermal Cells

The cells comprising the neural plate, i.e., the neuroectodermal cells, first form the neural tube and crests and then build the neural tissue as an outgrowth from the walls of the tube. These cells are the origin of the neuronal and glial cells.

Those cells which remain lining the neural tube change in shape and become **ependymal cells,** which are classified as a type of glial cells. The tube wall is called **ependyma** (Fig. 2-9).

Neural Crests

The neuroectodermal cells forming the neural crests develop **two processes** on opposite sides of their body. These later join,

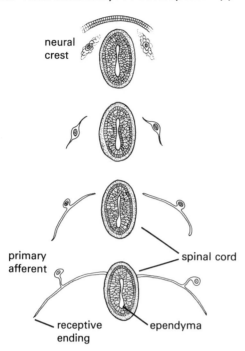

Fig. 2-9. Development of primary sensory neurons from neural crest.

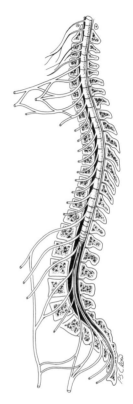

Fig. 2-10. Vertebral column cut open to show the spinal cord inside the vertebral canal.

reforming into one process shaped like a T (Fig. 2-9).

One of the ends grows toward an organ (e.g., muscle, skin) and becomes the receptive ending. The other end enters the spinal cord and transmits through a synapse into central neurons the impulse recorded at the receptive ending. It forms the **sensory peripheral path** from anywhere in the human body to the central nervous system (CNS). The neuronal cells making up the path are called *primary sensory neurons* or **primary afferent neurons.**

Neural crest cells also generate glial cells of the peripheral nervous system, melanoblasts, cells of the adrenal gland (chromaffin cells), as well as many other neuroendocrine cells.

Spinal Cord

The spinal cord of an adult human (Fig. 2-10) is roughly cylindrical, measuring ap-

proximately 12 × 9 mm in cross-section and about 41 cm (female) and 45 cm (male) in length. It tapers into a conical shape at its lower end. Its weight is around 38 g.

Connected to the spinal cord are the **sensory** and **motor processes.** Because of their rooting with the spinal cord, they are called **sensory** and **motor spinal roots** (Fig. 2-11). Each of these roots consists of several **rootlets** with thousands of cell processes.

The spinal cord is composed of segments. Each segment harbors two pairs of roots, one pair to the left and another to the right. Each pair consists of one **posterior** and one **anterior** root.

The sensory roots enter the spinal cord on the posterior surface and are therefore also called **posterior (dorsal) spinal roots.**

The cell bodies of each segmental dorsal

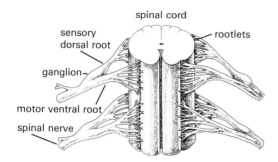

Fig. 2-11. Anterior view of two spinal cord segments with their roots.

root process are grouped together, forming a swelling called a **ganglion** (Gr. swelling). It is also called **dorsal root ganglion** or **spinal ganglion** and is sensory in nature. The sensory roots and ganglia are composed of primary sensory neurons.

The motor roots exit the spinal cord on the anterior surface and are therefore also called **anterior (ventral) spinal roots.**

The neuronal cell bodies of the processes forming the ventral roots are inside the spinal cord.

The human has 31 spinal cord segments (Fig. 2-12). According to their regional innervation, they are classified into

8 **cervical** (for the neck and arms);
12 **thoracic** (for a limited portion of the arm, thorax, and part of the abdomen);
5 **lumbar** (for part of the abdomen and legs);
5 **sacral** (for part of the legs and perineal region); and
1 **coccygeal** (for part of the perineal region).

The spinal cord can be viewed as the first center of **sensory input** from the body and the last center of **motor output** to the body. The rest of the central nervous system modulates these two centers.

It can be calculated that a body of 62 kg divided into 31 segments allots 2 kg per body segment. The weight of the spinal cord divided into 31 parts affords approximately 1 g per neural segment. This means that each 2 kg body segment is regulated

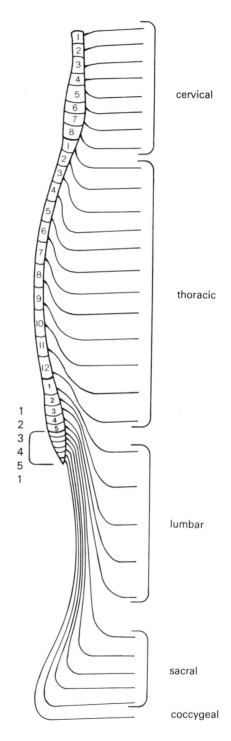

Fig. 2-12. Spinal cord segments.

by 1 g of spinal cord tissue, i.e., at a ratio of 2,000 to 1.

Medulla Oblongata

The **medulla oblongata** (or **medulla**) is a cone-shaped continuation of the spinal cord. It ends at the lower border of the thick belted prominence of the pons. Anterolaterally, on each side, there is an oval eminence in the shape of an olive. They are called the **inferior olives** (Fig. 2-13C).

Anteromedially, there is a fissure or groove called the **ventral median fissure.** Two prominences, called the **pyramids,** are situated along the medulla between the olives and the ventral median fissure.

Dorsomedially, there is a fold, or narrow fissure, by the name of the **dorsal median sulcus** (Fig. 2-13).

Dorsally, the medulla is hidden from view by the cerebellum (Fig. 2-14). When this is removed, one can observe that the lower half of the floor of the fourth ventricle is formed by the upper dorsal surface of the medulla.

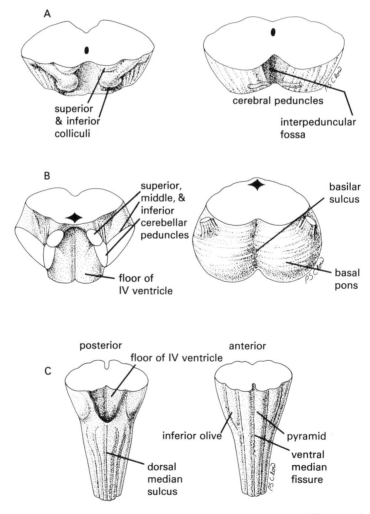

Fig. 2-13. Posterior and anterior views of (A) midbrain; (B) pons; (C) medulla oblongata.

The medulla oblongata can be considered the most vital center of the nervous tissue. Among other activities it regulates respiration, blood pressure, heart beat, and blood constants. Destruction of this region or neighboring neural tissue may mean death.

Pons

The **pons** in an anterior (ventral) view (Fig. 2-13B) is identified between the medulla and midbrain by its well-defined upper and lower borders. This belly-like portion of the pons is called the **basal pons.**

Anteromedially, there is a depression called the **basilar sulcus.** An anterolateral view reveals the prominent connections with the cerebellum.

The posterior portion of the pons is hidden from view by the cerebellum (Fig. 2-14). When removed, one can observe that the dorsal surface of the pons forms part of the floor of the fourth ventricle.

The pons shares with the medulla some of the control of vital functions.

Midbrain

The **midbrain** is smaller than the pons and difficult to see in a whole brain, as it is surrounded by the cerebral hemispheres, whose displacement is necessary to permit the observation of the surface features of the midbrain.

Ventrally, there are two masses diverging upward. These are the **left** and **right cerebral peduncles,** and the space occupied between them is called the **interpeduncular fossa** (Fig. 2-13A).

The upper border of the pons demarcates the lower border of the midbrain. Ontogenetically, the upper limit of the midbrain can be said to be where the cerebral peduncles became buried in the brain.

A dorsal view of the midbrain reveals in it four rounded eminences, two on each side, called the **quadrigeminal bodies.** These are also called the **superior colliculi,** in reference to the upper pair, and the **inferior colliculi,** to the lower pair (Fig. 2-13).

The colliculi are of service in attention and orientation reflex centers. The upper colliculi play a part in the processing of visual signals and the lower colliculi of auditory signals. The colliculi are a major relay center of visual, auditory and motor reflexes.

Brain Stem

The term **brain stem** includes the medulla, pons, and midbrain. The three of them together are like a trunk, or stem, for the **cerebrum** and the **cerebellum** (Figs. 2-14 and 2-15).

Cranial Nerves of the Brain Stem

There are 12 pairs of **cranial nerves.** The first 2 are connected with the cerebrum, and the remaining 10 (from III to XII) with the brain stem (Fig. 2-16), i.e., 2 with the midbrain (III, IV); 3 with the pons (V, VI, VII); and 5 with the medulla (VIII to XII).

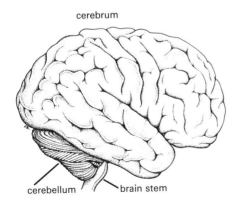

cerebrum

cerebellum   brain stem

Fig. 2-14. Right lateral view of the brain.

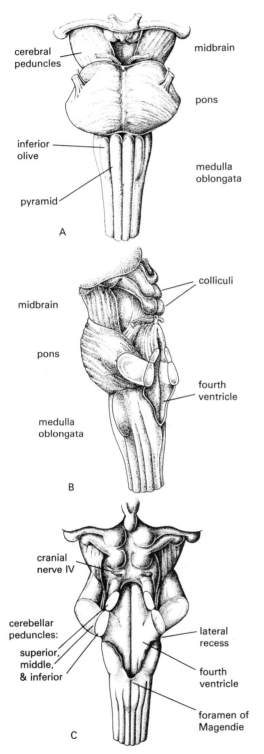

A

B

cranial
nerve IV

cerebellar
peduncles:

superior,
middle,
& inferior

C

Fig. 2-15. Brain stem. (A) Ventral view; (B)
lateral view; (C) dorsal view.

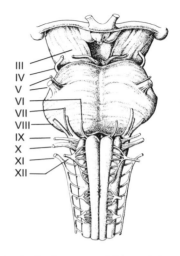

Fig. 2-16. Brain stem with cranial nerves.

Cerebellum

The **cerebellum** (Figs. 2-17 and 2-18), at
around 140 g, is much bigger than the
brain stem, which weighs only about 28 g.
Peculiar to the cerebellar surface are the
many thin foldings, which are called **folia**
(L. leaflets). The cerebellum consists of a
middle portion, called the **vermis,** and two
lateral **cerebellar hemispheres.**

The cerebellar mass is attached dorsally
to the brain stem by three pairs of peduncles. The **superior cerebellar peduncles**
attach to the midbrain; the **middle cerebellar peduncles,** the largest of the three,
attach to the pons; and the **inferior cerebellar peduncles** attach to the medulla
(Figs. 2-18 and 2-15).

The cerebellum closes the fourth ventri-

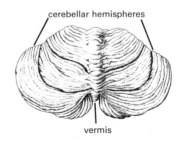

Fig. 2-17. Cerebellum, dorsal view.

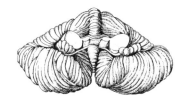

Fig. 2-18. Cerebellum, ventral view.

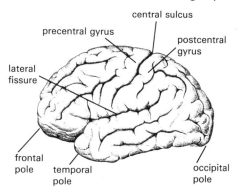

Fig. 2-19. Left hemisphere, lateral view.

cle posteriorly. Careful scrutiny reveals three holes, i.e., the lateral apertures, or foramina of Luschka, and the median aperture, or foramen of Magendie.

Cerebral Hemispheres

A lateral view of the brain (Fig. 2-19) displays only one **cerebral hemisphere.** Its surface shows folds, called **sulci,** with elevations, which are called **gyri,** between them. The **central sulcus** is limited by the **precentral** and **postcentral gyri.** A pronounced cleft on its lateral surface, i.e., the **lateral fissure,** accentuates the C-shape of the hemisphere.

Four principal portions or **lobes** can be identified in the cerebral hemispheres. They are called after the **cranial bones** which overlie them, i.e., the **frontal, parietal, occipital,** and **temporal lobes** (Fig. 2-20).

The three **poles** are **frontal, occipital,** and **temporal** (Fig. 2-19).

A frontal or superior view of the cerebral hemispheres shows that they are separated by an interhemispheric midsagittal or **longitudinal fissure** (Fig. 2-21). At the bottom of this fissure one encounters a dense mass of tissue, which links one hemisphere to the other. It is called the **corpus callosum** (L. *corpus* body; *callosus* hardened). Its texture is harder than the rest of the brain. It can be observed in a midsagittal section (Fig. 2-22) and (as well as the longitudinal fissure) in a coronal section of the brain (Fig. 2-23).

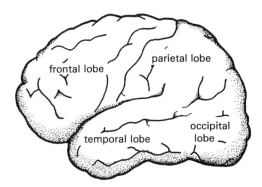

Fig. 2-20. Cerebral lobes.

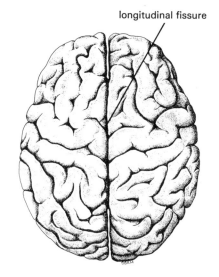

Fig. 2-21. Dorsal view of the cerebral hemispheres.

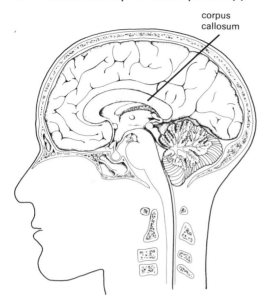

Fig. 2-22. Midsagittal section of the head displaying the right half.

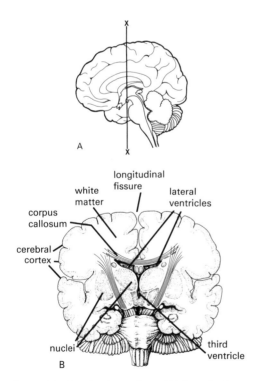

Fig. 2-23. Cerebral section. (A) Level of section; (B) coronal view.

Gray and White Matter

The grays and whites in the illustration of Figure 2-23 propose to imitate the shades of the **gray** and **white matter** of the real brain. The gray matter on the surface of the cerebral hemispheres is called the **cerebral cortex** and contains billions of neuronal cell bodies. The white matter contains mostly cell processes. It is located under the cerebral cortex and is seen as a large mass. These terms, i.e., the gray and white matter, will be used extensively in this text.

The Terms Ganglion and Nucleus

The terms **ganglion** and **nucleus,** which also will be used frequently from now on, ought to be introduced as well.

Today the definition of a ganglion is a swelling in the peripheral nervous system made up of a mass of neuronal cell bodies. Distinct from a ganglion, a group of neuronal cell bodies in the central nervous system is called a nucleus (Fig. 2-23).

In the course of time, the term ganglion has imparted different connotations. It was used by the old anatomists to indicate (1) a mass of nervous tissue, consisting mostly of neural cell bodies, protruding on the surface of the central nervous system; as well as (2) any neural swelling outside the central nervous system.

The old anatomists observed swellings on and around the base or core of the cerebrum and called them basal ganglia. The use of this term should be discontinued as it is misleading.

Diencephalon

The **diencephalon** (Figs. 2-23 and 2-24) is a paired structure on each side of the third ventricle. Parts of the lateral ventricles and the corpus callosum lie superiorly.

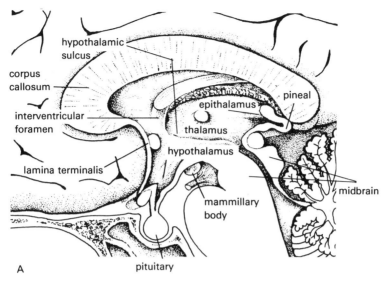

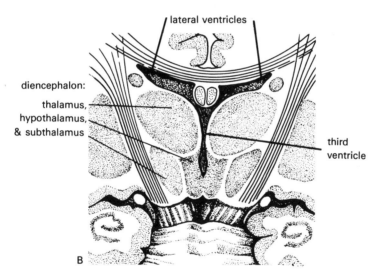

Fig. 2-24. Diencephalon with surrounding structures. (A) Enlarged view of Fig. 2-22; (B) enlarged view of Fig. 2-23.

The diencephalon and the third ventricle form the central core of the cerebrum.

The diencephalon is subdivided into four regions: the **thalamus, hypothalamus, subthalamus,** and **epithalamus.** Each of these regions is bilaterally represented.

On the medial surface of the diencephalon is the **hypothalamic sulcus,** which demarcates the thalamus (dorsally) and the hypothalamus (ventrally). This sulcus extends from the cerebral aqueduct to the interventricular foramen.

Thalamus

More than three-quarters of the diencephalon consists of the **thalamus** (Gr. *thalamos* (inner) chamber). A principal function of this structure is the processing of somatic sensory signals. It establishes numerous connections with the cerebral hemispheres.

Hypothalamus

Two distinct structures of the **hypothalamus** (Gr. *hypo* under) are the left and right **mammillary** (L. *mammilla* little breast) **bodies.** These two small rounded masses are seen protruding on the ventral surface close to another rounded midline mass, i.e., the **pituitary body** or **gland** (Figs. 2-24 and 2-25). The hypothalamus processes visceral signals.

Subthalamus

The **subthalamus** is also situated below the thalamus, but lateral to the hypothalamus. A function of the subthalamus is the processing of somatic motor signals.

Epithalamus

The **epithalamus** (Gr. *epi* on), whose function is visceral, may not be seen in a coronal section. It is located in the dorsoposterior part of the thalamus, and a midsagittal view (Fig. 2-24) allows it to be observed. Situated in the midline of the epithalamus is the **pineal body** or **gland** (L. *pinea* pine cone).

The diencephalon is limited caudally by the midbrain.

Lamina Terminalis

The **lamina terminalis** (Fig. 2-24) is the rostral end of the embryonic neural tube. In the developed brain it is a thin membrane constituting the anterior wall of the third ventricle.

This lamina is a telencephalic structure. Ontogenetically, it is the origin of the surrounding nervous tissue, which is intrinsic to the highest functions of the brain, such as judgment, control of social behavior, etc.

As a topographical mark the lamina terminalis is important in the study of the very complex region where it is situated. In the drawing of a midsagittal section, one can observe that the hypothalamus is posterior to the lamina terminalis; that it is continuous with the corpus callosum; and that the interventricular foramen is posterior to the upper part of the lamina terminalis.

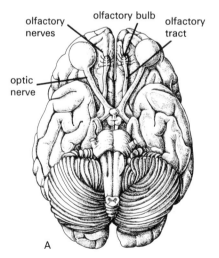
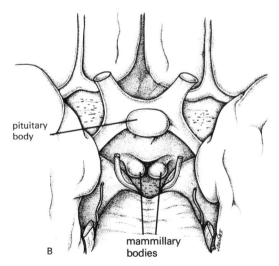

Fig. 2-25. (A) Ventral or basal view of the brain; (B) enlarged detail of A.

Cranial Nerves of the Cerebrum

The first pair of **cranial nerves** (Fig. 2-25), the **olfactory nerves,** are connected with a complex extension of the cerebral hemispheres, i.e., the **olfactory bulb** and **olfactory tract.** The second pair, the **optic nerves,** end up attached to the thalamus. Strictly speaking, the optic nerves are not true nerves, because they are a connection between the retina of the eye and the thalamus and hence do not connect with the periphery as do true nerves. The retina developed embryonically as a vesicular evagination of the diencephalon.

Cerebrum

The function of the cerebral hemispheres is to analyze, associate, integrate, and store sensory signals; retrieve past experiences of sensorial and motor nature; command motor behavior; control speech; make value judgments regarding the environment; build up principles, etc.

To understand the complex mechanisms involved in these processes, one must first comprehend the simpler phenomena underlying the processes.

The role of the cerebral hemispheres is to analyze all the sensory data picked up by the sense organs and channeled to the **cerebral cortex** through the diencephalon, mostly through the thalamus. Each specific type of **signal** (**tactile, visual,** etc.) travels its own specific path to specific cortical regions (the **tactile cortex,** the **visual cortex,** etc.).

The association of different signals is carried out in another cortical region, the **association cortex.** Also, the signals are processed once more through the thalamus, which in response sends stimuli to the association cortex.

The integration of all the signals employs yet another region of the cortex, i.e., the **integrative cortex,** which has connections with the other cortical regions. Also in such cases it is required that the integrated signals be processed again through the thalamus, which in turn sends stimuli to the integrative cortex.

The continuous sets of loops between the diencephalon and the cerebral hemispheres are integral to the higher functions of the nervous system and their importance cannot be exaggerated. The brain can be analyzed as a composite of many subsystems. However, at the level of its highest functions, the study of its parts does not convey its formidable sophistication as an integrated unit.

The weight of the cerebral hemispheres is approximately 1,100 g and that of the diencephalon less than 30 g. Belying its minute size, the diencephalon is the most complex structure of the human nervous system and hence of the entire body.

Neuraxis

The term **neuraxis** most commonly refers to the axis of the central nervous sys-

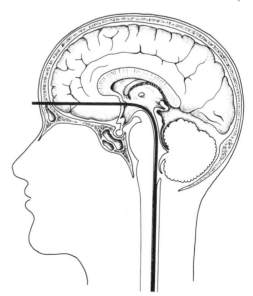

Fig. 2-26. Axis of the CNS.

tem. In a sagittal section of the nervous system, one can observe the neuraxis curving at the level of the brain (Fig. 2-26). This axis constitutes the reference for the topographical terms ventral and dorsal, as exemplified in phrases like "the cerebellum is dorsal to the pons;" "the hypothalamus is ventrally located" (i.e., dorsally and ventrally, respectively, in relation to the neuraxis).

Due to the change in the orientation of the neuraxis at the level of the brain, the terms dorsal and ventral do not correlate with anterior and posterior.

The terms dorsal and ventral are most frequently used in the study of brain topography, as they remain reliable in spite of three major variables, i.e.,

1. individual differences in shape of human brains;
2. changes in brain stem orientation due to variations of head position; and
3. distortion of brain structures during postmortem fixation procedures due to the softness of brain tissue.

Other terms that require special attention are:

roof (dorsal closure) / **floor** (ventral closure) } of { fourth ventricle / aqueduct / third ventricle

Basal pons means the most ventral region of pons.

Base of the brain means the lower surface of the brain.

The transverse (cross-sectional) planes are any planes cutting across the central nervous system perpendicular to the neuraxis.

Suggested Readings

Carpenter MB: Human Neuroanatomy. Seventh Edition. Williams and Wilkins, Baltimore, pp. 49–70, 1976.

Cowan WM: The development of the brain, Sci Am 241(3):107–117, 1979.

Heimer L: The Human Brain and Spinal Cord, Springer-Verlag, New York, pp. 9–36, 1983.

Lemire RJ, Loeser JD, Leech RW, Alvord EC, Jr.: Normal and Abnormal Development of the Human Nervous System, Harper and Row, Hagerstown, 1975.

Lou HC: Developmental Neurology, Raven Press, New York, 1982.

Lund RD: Development and Plasticity of the Brain, Oxford University Press, New York, 1978.

Moore KL: The Developing Human: Clinically Oriented Embryology. Second Edition. WB Saunders, Philadelphia, 1977.

O'Rahilly R, Gardner E: The initial development of the human brain, Acta Anat 104:123–133, 1979.

Sidman RL, Rakic P: Development of the human central nervous system. In Haymaker W, Adams RD, Eds: Histology and Histopathology of the Nervous System, Charles C Thomas, Springfield, pp. 3–145, 1982.

Volpe JJ: Neurology of the Newborn. WB Saunders, Philadelphia, pp. 3–59, 1981.

3

Coverings of the Brain

The physical consistency of the central nervous system is soft and must therefore be adequately wrapped and protected. One type of covering is bony—the skull for the brain and the vertebral column for the spinal cord—and another is membraneous—the dura mater, arachnoid mater, and pia mater.

The Skull

The **skull** (Figs. 3-1 and 3-2) forms the entire bony framework of the head and has two main regions, the brain case or **cranium** with its cranial cavity and the **skeleton of the face.** The cranium consists of (1) the **dome** or **vault;** and (2) the **base.** The following bones make up the cranium:

frontal bone (one)—dome and base
parietal bones (two)—dome
occipital bone (one)—dome and base
temporal bones (two)—dome and base
sphenoid bone (one)—base
ethmoid bone (one)—base

The bones that are paired, i.e., the pari-

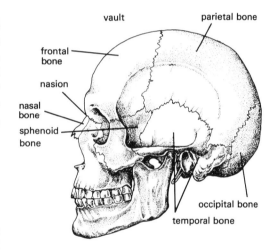

Fig. 3-1. Lateral view of the skull.

etal and temporal bones, are located on the left and right sides of the cranium.

The frontal and occipital bones are in the anterior and posterior region of the cranium and join the parietal bones anteriorly and posteriorly, respectively. Between the frontal and two temporal bones the brain case is completed with the ethmoid and sphenoid bones, which are readily ob-

31

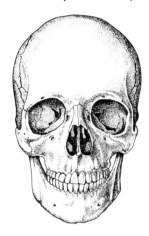

Fig. 3-2. Frontal view of the skull.

the cranium. On the surface of the occipital bone one can palpate the **external occipital protuberance** or **inion** (Fig. 3-4), another important craniometric point.

In the occipital bone there is a large opening, the **foramen magnum,** through which the spinal cord enters the cranium as the brain stem. There are two **condyles**

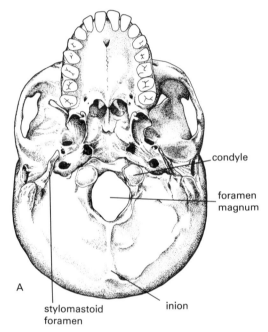

A

Fig. 3-4. (A) Inferior view of the cranium; (B) posterior view of the cranium.

served in an internal view of the cranium (Fig. 3-3).

The frontal bone constitutes the forehead and the upper margins of the orbits and articulates with the nasal bone. The midsagittal point of this frontonasal articulation is called **nasion,** an important craniometric point.

The parietal bones make up much of the top and the sides of the cranium.

The occipital bone (Fig. 3-4) forms the posterior and a large part of the base of

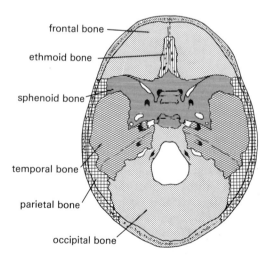

Fig. 3-3. Schematic representation of the internal surface view of the base of the cranium.

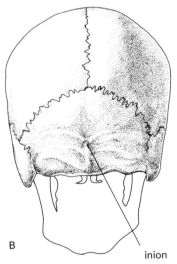

B

Fig. 3-4. (A) Inferior view of the cranium; (B) posterior view of the cranium.

(knuckles), one on each side of the foramen magnum, for articulation with the first vertebra, the so-called **atlas.**

The temporal bones (Figs. 3-5 and 3-6) have two major portions: the **squamous** portion or **squama;** and the **petrous** (L. *petra* stone) portion, which contains the sense organs of position and hearing.

Two downward protrusions of the temporal bones are the sharply pointed **styloid process** and the rounded **mastoid process.**

The sphenoid bone (Fig. 3-7), visible on the internal surface of the base of the cranium, has a middle portion or body and two pairs of wings extending laterally. The sphenoid bone articulates with the other seven cranial bones (Fig. 3-3).

The body of the sphenoid bone shows a depression shaped like a saddle. This is the

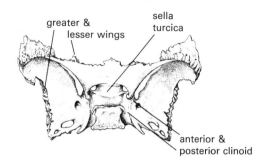

Fig. 3-7. Internal surface view of the sphenoid bone.

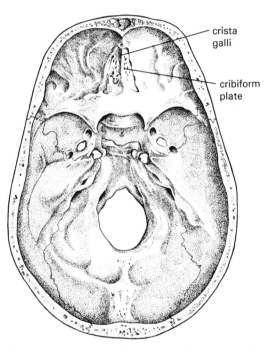

Fig. 3-8. Internal surface view of the base of the cranium.

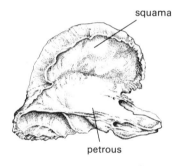

Fig. 3-5. Internal surface view of the temporal bone.

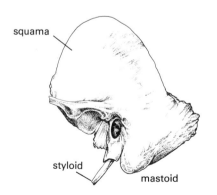

Fig. 3-6. External surface view of the temporal bone.

sella turcica, which is limited by the **anterior** and **posterior clinoid processes,** four tiny prominences. The sella turcica houses the pituitary gland.

Looking at the base of the cranium internally (Fig. 3-8), one observes the ethmoid bone surrounded anteriorly mostly by the frontal bone and posteriorly by the sphenoid. The ethmoid bone reveals in the midline, protruding upward, a sharp crest, the **crista galli** (L. cock's comb). On the sides of this crest is the **cribiform plate,** which consists of two narrow plates of bone with many holes.

Fontanelles

The cranial bones are covered by a tough, fibrous membrane, called the **periosteum.** In the cranium there is an **external periosteal membrane** or **pericranium** and an **inner periosteal membrane** or **endocranium.** In the newborn the **cranial ossification** is not yet completed, leaving some spaces covered only with the periosteal membranes. These spaces are called **fontanelles** (Figs. 3-9 and 3-10). The four most important ones are

1. the **anterior fontanelle**—between the frontal and parietal bones; closes at 18 months;
2. the **posterior fontanelle**—between the occipital and parietal bones; closes at two months;
3. the **anterolateral fontanelle**—between the frontal, parietal, sphenoid, and temporal bones; closes at two months;
4. the **posterolateral fontanelle**—between the parietal, occipital, and temporal bones; closes within 2 years.

In recognition of their importance as landmarks, the very closing points of the four fontanelles have special names: (1) **bregma** (anterior), (2) **lambda** (posterior), (3) **pterion** (anterolateral), and (4) **asterion** (posterolateral).

Sutures

When the ossification is completed, the articulations of the cranial bones have become immobile points appearing like seams or, as they are fittingly called, **sutures** (Fig. 3-11).

With the two parietal bones the frontal forms the **coronal suture.**

The two parietal bones make up the **sagittal suture.**

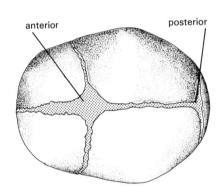

Fig. 3-9. Fontanelles.

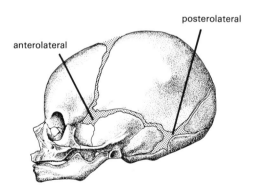

Fig. 3-10. Fontanelles.

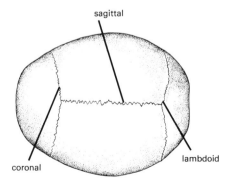

Fig. 3-11. Superior view of the cranium.

Together the two parietal bones shape with the occipital bone the **lambdoid** (Gr. letter *lambda*) **suture.**

Other sutures are named after the two conjugated bones involved (e.g., the **parietotemporal suture**).

Cranial Air Sinuses

Some of the cranial bones (Fig. 3-12) (frontal, sphenoid, ethmoid, mastoid) contain air spaces or **sinuses.** These cavities are lined with mucous membranes. Inflammation of these sinuses may occur.

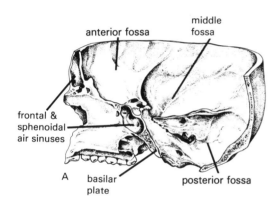

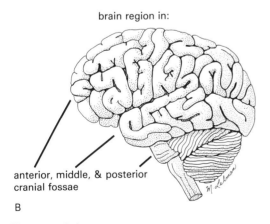

Fig. 3-12. (A) Internal view of right half of cranium with skull cap removed; (B) lateral view of brain.

Cranial Fossae

The interior surface of the base of the skull is shaped into three levels or platforms, namely the **anterior, middle,** and **posterior cranial fossae** (Fig. 3-12).

The anterior cranial fossa is formed mostly by a part of the frontal bone; the middle cranial fossa by the sphenoid and temporal bones; and the posterior cranial fossa mostly of the occipital bone.

These three levels support the three levels of the base of the brain. The frontal lobe rests on the anterior cranial fossa; the temporal lobe on the middle cranial fossa; and the brain stem and cerebellum on the posterior cranial fossa.

The pituitary gland is situated in the sella turcica. The bony slope, formed by the occipital and sphenoid bones, anterior to the foramen magnum, is where the base of the medulla and pons is located. This bony slope is the **basilar plate** or **clivus.**

Foramina of the Base of the Skull

The cranium needs to have openings for the passage of the vessels and cranial nerves. These openings are found on the base of the skull (Fig. 3-13). We have already mentioned the foramen magnum through which the medulla oblongata continues with the spinal cord.

Table 3-1 presents a listing of the most important foramina, their position and the structures which pass through them.

Meninges and Meningeal Spaces

There are three connective tissue **membranes** or, to use the Latin term, **meninges,** covering the brain. Their names are

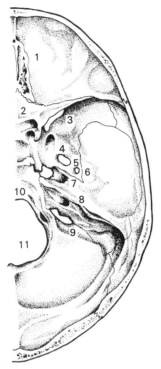

Fig. 3-13. Internal surface view of the base of the cranium (right half). See Table 3-1 for numbers in figure.

dura mater, arachnoid mater, and **pia mater.**

The word mater (L. mother) alludes to the mother or membrane-like scum of old vinegar or wine, whose appearance they call to mind. The Latin word *durus* means "hard, tough." The term *arachnoid* is Greek and means "resembling a spider-web." The Latin term *pius* means "soft, tender."

The arrangement of the brain coverings and the interspaces from the outside inward is shown in Table 3-2 and Figure 3-14.

The internal periosteum fuses with the dura. The term dura is commonly used to include the periosteum because of their fusion. Another less common term is **pachymeninx** (Gr. *pachys* thick; *meninx* membrane). The dura apposes to the arachnoid but does not attach itself; between these layers there is what is called a potential **subdural space** visible with the aid of a microscope in histological preparations in normal conditions. Some veins course across, bridging over this space. Although in normal conditions the dura and arach-

Table 3-1. Foramina of the Base of the Skull

Opening	Position	Numbers of Fig. 3-13	Structure(s) (cranial nerves and vessels)
Olfactory foramina	Cribiform plate	1	I olfactory nerves
Optic foramen	Sphenoid	2	II optic nerve, ophthalmic artery
Superior orbital fissure ˮ	Between small and great wing of sphenoid	3	III, IV, V-1, VI
Foramen rotundum	Great wing	4	V-2
Foramen ovale	Great wing	5	V-3
Foramen spinosum	Great wing	6	Middle meningeal artery and vein
Carotid canal	Petrous of temporal and sphenoid	7	Internal carotid artery
Internal acoustic meatus	Petrous of temporal	8	VII and VIII
Jugular foramen	Between petrous of temporal and occipital	9	IX, X, and XI, continuation of sigmoid sinus into jugular vein
Hypoglossal canal	Occipital	10	XII
Foramen magnum	Anterolateral edge of foramen magnum Occipital	11	Spinal cord—medulla, XI, vertebral arteries, anterior and posterior arteries
Stylomastoid foramen	Temporal (external surface)		VII

Table 3.2 Brain Coverings and
Interspaces

Layer	Space
External periosteum 1	None
Bone 2	None
Internal periosteum 3	None
Dura mater 4	Subdural
Arachnoid mater 5	Subarachnoid
Pia mater 6	Subpial
Brain surface 7	

Numbers are from Fig. 3-14.

noid layers are apposed, they have the affinity to easily become separated if fluid exudates or blood extravasates reach this space (e.g., **subdural hematoma** in trauma), hence making the potential subdural space a reality. The accumulation and retention of blood in the subdural space may reach proportions that are able to compress the underlying nervous tissue with fatal consequences.

Threads of connective tissue, i.e., **arachnoid trabeculae,** can be observed in the subarachnoid space. The pia and arachnoid are also called **leptomeninges** or **slender membranes,** which in essence are one split but continuous membrane, the **pia-arachnoid membrane.**

Below the mesothelial cell layer of the pia there is the so-called **basement membrane.**

The pia follows the brain surface. Furthermore, any vessel penetrating the brain is surrounded by a pial cuff. This pial arrangement makes the pia undetachable from the brain as a whole.

Subarachnoid Cisterns

The distance between the pia and arachnoid membrane, i.e., the size of the subarachnoid space, varies in different regions. Larger such spaces are called **subarachnoid cisterns** (Fig. 3-15). Five of the cisterns related to the brain stem are

1. the **cisterna magna** or **cerebellomedullary cistern;**
2. the **superior cistern,** dorsal to the midbrain; it is also called the cistern of the great cerebral vein;
3. the **pontine cistern,** beneath the base of the pons;
4. the **interpeduncular cistern** between the two cerebral peduncles; and
5. the **cisterna ambiens** on the sides of the midbrain.

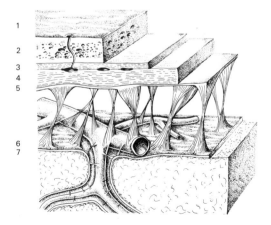

Fig. 3-14. Coverings of the brain. See Table 3-2 for numbers in figure.

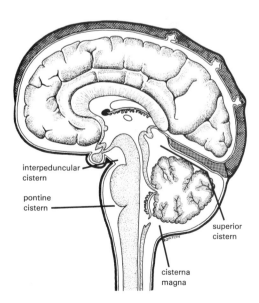

interpeduncular cistern

pontine cistern

superior cistern

cisterna magna

Fig. 3-15. Sagittal section of the brain.

Four of the **cerebral cisterns** are named according to their location: **cisterns of the optic chiasm, of the lamina terminalis, of the corpus callosum,** and **of the lateral fissure.**

Meningeal Foldings

Between the two cerebral hemispheres, in the space called the **cerebral sagittal fissure,** a folding of the dura and arachnoid is found. It is called **falx cerebri** (Fig. 3-16), owing to its sickle shape. It attaches anteriorly to the crista galli of the ethmoid (Figs. 3-17 and 3-18).

Between the posterior region of the cerebral hemispheres above and the cerebellum below, in the space called the **transverse fissure** (Fig. 3-17), another folding of the meninges is found. It is called the **tentorium cerebelli,** as it appears like a tent of the cerebellum.

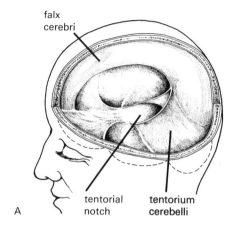

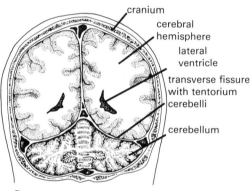

B

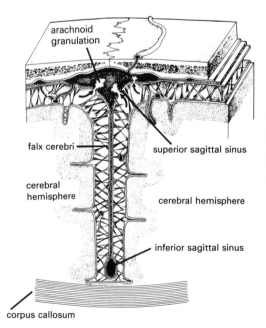

Fig. 3-16. Schematic cross-sectional view of sagittal fissure with falx cerebri.

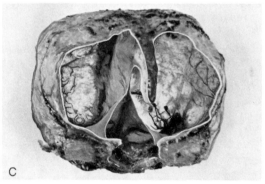

C

Fig. 3-17. (A) Meningeal foldings; (B) coronal section of the head; (C) photograph of freeze-dried dura mater.

The edge of the tentorium cerebelli embraces the midbrain and ends attaching to the anterior clinoid processes of the sphenoid. The tentorial edge is sharp and hard. The space left for the passage of the mid-

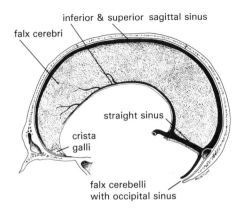

falx cerebri

inferior & superior sagittal sinus

straight sinus

crista galli

falx cerebelli with occipital sinus

Fig. 3-18. Dural venous sinuses in falx cerebri and falx cerebelli.

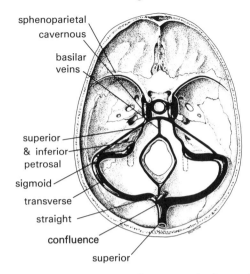

sphenoparietal

cavernous

basilar veins

superior & inferior petrosal

sigmoid

transverse

straight

confluence

superior

brain is called **tentorial notch** or **incisure of the tentorium.**

The **falx cerebelli** (Fig. 3-18) extends in the midline on the posterior cranial fossa between the cerebellar hemispheres.

Posteriorly, the falx cerebri meets at right angles with the tentorium cerebelli.

The attachments of the dura on the clinoid processes form a diaphragm, called **diaphragma sellae,** on top of the pituitary gland.

Dural Venous Sinuses

The dura is detached from the periosteum where it forms the **meningeal foldings.** At the base of these foldings are **dural venous sinuses,** which are filled with venous blood. The one found at the base of the falx cerebri is called the **superior sagittal sinus** (Figs. 3-16 and 3-18).

The ones found at the base of the tentorium cerebelli are the **transverse sinuses** and the **superior petrosal sinuses.** The one located in the falx cerebri is the **occipital sinus** (Figs. 3-18, 3-19, and 3-20).

There are other dural venous sinuses. The **inferior sagittal sinus** is situated in the free edge of the falx cerebri. The

Fig. 3-19. Dural venous sinuses on the base of the cranium.

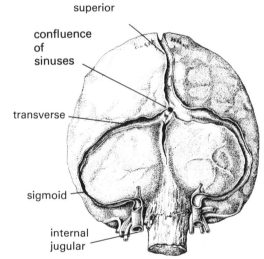

superior

confluence of sinuses

transverse

sigmoid

internal jugular

Fig. 3-20. Posterior view of the brain covered by the dura; the dural sinuses are displayed open.

straight sinus lies in the junction of the tentorium cerebelli with the falx cerebri. The junction of the straight, superior sagittal, transverse, and occipital sinuses is called **confluence of the sinuses** or **torcular Herophili** (Figs. 3-18, 3-19, and 3-20).

Upon reaching the petrous region, the

transverse sinus continues downward as the **sigmoid sinus** (so called because of its S-shape) and exits the cranium through the jugular foramen to become the internal jugular vein (Fig. 3-20).

The **cavernous sinuses** are placed on each side of the body of the sphenoid bone (Fig. 3-19). Venous communications between the cavernous sinuses form the **circular sinus.**

Venous communications between the cavernous sinus and jugular vein form the **inferior petrosal sinus.**

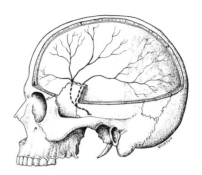

Fig. 3-21. Lateral view of the cranium with part of the bone removed to show the middle meningeal artery and its branches running on the dura mater.

Vascular Supply of the Brain and Meninges

In the first chapter we stressed the importance of good knowledge of the vascular supply to the nervous system. In fact, the clinician encounters more neurological cases that are due to vascular problems than to any other single cause.

At this stage of learning it is timely to become acquainted with the basis of the blood supply of the brain and meninges. The term **intracranial vessels,** in distinction to the **extracranial vessels,** refers to the vessels inside the cranium. The arteries inside the cranium are divided into two groups: **meningeal arteries** and **brain arteries.**

Meningeal Arteries

Meningeal arteries are those found sandwiched between the dura and the endosteum. The **left** and **right middle meningeal arteries** (Fig. 3-21) are the biggest ones; they are branches of the **maxillary artery.** They enter the cranium through the foramen spinosum. Traumatic injuries to the head may rupture the meningeal arteries and produce hemorrhage (**epidural** or **extradural hematoma**). If enough bleeding occurs, death due to brain compression ensues.

Brain Arteries and Blood Circulation

The **arteries to the brain** (two **vertebral** and two **internal carotids**) perforate the dura and arachnoid. They spread many branches in the subarachnoid space, forming a well-developed vascular network on the surface of the brain. From here nutrient vessels penetrate the brain, carrying with them a coating of pia mater. The blood from the brain capillaries continues through the venules and veins, which empty in the dural venous sinuses. These send out their blood extracranially via the internal jugular vein (through the jugular foramen).

It is usual to refer to the two vertebral arteries and their branches as the **vertebral system** and to the two internal carotids and their branches as the **internal carotid system.**

Vertebral System

The vertebral arteries (Figs. 3-22 and 3-23) pierce the dura mater and arachnoid just below the level where they pass through the foramen magnum, in the subarachnoid space upward, forward, and

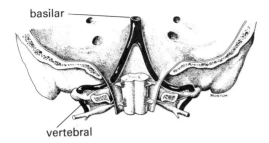

basilar

vertebral

Fig. 3-22. Vertebral arteries entering the cranium and becoming the basilar artery.

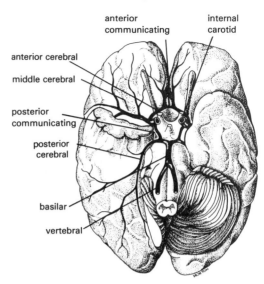

anterior communicating

internal carotid

anterior cerebral

middle cerebral

posterior communicating

posterior cerebral

basilar

vertebral

Fig. 3-23. Vertebrobasilar and internal carotid systems.

medially. At the lower border of the pons, the two arteries fuse and form the **basilar artery,** which ascends along the base of the pons and ends dividing into the **left** and **right posterior cerebral arteries.**

Through its branches the vertebral arterial system supplies all the blood to the medulla, pons, midbrain, and cerebellum as well as it contributes blood to the spinal cord and some regions of the brain.

Internal Carotid System

The left and right internal carotid arteries enter the cranium through the **carotid canal** of the temporal bone and reach the floor of the cavernous sinus. There they course forward and ascend on their anterior wall until they reach the dura and arachnoid, which they perforate. They then bend again posterolaterally within the subarachnoid space. This double bending of the internal carotids is called the **carotid siphon.**

After all its bendings the internal carotid divides into the **anterior** and **middle cerebral arteries.**

Communicating Arteries—Circle of Willis

The existence of three **communicating arteries,** one **anterior** and two **posterior** (Figs. 3-23 and 3-24), permits the circula-

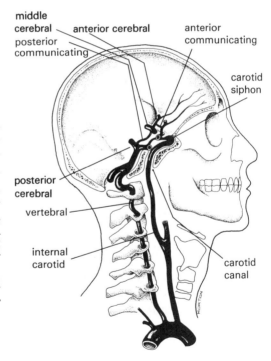

middle cerebral

anterior cerebral

anterior communicating

posterior communicating

carotid siphon

posterior cerebral

vertebral

internal carotid

carotid canal

Fig. 3-24. Circle of Willis.

tion of blood in any direction within the arteries. The anterior communicating artery joins the two anterior cerebral arter-

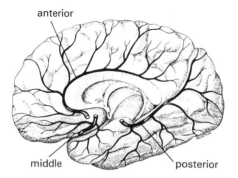

Fig. 3-25. Inferior and medial surfaces of the right hemisphere with its arterial supply.

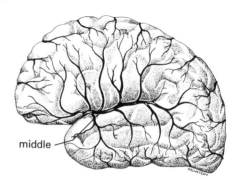

Fig. 3-26. Lateral surface of the left hemisphere with its arterial supply.

ies. The two posterior communicating arteries join the internal carotids with the posterior cerebral arteries. These junctions close a ring of nine arteries called the **circle of Willis,** composed of: one anterior communicating, two anterior cerebral, two internal carotid, two posterior communicating, and two posterior cerebral arteries.

The surface of the cerebral hemispheres is covered by the three above mentioned arteries: the anterior, middle, and posterior cerebral arteries. An image of their regional distribution is depicted in Figures 3-25 and 3-26.

Environment of the Nervous System

The nervous system requires its own environment. The medium in which it bathes itself is the **cerebrospinal fluid (CSF).** Among others, the CSF provides the following benefits to the nervous system:

1. It affords a cushioning (buoyant) effect during rapid movements of the body.
2. It buffers the effects of the changes in blood composition.
3. It acts as a sink for the removal of waste products.
4. It buffers the intracranial pressure.
5. It buffers the metabolic temperature.

6. It prevents noxious elements to and from the blood from coming in contact with the neural tissue.
7. It distributes substances (hormones) through the nervous system.

The volume of the CSF is 90 to 150 ml in the adult man. It is a clear water-like fluid with a composition different from that of blood, especially in regards to protein (very little) and cells (0 to 5 per mm³).

Formation of CSF—Choroid Plexuses—Blood-Brain Barrier

The vessels of the nervous system have two types of functions. One type is inherent to blood supply, and the other type to the formation of CSF as required by the nervous system. For this purpose the **tela choroidea,** which is composed of vessels with their pial connective tissue layer, penetrates the ventricles and becomes coated with a layer of modified ependymal cells called **choroidal epithelium.** These intraventricular vessels coated by connective tissue and choroidal epithelium are the **choroidal plexuses** of the lateral, third, and fourth ventricles. The profuse choroid plexus of the atrium of the lateral ventricle is known as **glomus choroideum.**

The cells constituting the walls of the capillaries irrigating the nervous system, i.e., the **endothelial cells,** are tightly joined. These **tight junctions** act as a barrier for the passage of large molecules from the blood to the brain. It is called **blood-brain barrier (BBB).**

The endothelial cells of the capillary vessels of the choroidal plexuses become modified. Unlike the endothelial cells of the vessels supplying the nervous tissue, these cells have fenestrations (which exhibit a diaphragm) permeable to macromolecules.

It has been suggested that the choroidal endothelial cells become modified by the influence of the choroidal epithelial cells.

The choroidal epithelial cells are a barrier to macromolecules. The CSF is filtered through the complex endothelial cells–connective tissue and epithelial cells of the choroid plexus. The choroid plexus is a modified blood-brain barrier.

The barrier is necessary for many chemicals between the blood and the brain. Nevertheless, the brain must somehow be aware of the chemical composition of the blood. For this purpose there are discrete chemoreceptor areas in the walls of the third and fourth ventricles where the capillaries irrigating them do not have such a barrier.

Circulation and Absorption of the CSF

The fluid circulates from the lateral ventricles to the foramina of Monro to the third ventricle to the aqueduct to the fourth ventricle to the foramina of Luschka and Magendie to the subarachnoid space (Fig. 3-27).

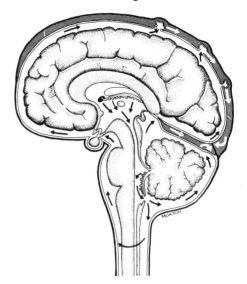

Fig. 3-27. Circulation and absorption of the CSF.

Positions and movements of the body, vascular pulsative movements, diffusion, and convection currents move the CSF through the subarachnoid space.

The fluid is emptied into the dural venous sinuses, especially the superior sagittal sinus, through the **arachnoid villi,** which protrude inside the sinus. Hydrostatic and osmotic pressures regulate the rate of absorption. Although active cellular mechanisms have also been claimed to participate in the absorption rate, it remains a subject of debate.

The arachnoid villi grow in size with age and eventually become **arachnoid granulations** or **pacchionian bodies** (see Fig. 3-16).

Some production and absorption of CSF have been demonstrated along the walls and vessels of the subarachnoid space. The production of CSF has been found to be between 500 and 750 ml per day, which hence is several times its total volume. This implies a very active circulation and renewal of fluid.

When there is an excess of CSF the condition is known as **hydrocephalus** and, specifically, **external hydrocephalus** if the excessive CSF is situated in the sub-

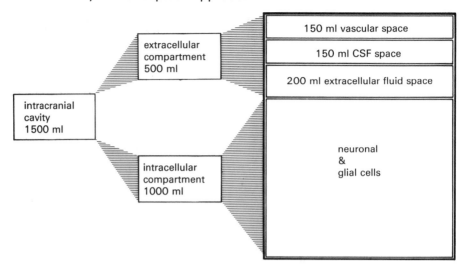

Fig. 3-28. Intracranial compartments.

arachoid space and **internal hydrocephalus** if in the ventricles, which become dilated.

The CSF is colorless and has specific gravity of 1.003 to 1.008. The few cells it contains are lymphocytes. If the number of cells is greater than $10/mm^3$, it is indicative of disease. The protein content is very low, 15 to 45 mg/dl, and the glucose content is half of that of blood.

Intracranial Compartments— Intracranial Pressure

In rough figures, the average volume of the intracranial cavity (Fig. 3-28) is 1,500 ml. This cavity is divided into two major distinct compartments:

1. the **intracellular compartment** (1,000 ml), consisting mostly of neurons and glial cells; and
2. the **extracellular compartment** (500 ml), which in turn is subdivided into
   A. the **vascular space** (150 ml);

B. the **CSF space** (150 ml), consisting of brain ventricles and the subarachnoid space; and
C. the **extracellular space (ECS)**, which is the space between neurons and glial cells and which is filled with **extracellular fluid (ECF)**.

The CSF and ECF are in continuous exchange by diffusion and convection currents.

The subarachnoid pressure reading is a relative indicator of the intracranial pressure, which is important in clinical diagnosis. Increased intracranial pressure may produce herniation of brain tissue in the foramen magnum or the tentorial notch.

Suggested Readings

Agnew WF, Yuen TGH, Achtyl TR: Ultrastructural observations suggesting apocrine secretion in the choroid plexus. A comparative study, Neurol Res 1:313–332, 1980.

Alksne JF, Lovings ET: Functional ultrastructure of the arachnoid villus, Arch Neurol 27:371–377, 1972.

Browder J, Kaplan HA: Cerebral Dural Sinuses

and Their Tributaries, Charles C Thomas, Springfield, 1976.

Carpenter MB: Human Neuroanatomy. Seventh Edition. Williams & Wilkins, Baltimore, pp. 1–20, 1976.

Davson H, Hollingsworth G, Segal MB: The mechanism of drainage of the cerebrospinal fluid, Brain 93:665–678, 1970.

Dohrmann GJ: The choroid plexus: a historical review, Brain Res 18:197–218, 1970.

Dohrmann GJ, Bucy PC: Human choroid plexus: a light and electronic microscopic study, J Neurosurg 33:506–516, 1970.

Jennett B, Teasdale G: Management of Head Injuries, FA Davis Co., Philadelphia, 1981.

Rapoport SI: Blood-Brain Barrier in Physiology and Medicine, Raven Press, New York, 1976.

Wood JH Ed.: Neurobiology of Cerebrospinal Fluid, Plenum Press, New York, 1980.

4

Components of the Nervous System

The basic structural unit of all tissues is the cell. The cells typical of the nervous tissue are the neurons and the glial cells.

Apart from these two populations of cells one finds in the nervous tissue: extracellular fluid; cerebrospinal fluid (CSF); connective tissue composing the membrane coverings; and blood and blood vessels.

Neurons

The original and still valid meaning of **neuron** (Fig. 4-1) is "nerve cell."

The neurons are the cells of the body best equipped to sense and react to the chemical and physical changes occurring in their surroundings. They permeate the entire human body and communicate with each other regarding their conditions and reactions. Reception, conduction, and transmission are aspects of neural function.

To detect, conduct, and transmit stimuli to another cell or cells, neurons grow two types of processes from their bodies, namely, **axons** and **dendrites** (Gr. *dendron* tree).

Dendrites

Those processes that are concerned mainly with the reception of stimuli from their environment are short but have many branches, **dendrites,** to facilitate the pick-up.

Note: In one stage of their ontogenetic development, the peripheral sensory cells had a dendrite-shaped process and an axon-shaped process. Later both types of processes were shaped like axons. In general, one may refer to them as axons, while a more discriminating scientific awareness of their differences can produce insights into implications that are beyond the apparent similarities in shape.

Axons

Axons or **neurites,** i.e., processes concerned with the conduction and transmis-

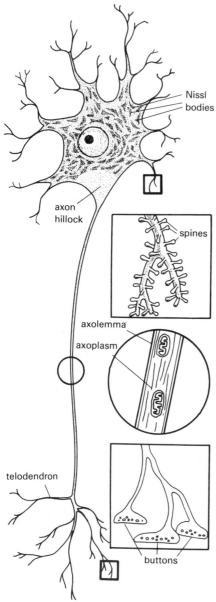

Fig. 4-1. Neuron.

The axon originates from a conical region of the cell body called **axon hillock.** The membrane of the axon is named **axolemma** and the cytoplasm of the axon, **axoplasm.**

A consequence of the communication between neurons is the development of small protrusions, i.e., **spines,** on the surface of the dendrites and **bulbs,** or **buttons (boutons),** at the ends of the axons **(end bulbs)** or along the axons **(boutons en passant).**

The growth in size of axonal and dendritic processes is sometimes 1,000 times that of the body of the neuron, thus greatly increasing its neuronal surface area.

To keep these processes alive, the neuron cell body needs to synthesize huge quantities of proteins. The neurons develop a large granular **endoplasmic reticulum** (Fig. 4-2) with free **ribosomes.** This is also known as **Nissl bodies** and is the region which participates in protein synthesis. It is found in the cell body and dendrites but not in the axon nor in the axon hillock.

The neurons also develop a large **nucleolus,** which plays a role in the synthesis of **ribonucleic acid (RNA).**

The proteins synthesized in the cell body of the neuron need to travel along the axon to supply it. This creates a movement of plasma called **axoplasmic flow,** which serves **axonal transport.** Two different rates of speed have been recognized, one slow, 2 to 3 mm/day, and another fast rate, 200 to 400 mm/day. Also, axonal transport in the opposite direction, from the axon to the cell body, has been described.

The body of the neuron is its metabolic center and the source of life for itself and its processes.

The cytoplasm of the neuron contains **organelles** common to any cell. The microtubules of the neurons are known as **neurotubules.** Their filamentous structures are described as **neurofilaments** when seen by electron microscopy or as **neurofibrils** when seen by light microscopy.

sion of the stimulus-signal to another cell or cells stretch from a length of a few micra to more than a meter, depending on the distance to their target. When the target consists of many cells, the axon gives out collateral branches. The terminal branches of an axon are called **telodendria.**

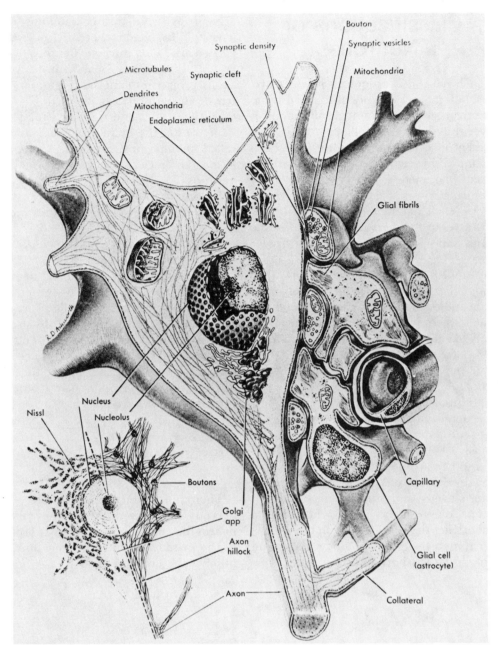

Fig. 4-2. Body of neuron. (Willis WD Jr, Grossman RG: Medical Neurobiology. Third Edition. CV Mosby Co., St. Louis, 1981.)

The cytoplasm may contain pigment granules like **lipofucsin (lipochrome)** or, less commonly, **melanin.**

The **centrosome,** which is an organelle involved in cell division, is atrophic or absent in mature neurons because the neurons do not undergo mitosis.

The neuron cell bodies are surrounded mainly by a mesh of neuronal and glial processes called **neuropil.**

Classifications of Neurons

Each neuron is unique in its structure, metabolism, and functional role. To facilitate their study, different classifications of these hundreds of millions of neurons present in every human adult have been attempted by scientists, who have used different parameters by which to classify them.

One such parameter is the number of processes of the neuron, as evident in the terms **unipolar, bipolar,** and **multipolar** (Fig. 4-3).

Unipolar neurons have only one process, either a dendrite and no axon, or an axon and no dendrite. Cells with dendrites and without axons are called **amacrine cells** like the amacrine cells of the retina.

Bipolar cells have an axon and a dentritic process like the bipolar cells of the retina.

Multipolar cells have an axon and several dendritic processes. Most neurons in the central nervous system (CNS) are multipolar.

Another accepted method of classification divides neurons into **sensory neurons, interneurons,** and **motor neurons.**

The length of the axon is the criterion underlying the classification in the following terms: **Golgi type I** (long axon) and **Golgi type II** (short axon).

Neurons with axons confining their length to the region where the cell body is located are called **intrinsic neurons** (to the region) or **local neurons.** Neurons whose axons project into another region are **extrinsic** to the region they reach. Neurons that connect left and right structures, like structures in the brain or spinal cord, are called **commissural neurons.** Axons projected a distance away belong to **projection neurons.**

Following another method of classification, a neuron can be named after the region where it is located, e.g., **motor horn neuron** in the anterior horn region.

Furthermore, neurons may be named after their shape, e.g., **pyramidal neurons** (after the shape of their cell body) and **stellate** (star-shaped) **neurons.** They are also sometimes named after their discoverer, e.g., cell of Purkinje, cell of Martinotti.

To exemplify the usage of these classifications, one can describe one and the same neuron as being a multipolar motor pyramidal neuron of Golgi type I.

Glial Cells

The other distinct group of cells of the nervous system is called **glia,** or **glial** or **neuroglial cells.** They comprise two-thirds of the mass of the neural tissue and outnumber the neurons 10 to 1.

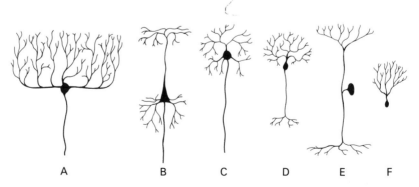

Fig. 4-3. Types of neurons: (A) Purkinje; (B) pyramidal; (C) stellate; (D) multipolar; (E) bipolar; (F) amacrine.

The various functions of the glia remained obscure until the sixties. Since then researchers keep unveiling new functions of these cells.

Glial cells are purported to be

1. mechanically supportive elements of neurons;
2. insulators of neurons;
3. phagocytic defense mechanisms;
4. secretory;
5. modifiers of electrical activity in neurons;
6. regulators of metabolism in neurons;
7. developmental assistants in neural circuitry; and
8. producers of myelin.

Glial cells retain the ability to divide throughout life.

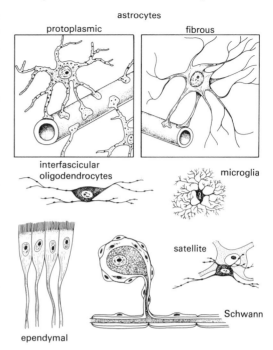

Fig. 4-4. Types of glial cells.

Central Nervous System Glial Cells

Basically, there are four types of glial cells in the CNS: **astroglia, oligodendroglia, microglia,** and **ependymal cells** (Fig. 4-4).

Astrocytes

Astrocytes are mature **astroglial cells.** There are two types, i.e., **protoplasmic** and **fibrous astrocytes.** Protoplasmic astrocytes with processes rich in plasma are most numerous in the gray matter. Fibrous astrocytes, which have processes with abundant glial filaments, are most numerous in the white matter.

The tips of the astrocytic processes are called **end feet** and attach to the blood vessels, covering 90 percent of the surface of the vessels. The end feet are also found next to the surface of neurons.

Astrocytes react to injury of the CNS by swelling or hypertrophy. They may even form scars and become a cause of seizures.

Oligodendrocytes

Oligodendrocytes are mature oligodendroglial cells. *Oligo* in Greek means "few" and the term indicates that they are cells with few processes.

When located around the neuron cell bodies, these cells are called **perineuronal oligodendrocytes,** or **satellite cells,** and when situated in rows covering the axons, they are called **interfascicular oligodendrocytes.** They engender the lipoprotein myelin around the axon.

Microglia

Microglia, which originate from mesodermal cells, are small in comparison with other glial cells. They appear to be inactive cells, but inflammatory or degenerative processes of the CNS mobilize them. Through these processes they proliferate in number and size and become macrophages which phagocytise debris.

Dormant microglial cells are modified **perivascular cells (pericytes),** which are undifferentiated mesodermal cells around the vessels. Following an injury these cells, together with blood-derived monocytes, are believed to become phagocytic **scavenger cells,** or **gitter cells,** in the brain. Also in consequence to an injury, the oligodendrocytes change their structural shape, contributing to the appearance of **extraneous cells** in the brain.

Ependymal Cells

Ependymal cells have important secretory and absorptive functions. They are arranged in a single layer called the **ependyma,** which lines the central canal and ventricular cavities. They have **cilia** projecting into the ventricle and short processes. Some ependymal cells, known as **tanycytes,** retain long processes.

The vessels protruding into the ventricles are coated with a layer of special epithelial ependymal cells, i.e., choroidal epithelial cells. Each such cell, instead of a short process, has a wavy cell surface in its base near the vessel wall, vesiculated microvilli, and some cilia oriented toward the ventricular cavity. These microvilli have selective secretory and absorptive properties. The ventricular vessels and their coating form the **choroid plexuses** (Fig. 4-5).

Peripheral Nervous System Glial Cells

There are two types of glial cells in the peripheral nervous system (PNS), namely, **Schwann cells** and **satellite cells.**

Schwann cells are aligned in rows along the axons. They are in their structure and functional arrangement equivalent to the interfascicular oligodendrocytes. Satellite cells are grouped around the cell bodies of neurons, together forming a capsule of cells for each cell body. They are equivalent to the perineuronal oligodendrocytes of the CNS.

The Schwann cells and satellite cells of the PNS should be considered a group of cells of their own based on their origin (neural crest) and distinct characteristics.

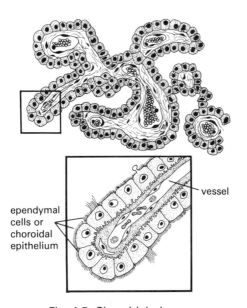

ependymal cells or choroidal epithelium

vessel

Fig. 4-5. Choroidal plexus.

Endings or "Terminals" in the PNS

Sensory and **motor endings** are two distinct groups in the PNS.

Sensory Endings

The sensory endings pick up a stimulus either directly from their environment as **simple receptors** or indirectly through specialized cells, as **encapsulated receptors** or **receptor organs.**

Receptors

A **receptor** is a biologic transducer which picks up one form of energy, or stimulus, and transforms it into another form of energy. We have receptors throughout the body.

Structurally, a receptor consists of a mere portion of a cell or cells or as much as a whole cell or a group of cells.

In broad terms, all peripheral sensory endings are sensory receptors either directly or indirectly.

Motor Endings

Motor endings are neural endings that transmit impulses to the effector cells.

Effectors

Effectors are cells or organs that respond to an impulse from the nervous system. Muscles and glands are effectors.

Classifications of Sensory Endings or Receptors

One method of classification of sensory endings is shown in Table 4-1.

The following are some other classification methods:

1. **Somatic sensory endings**—from the soma or body—and **visceral sensory endings**—from the viscera;
2. **superficial** and **deep sensory endings;**
3. according to their function, e.g., **mechanoreceptors, thermoreceptors, chemoreceptors (chemoceptors), nociceptors,** and **visceroceptors;**
4. according to the structure surrounding the endings: **free endings** and **encapsulated endings.**

Table 4-1. Classification of Sensory Endings or Receptors

Exteroreceptors
Localized in the body surface
Receive information from the exterior, i.e., the environment
Sight, hearing, smell
Pick up distant stimuli **(teloreceptors)**
Touch, pressure, temperature
Stimulated by contact
Proprioceptors
Localized in the locomotor apparatus (muscles, tendons, and joints)
Receive information regarding posture and movement
Interoceptors
Visceral activities, e.g., digestion, excretion, circulation
Located in viscera and blood vessels
Also known as **visceroceptors**

Free Endings—Nonencapsulated Endings

Most free endings (Fig. 4-6) form arborizations between the tissue cells. The most undifferentiated type is almost exclusively related to the perception of subtle changes around the endings and nociceptive stimuli.

Other free endings may be found coiled around hair follicles. They are very sensitive to touch. Also, they may shape into discs and attach to special dermal cells known as **Merkel's cells** that form the **tactile discs of Merkel.**

Encapsulated Endings

Many encapsulated endings have been described, e.g., the **end bulb of Krause,** found in hairy skin and considered equivalent to the corpuscle of Meissner. However, only five encapsulated endings will be dealt with here: the **end organs of Ruffini,** the **tactile corpuscles of Meissner,** the **Pacinian corpuscles,** the **neuromuscular spindles,** and the **neurotendinous organs of Golgi.**

Ruffini Endings. The **end organs of Ruffini** (Fig. 4-6) are found in the dermis.

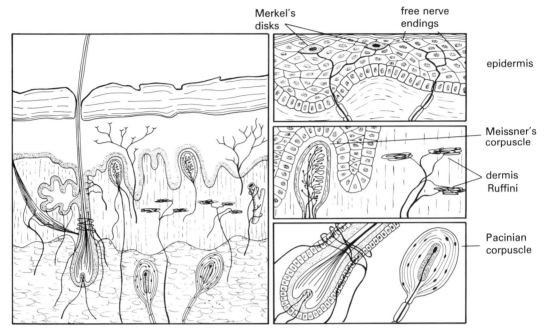

Fig. 4-6. Skin nerve endings.

These nerve terminals are intimately associated with collagen fibrils in the capsule. They are slowly adapting tactile and pressure receptors.

Corpuscle of Meissner. The **tactile corpuscles of Meissner** (Fig. 4-6) are found mostly in hairless portions of skin, in its dermal layer. The corpuscles consist of many epitheloid cells, neural endings spiralling around them, and a covering of a thin connective tissue sheath. They are highly discriminative tactile receptors.

Pacinian Corpuscle. The **Pacinian corpuscles** (Fig. 4-6) are considered specialized receptors for vibration and are widely distributed in the connective tissue. A Pacinian corpuscle consists of a cylindrical core housing the neural ending. It is covered by many layers of connective tissue cells.

Neuromuscular Spindles and Neurotendinous Organs of Golgi. Two other encapsulated and highly specialized receptors of stretch are the **neuromuscular spindles** and the **neurotendinous organs of Golgi.**

The muscles of locomotion, or striated muscles, are composed of two groups of muscle fibers: the real effectors of body movement or **extrafusal fibers;** and much smaller fibers grouped in little bundles, encapsulated and attached by their two ends to an extrafusal fiber. These are called **intrafusal muscle fibers,** because they are located inside a capsule.

Neuromuscular Spindles. Intrafusal muscle fibers with their neural endings are called **neuromuscular spindles** (Figs. 4-7A, B, and C).

The components of a neuromuscular spindle are shown in Table 4-2.

The spindle is attached to the extrafusal fiber. When the extrafusal fiber lengthens, it lengthens the spindle. This, in turn, excites the afferent endings. The stimulus-impulse travels to the CNS and activates α motor neurons, which innervate extrafusal fibers and make them contract, relaxing the spindle and stopping its impulses. This

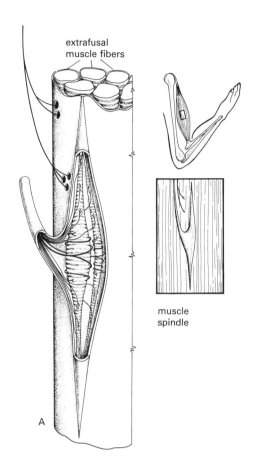

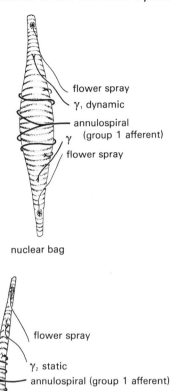

Fig. 4-7(A) Neuromuscular spindle. (B) Nuclear bag with nerve endings. (C) Nuclear chain with nerve endings.

is a reflex to regulate muscle tone.

The γ motor neurons terminate with **fusimotor fiber endings** in the intrafusal muscle fibers to adjust the sensitivity of the spindle by adjusting the length of the spindle.

Neurotendinous Organs. The **neurotendinous organs of Golgi** (Fig. 4-8) are found near the attachment of tendons to muscles. They are composed of a few collagenous fibers wrapped by a sensory ending and enclosed in a thin connective tissue capsule.

One function of these sensor organs is to counteract the role of the neuromuscular

Table 4-2. Components of a Neuromuscular Spindle

Muscle fibers
 Intrafusal, 2–10
  Nuclear bag—thickening in the midregion with many nuclei
  Nuclear chain—homogeneous with a chain of nuclei
Innervation—endings
 Afferent endings; sensory
  Primary afferent endings—annulospiral in midregion of fibers
  Secondary afferent endings—flower spray at the side of the midregions
 Efferent endings, motor
  γ; size: 3–7 μ
Capsule
 Thin connective tissue

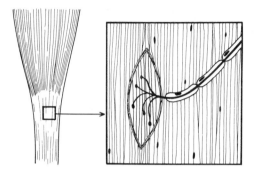

Fig. 4-8. Neurotendinous organ.

Efferent Endings

The axons projecting from the CNS toward the rest of the body and forming part of the efferent peripheral nervous system end in somatic (skeletal) muscles, if the axons are somatic. It was mentioned above that α motor neurons end in extrafusal muscle fibers and γ motor neurons in intrafusal muscle fibers. Their endings are thus of two types, i.e., α and γ **motor neuron endings.**

The nerve ending, together with the muscle fiber region where it establishes relation, is called interchangeably: **nerve muscle synapse, nerve muscle junction, neuromuscular junction, myoneural junction, end plate synapse,** and **motor end plate** (Fig. 4-9). All these names are synonyms for (1) the neural ending; (2) the portion of the muscle fiber that receives

spindles. When the tendon becomes too stretched, due to excessive contraction of the muscle, the excited neurotendinous spindles send an impulse to the CNS. This impulse inhibits the α motor neurons contracting the muscle, and as a result the force of the muscle contraction is reduced.

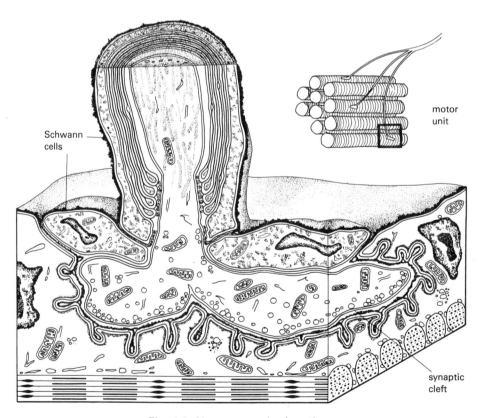

Fig. 4-9. Neuromuscular junction.

the ending and is shaped like a trough or plate, which may have foldings; and (3) a gap or cleft between them called the **synaptic** or **myoneural cleft.**

Motor Unit

A motor neuron sends the axon to the muscle where it branches out, giving off endings to 1 to 100 fibers. A motor neuron and the muscle fiber or fibers it innervates are together called a **motor unit** (Fig. 4-9).

Endings in the CNS: Synapse

The vast majority of neurons send their processes within the CNS to establish communication with other neurons. The junction were two neurons communicate is called a **synapse.** It has been calculated that there are at least 10^{14} synapses in the adult human.

Synapses are made by the coupling of any of the three regions of two neurons, i.e., axon, soma, and dendrite (Fig. 4-10), which render the basis for their various names, e.g., axodendritic, axosomatic, axoaxonic, and dendrodendritic synapses. The first three are the most common. In fact, examples of some of the other types have not even been found yet in the human nervous system.

Three regions are distinguished in a synapse (Fig. 4-11); (1) the **presynaptic region,** (2) the **synaptic cleft,** and (3) the **postsynaptic region.**

A number of elements and related terms in each region are self-explanatory:

1. **presynaptic terminal, presynaptic membrane, presynaptic vesicles,** etc.
2. **postsynaptic terminal, postsynaptic (subsynaptic) membrane, postsynaptic cytoplasmic densities,** etc.

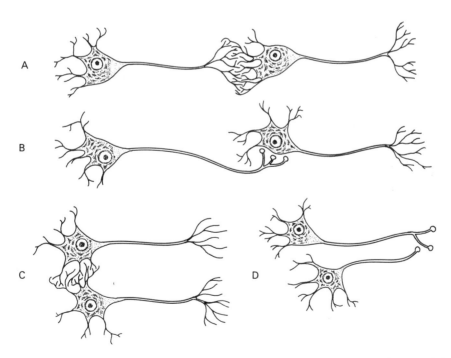

Fig. 4-10. Types of synapses: (A) axodendritic; (B) axosomatic; (C) dendrodendritic; (D) axoaxonic.

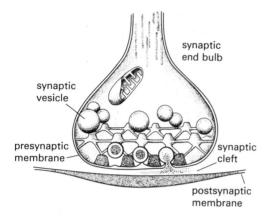

Fig. 4-11. Synapse.

The **presynaptic vesicles,** containing a chemical transmitter substance, attach to the presynaptic membrane and release the chemical into the cleft. The chemical transmitter released may be altering or stabilizing the **postsynaptic membrane,** thus qualifying the synapses as **excitatory** or **inhibitory,** respectively.

Those using chemical transmitters are **chemical synapses,** which constitute the majority. **Electrical synapses** or gap junctions transmit impulses electrically. The gap junctions have ultramicroscopic channels through which neurons are in communication with each other, providing synchronized firing. The neurons are said to be coupled.

The number of endings received by a neuron varies greatly, oscillating from a few endings to several hundred-thousand. Also the number of endings sent out by an axon varies, ranging from a few endings to several thousand.

Neuron Theory Versus Reticular Theory

The neuron theory defended the concept that the nervous system is composed of neurons that are independent structural and functional units, isolated from each other by gaps, or synaptic clefts.

The reticular theory, on the other hand, held that the nervous system consists of nerve cells forming a continuous reticulum or **syncytium.**

Although the neuron theory is well-established and the reticular theory abandoned, some modifications are being introduced following the recognition of electrical synapses.

Other concepts related to the neuron theory were developed. For example, **polarity of conduction,** i.e., the conduction of a stimulus in a fixed pattern (dendrite to cell body to axon to dendrite) is being reexamined subsequent to the recognition of other patterns of synaptic contacts.

Nerve Fibers

The axons are covered by glial cells. Only the sites of synapses are free from this glial lining.

The axons in the CNS are covered by glial cells and in the PNS by **Schwann cells.** An axon with its glial cells covering is called a **nerve fiber.**

Depending on the existence or nonexistence of a lipidoproteic material called **myelin,** the fibers are classified as **myelinated** and **unmyelinated (nonmyelinated) fibers,** respectively.

In myelinated fibers (Fig. 4-12) the apposed plasma membranes are arranged spirally around the axon. In the region of

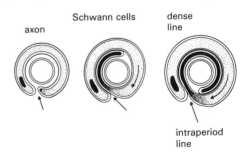

Fig. 4-12. Myelination.

contact between the inner surfaces of the plasma membrane, a dense substance, known as the **dense line,** or **major dense line,** is observed. In the region of contact between the outer surfaces of the plasma membrane runs a thin line, known as the **intraperiod line** (Fig. 4-13).

In general terms, myelin is the spiraled membrane with its entrapped material.

Outside the myelin are the **glial cytoplasm,** the **glial nucleus,** and the external **glial membrane,** which is also called **gliolemma** (Fig. 4-14).

A longitudinal sectional view of a peripheral myelinated fiber displays the interruptions of myelin between contiguous Schwann cells; these nodal gaps or clefts are the **nodes of Ranvier** (Figs. 4-14, 4-15, and 4-16) that, by definition, exist only in myelinated fibers.

The axons are not naked at the nodal cleft, but covered by interdigitations of the

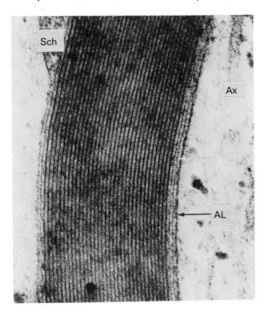

Fig. 4-13. Myelin layers. Ax, axon; AL, axolemma; Sch, Schwann cytoplasm.

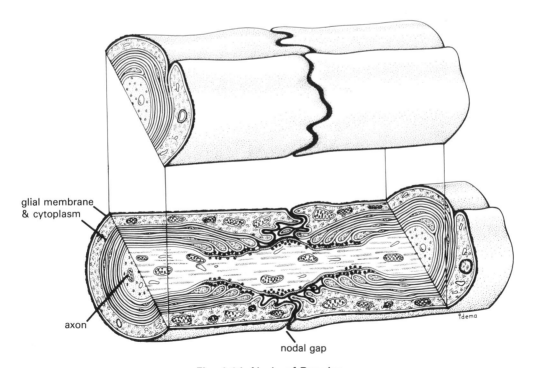

Fig. 4-14. Node of Ranvier.

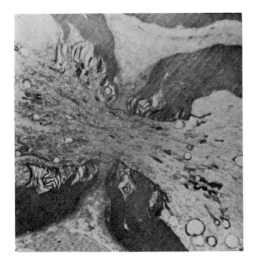

Fig. 4-15. Node of Ranvier.

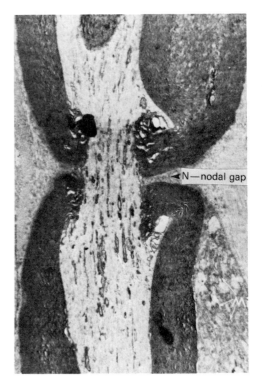

Fig. 4-16. Node of Ranvier. N, nodal gap.

Schmidt-Lantermann
cleft

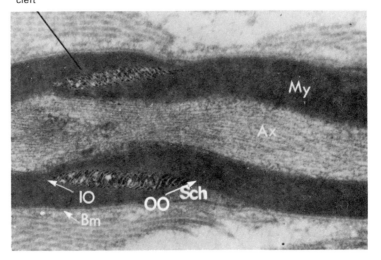

Fig. 4-17. Schmidt-Lantermann cleft. IO, inner opening; OO, outer opening; Sch, Schmidt-Lantermann cleft; My, myelin; Bm, basal membrane; Ax, axon.

outer portion of contiguous glial cells.

Another feature of myelinated fibers are the **Schmidt-Lantermann clefts** or **incisures** (Figs. 4-17 and 4-18). These appear as funnel-shaped gaps in the myelin and are due to a localized form of expansions of the dense lines.

In the case of unmyelinated fibers (Figs. 4-19 and 4-20), a row of glial cells encloses one or several axons.

Recent findings indicate that the unmyelinated fibers of the CNS are covered by astrocytes and not by oligodendrocytes as previously believed.

The caliber of fiber diameter ranges from .5 to 22 μ: fibers of .5 to 1.5 μ caliber are unmyelinated; myelinated fibers range between 1 and 22 μ. The thicker the axon, the thicker the myelin and the longer the **internodal length,** i.e., the distance between nodal clefts.

Classifications of Fibers in the PNS

There are several classifications for the millions of nerve fibers constituting the

PNS. Four of them have already been introduced: (1) sensory or motor—afferent or efferent; (2) somatic—visceral; (3) spinal—cranial; and (4) myelinated—unmyelinated.

A certain correlation has been found between the speed of the impulse recorded in fibers and their caliber: the greater the caliber, the faster the conduction.

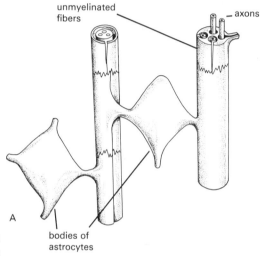

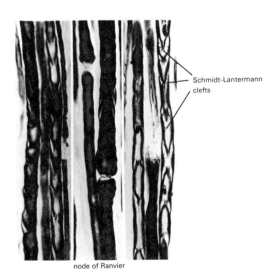

Fig. 4-18. Nerve fibers.

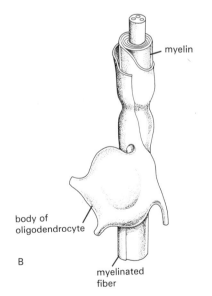

Fig. 4-19. Fibers of CNS.

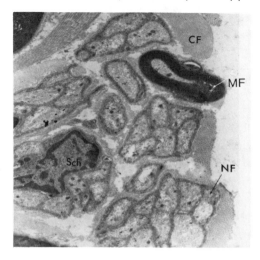

Fig. 4-20. One myelinated and many unmyelinated fibers. CF, collagen fiber; MF, myelinated fibers; NF, nonmyelinated fibers; Sch, Schwann cell nucleus.

Table 4-3. Fiber Diameter and Speed of Signal Conduction

Group	Diameter (μ)	Speed of Conduction (meters/second)
A ($\alpha, \beta, \gamma, \delta$)	1–20	5–120
B	1–3	3–15
C	0.5–1.5	0.6–2

Table 4-4. Somatic Afferent Fiber Receptors

Number	Receptors	Letter Equivalent
Ia	Annulospiral ending of neuromuscular spindle	A_α
b	Neurotendinous spindle	
II	Flower spray ending of neuromuscular spindle; touch and pressure receptors	$A_{\beta\&\gamma}$
III	Pain and temperature receptors	A_δ
IV	Pain and temperature receptors	C

As shown in Table 4-3, the letters A, B, and C have been used to designate three functionally differentiated groups of fibers where a correlation between their diameter and functional characteristics is established. Group A is further divided into four subgroups, α, β, γ, and δ.

Another classification specific to somatic afferent fibers uses numbers (Table 4-4).

Peripheral Nerves

A bundle or bundles of fibers wrapped in a connective tissue sheath is a **peripheral nerve** (Figs. 4-21 and 4-22).

The spinal and cranial nerves in a proximo-distal direction to the CNS branch off into progressively smaller peripheral nerves, also called **peripheral nerve branches.** The most distinct sheaths wrapping the fibers are the ones called **perineurium,** which consists of two or more layers of connective tissue cells encircling each bundle of fibers.

Within each bundle, between the fibers, collagen fibers and a few fibroblasts are sit-

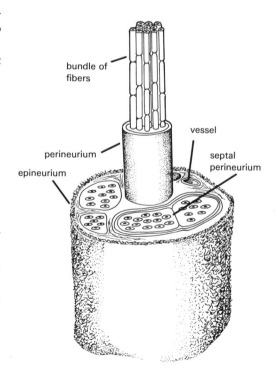

bundle of fibers

vessel

perineurium

septal perineurium

epineurium

Fig. 4-21. Nerve sheaths.

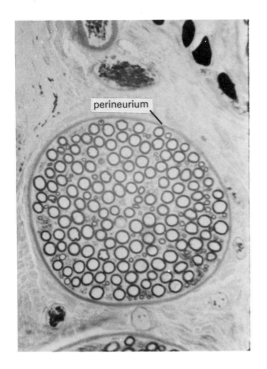

Fig. 4-22. Cross-section of nerve bundle.

uated. This is called **endoneurium.**

Between bundles of fibers there is loose connective tissue, i.e., the **epineurium,** infiltrated with droplets of fat.

When a nerve bundle reaches a region in the body where it branches off into smaller bundles, the innermost perineural layer builds a partition layer, the so-called **septal perineurium.**

Response of Nervous System to Injury

Due to previously mentioned properties of neurons and glial cells, an insult to the nervous system makes the neurons potential losers. They may suffer degenerative changes in their structure, which might end in cell death and **phagocytosis.** Principally, such changes are: eccentric position of the nucleus, swelling of the cell body, and finely granular dispersion of the Nissl substance or **chromatolysis.** Some glial cells, e.g., astroglia and microglia, become apparent winners. They may develop structural growth and proliferation. However, this imbalanced neuron-glia relationship places the nervous system as a whole in jeopardy.

Types of Degeneration

It has long been obvious and common knowledge that a deadly localized lesion of a tissue of the body will degenerate that tissue locally. The primary or initial cause is the injury. The degeneration of cells or tissue localized in the area receiving the insult is called the **primary** or **initial degeneration.**

In the last century it was discovered that a lesion in one region of the body (e.g., in the shoulder) could show degeneration of neural cells in another part of the body (along the arm) days or weeks later. This type of degeneration, distal from the injured area, secondary to the initial or pri-

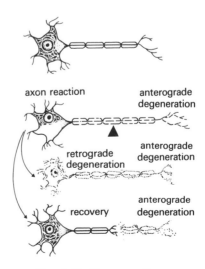

Fig. 4-23. Degeneration.

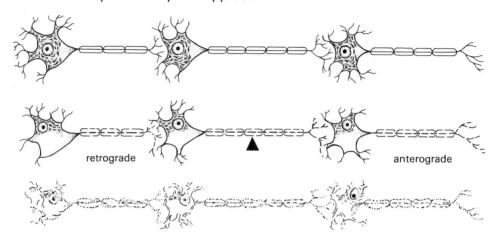

Fig. 4-24. Transneuronal degeneration.

mary degeneration, was named **secondary degeneration.**

The cause of such secondary degeneration of nervous tissue is that axons that become disrupted from their cell bodies die. The cell bodies are the center of life for their processes. This explanation was advanced by Waller in 1850. Later it was discovered that if a nerve is cut, not only is a degeneration of the distal (anterior) portion of the axons inflicted, as described by Waller, but changes also occur in the proximal portion attached to the cells. Such proximal axonal changes may be transitory and the cell with the retained portion of the axon may recover.

To distinguish these two phenomena of secondary degeneration, the following distinct terms are used (Fig. 4-23):

1. **Anterograde** or **Wallerian degeneration** for the degenerative changes occurring in the distal severed portion of the axon, i.e., the portion disconnected from the rest of the neuron.
2. A. **Retrograde degeneration** for degenerative changes occurring in the cell body and the proximal portion of the axon.
   B. **Axon reaction** for reactive changes occurring in the cell body and the proximal portion of the axon.

It happens in certain areas of the nervous system that the degeneration of a neuron is transmitted to the neuron with which it makes a connection. This describes **transneuronal degeneration.** It is a type of neuronal degeneration similar to what befalls skeletal muscle fibers, which degenerate when they become disconnected from their nerve fibers (Fig. 4-24).

Suggested Readings

Angevine JB: The nervous tissue. Chapter 12 in Bloom W, Fawcett DW, Eds.: A Textbook of Histology. Tenth Edition. WB Saunders, Philadelphia, 1975.

Barr ML, Kiernan JA: The Human Nervous System. Fourth Edition. Harper and Row, Philadelphia, pp. 13–58, 1983.

Carpenter MB: Human Neuroanatomy. Seventh Edition. Williams and Wilkins, Baltimore, pp. 71–158, 1976.

Elias H, Pauly JE: Human Microanatomy. Third Edition. FA Davis Co., Philadelphia, pp. 77–98, 1966.

Escourolle R, Poirier J: Manual of Basic Neuropathology. Second Edition. WB Saunders, Philadelphia, pp. 1–17, 1978.

Grafstein B, Forman SD: Intracellular transport in neurons, Physiol Rev 60:1167–1283, 1980.

Halperin JJ, La Vail JH: A study of the dynamics of retrograde transport and accumulation of horseradish peroxidase in injured neurons, Brain Res 100:253–269, 1975.

Heimer L: The Human Brain and Spinal Cord, Springer-Verlag, New York, pp. 127–150, 1983.

Heimer L, Robards MJ, Eds.: Neuroanatomical Tract-Tracing Methods, Plenum Press, New York, 1981.

Iggo A: Cutaneous receptors. In Hubbard JI Ed.: The Peripheral Nervous System, Plenum Press, New York, pp. 347–420, 1974

Iggo A, Andres KH: Morphology of cutaneous receptors, Ann Rev Neurosci 5:1–31, 1982.

Krnjevic K: Chemical nature of synaptic transmission in vertebrates, Physiol Rev 54:418–540, 1974.

Morell P, Norton WT: Myelin, Sci Am 242(5):88–117, 1980.

Peters A, Palay SL, Webster HdeF: The Fine Structure of the Nervous System, the Neurons and Supporting Cells, WB Saunders, Philadelphia, 1976.

Schwartz JH: The transport of substances in nerve cells, Sci Am 242(4):152–171, 1980.

Sears TA, Ed.: Neuronal-Glial Cell Interrelationships. Dahlem Workshop Reports, Vol. 20, Springer-Verlag, New York, 1982.

Shepherd GM: The Synaptic Organization of the Brain. Second Edition. Oxford University Press, New York, 1979.

Snell RS: Clinical Neuroanatomy for Medical Students, Little, Brown and Co., Boston, pp. 43–138, 1980.

Stevens CF: The neuron, Sci Am 241(3):54–65, 1979.

Varon SS, Somjen GG, Eds.: Neuron-glia interactions, Neurosci Res Program Bull 17:1–239, 1979.

II
Regional Anatomy

5

Spinal Cord and its Coverings

Vertebral Column

The **vertebral column** constitutes the bony case to the spinal cord, whose length it exceeds.

The column is composed of 7 **cervical,** 12 **thoracic,** and 5 **lumbar vertebrae** in addition to the **sacrum** (5 fused vertebrae) and the **coccyx** (4 small fused vertebrae) (Fig. 5-1).

There are two essential parts of the vertebral column (Fig. 5-2): (1) anteriorly, the **vertebral bodies** with their **intervertebral discs,** which are weight bearing; and (2) posteriorly, the **vertebral arches,** which form a protective covering of the spinal cord.

An **anterior** and a **posterior longitudinal ligament** attach to the front and back of the vertebral bodies, respectively, reinforcing the discs in these regions.

The intervertebral disc (Fig. 5-3) consists of an outer fibrous ring and a core of pulpy cartilage, the **nucleus pulposus.** Under excessive pressure, the fibrous ring may rupture and the nucleus pulposus may extrude, resulting in what is commonly known as a **ruptured, herniated** (or, misleadingly, **slipped**), **disc.** The disc usually ruptures lateral to the posterior longitudinal ligament.

The vertebral arches (Fig. 5-4) are composed of the **pedicles** and **laminae,** which meet in the posterior midline and project backward as the **spinous process.** The hole thus framed behind the vertebral body is the **vertebral foramen,** and the succession of these foramina forms the vertebral canal.

Attached to the laminae are the **ligamenta flava** (Fig. 5-2).

The pedicles of adjacent vertebrae frame the **intervertebral foramina** (Fig. 5-2). These holes serve as points of exit and entrance to spinal nerves and vessels.

A side view of two vertebrae shows the participation of the region where disc herniation in the intervertebral foramen commonly occurs.

The **sacral foramina** are intervertebral

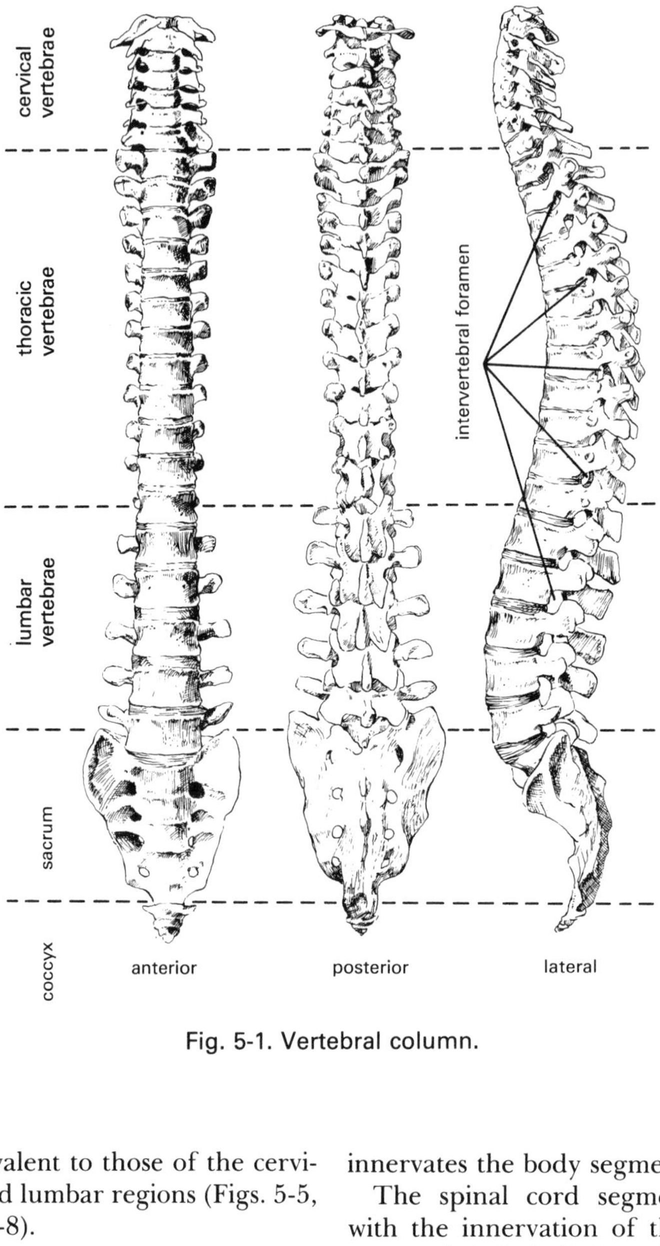

cervical vertebrae

thoracic vertebrae

intervertebral foramen

lumbar vertebrae

sacrum

coccyx

anterior   posterior   lateral

Fig. 5-1. Vertebral column.

foramina equivalent to those of the cervical, thoracic and lumbar regions (Figs. 5-5, 5-6, 5-7, and 5-8).

External Surface and Shape of the Spinal Cord

The 31 spinal cord segments together shape the spinal cord into a cylinder which

innervates the body segments.

The spinal cord segments concerned with the innervation of the upper limbs are cervical 5, 6, 7, 8, and thoracic 1 (C5 to T1).

The spinal cord segments concerned with the innervation of the lower limb are lumbar 1, 2, 3, 4, 5, sacral 1, 2, and 3 (L1 to S3).

Two regions of the spinal cord, C5 to T1 and L1 to S2, are larger than the other segments and are known as the **cervical** and **lumbar enlargements** of the spinal

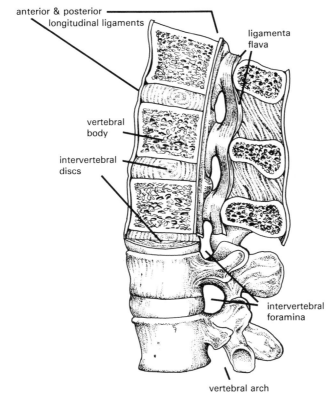

anterior & posterior
longitudinal ligaments

ligamenta
flava

vertebral
body

intervertebral
discs

intervertebral
foramina

vertebral arch

Fig. 5-2. Section of vertebral column.

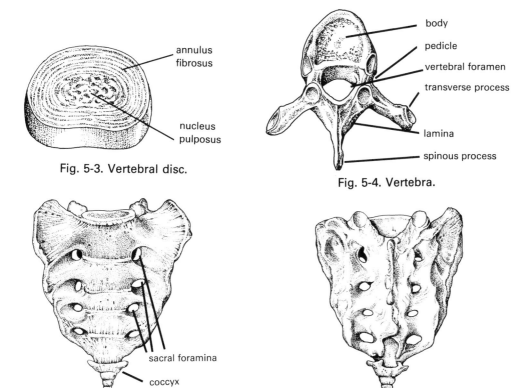

annulus
fibrosus

nucleus
pulposus

Fig. 5-3. Vertebral disc.

body

pedicle

vertebral foramen

transverse process

lamina

spinous process

Fig. 5-4. Vertebra.

sacral foramina

coccyx

Fig. 5-5. Anterior view of sacrum.

Fig. 5-6. Posterior view of sacrum.

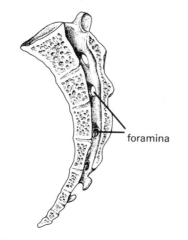

foramina

Fig. 5-7. Sagittal section of sacrum.

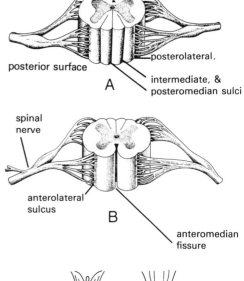

posterior surface

posterolateral,

intermediate, & posteromedian sulci

A

spinal nerve

anterolateral sulcus

B

anteromedian fissure

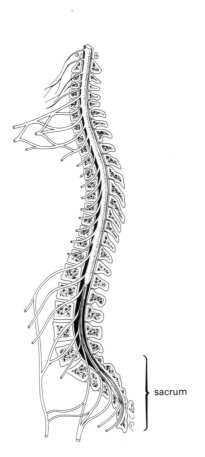

sacrum

Fig. 5-8. View of spinal cord within vertebral column.

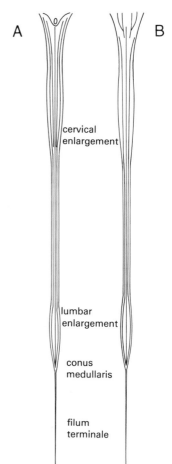

A

B

cervical enlargement

lumbar enlargement

conus medullaris

filum terminale

Fig. 5-9. Posterior (A) and anterior (B) views of spinal cord.

cord (Fig. 5-9).

Below the lumbar enlargement, the cord rapidly narrows to a cone-shaped termination, the **conus medullaris.**

The surface of the cord shows a number of longitudinal grooves, which are very helpful landmarks. Among them are the **anteromedian fissure,** which is the most prominent of all, and the **posteromedian sulcus.** More laterally are the **anterolateral** and **posterolateral sulci,** which demarcate the region of exit and entrance of the spinal roots. In the upper half of the cord (segments C1 to T6), another groove is situated between the posteromedian and posterolateral sulci, namely, the **posterior intermediate sulcus** (Fig. 5-9).

The terms ventral, ventro-, dorsal, and dorso- may be found in other textbooks replacing anterior, antero-, posterior, and postero-, which are used here. They are interchangeable.

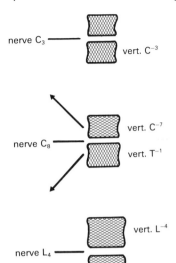

Fig. 5-10. Spinal nerves. Intervertebral relations.

Spinal Roots and Rootlets

The posterior and anterior roots fan out into bundles, **rootlets,** which are attached along the length of their cord segment.

The identification of the different cord segments can be ascertained by identifying their roots and rootlets. The **posterior root ganglion** is located in the region of the intervertebral foramen. The sensory fibers composing the distal pole of the ganglion join the **anterior root fibers** forming the spinal nerve (Fig. 5-9).

The identification of a spinal nerve can be settled by identifying its intervertebral foramen.

Given the number of vertebrae and the number of cord segments, and given the fact that cervical nerve C8 corresponds to intervertebral foramen formed by vertebrae C7 to T1, one can make the following rule of thumb: any nerve **above** C8 exits (enters) **above** its corresponding vertebral number; and any nerve **below** C8 exits (enters) **below** its corresponding vertebral number, e.g., lumbar spinal nerve IV exits below lumbar vertebra 4. The intervertebral foramen is formed by L4 and L5 (Fig. 5-10).

Meningeal Coverings of the Spinal Cord and Spaces

There is one major difference between the meningeal coverings of the brain and those of the spinal cord. In the spinal cord, the dura and the periosteum separate, leaving the epidural space, which is filled with venous plexuses and fat.

The cause of this epidural space at the spinal cord level is the increasing disproportion of growth between the cord and the column. In the case of the brain and the cranium, their growth is proportional.

It can be conceived that the brain in its

Table 5-1. Meningeal Coverings of the
Spinal Cord and Spaces

Structure	Space
Bone	
Periosteum	
Fat and veins	Epidural space
Dura	
	Subdural space (not visible)
Arachnoid	
	Subarachnoid space with CSF
Pia	
	Subpial space
CNS	

developmental growth pushes the dura
against the cranial periosteum and, fusing
both layers, squeezes the epidural venous
plexuses into discrete regions, which form
the dural sinuses. This process is possibly
not mechanical and its true nature is in
question.

In Table 5-1 the structural layers and
spaces are shown in a cross section of the
column with its contents (Figs. 5-11 and
5-12).

These coverings exhibit two peculiarities
in regards to the regional bony configuration: the **intervertebral foraminal recesses
of the meninges** (Fig. 5-13) and the **lumbar cistern** (Fig. 5-14).

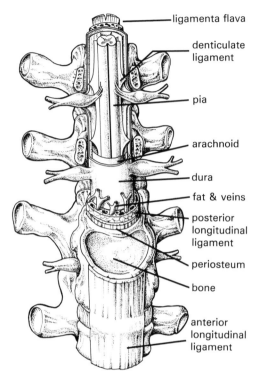

Fig. 5-11. Coverings of spinal cord.

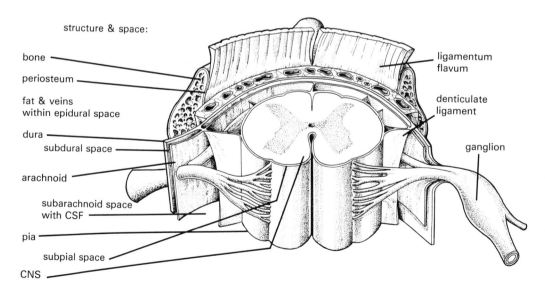

Fig. 5-12. Coverings of spinal cord.

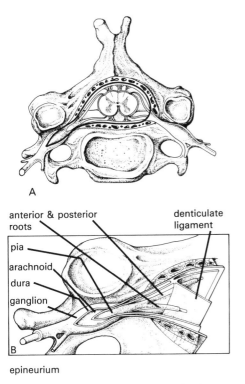

A

anterior & posterior
roots

denticulate
ligament

pia

arachnoid

dura

ganglion

B

epineurium

Fig. 5-13. (A) Intervertebral foraminal recess.
(B) Detailed view of A.

Intervertebral Foraminal Recesses of the Meninges

The roots with their rootlets are situated in the subarachnoid space. Along their length they are invested with a layer of pia that is continuous with the arachnoid. Reaching the spinal nerve, the pia continues as the inner and the arachnoid as the outer **perineurial connective tissue layers,** respectively.

The dura also forms a cuff to the distal end of the roots and the ganglion. It attaches to the periosteum at the level of the intervertebral foramen and continues outward over the outer layers of the perineurium as the epineurium.

The subarachnoid space is continuous

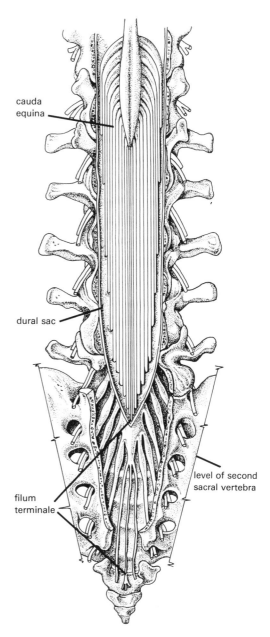

cauda
equina

dural sac

filum
terminale

level of second
sacral vertebra

Fig. 5-14. Lumbar cistern.

with the perineurial space between the inner and outer perineurial layers. The subpial space is continuous with the endoneurial space.

Lumbar Cistern

To understand the shape of the lumbar cistern, one must remember the disproportion between vertebral longitudinal growth and that of the cord. The vertebral canal continues through the sacrum down to the coccyx. The dura and arachnoid descend to the level of the second sacral vertebra, ending in a bag-shaped formation, the so-called **dural sac,** which contains the cerebrospinal fluid (CSF).

The pia mater, attached to the cord, continues at the tip of the conus medullaris downward as a thread of ependymal, glial, and connective tissue. At the level of the second sacral vertebra, it becomes invested with more connective tissue from the arachnoid and the layers of the dural sac. With this reinforcement it proceeds downward and reaches the dorsum of the coccyx, where it attaches. This thread is the **filum terminale** (Figs. 5-14 and 5-15).

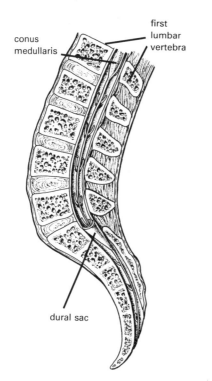

conus medullaris

first lumbar vertebra

dural sac

Fig. 5-15. Lumbosacral vertebral canal region.

The aforementioned discrepancy in cord versus vertebral lengths (cord: 44 cm; column: 70 cm) accounts for the lower roots being much longer than the upper roots.

The descending last lumbar and sacral roots seen inside the dural sac is graphically called the **cauda equina** (L. horse's tail).

The lumbar cistern containing the CSF can be punctured to have samples taken of this fluid for clinical diagnosis or to have chemicals injected for clinical diagnosis or treatment.

Punctures can be performed between vertebrae L3 and L4; L4 and L5; and L5 and S1 without risk of damaging the cord. In adults the preferred level is L3 to 4. The fact that infants may have the cord end at a lower than normal level, and that the largest dimension of the sac is at the level L5 to S1, makes this level the preferred one for infants.

Two different types of caudal punctures, i.e., the subarachnoid lumbar puncture and the transsacral epidural puncture, are illustrated in Figure 5-16.

Note: In cases of intracranial pressure, lumbar puncture is contraindicated because of the risk of brain herniation through the foramen magnum and subsequent death.

Topographical Relation of Cord Segments to Vertebrae

It is important for the clinician to know which cord segment is covered by which vertebra. The whole spinal cord occupies less than the two upper thirds of the vertebral canal. Normally, the tip of the cord is at the level of the L1 vertebra (Fig. 5-17).

Table 5-2 shows some useful cord seg-

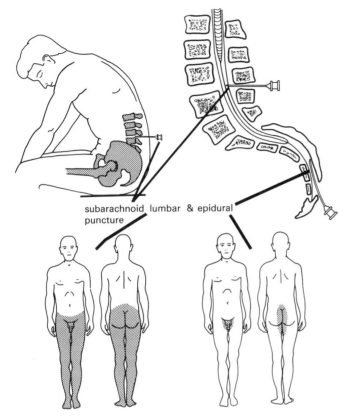

subarachnoid lumbar & epidural
puncture

Fig. 5-16. Caudal punctures.

Table 5-2. Relationships of Spinal Cord Segments—Vertebral Body Segments

Cord Segment	Vertebral Body	Spinous Process
C8	C6–7	C6
T6	T4–5	T3–4
L1	T11	T10
Sacral	L1	T12–L1

ment–vertebral body segment relationships.

A simplified rule of cord segments–vertebral body segments relation is cervical cord segments are located within the cervical vertebrae; thoracic cord segments within the first 10 thoracic vertebrae; lumbar cord segments within the last 2 thoracic vertebrae; and sacral segments within the first lumbar vertebra.

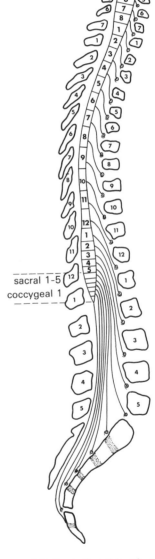

sacral 1-5
coccygeal 1

Fig. 5-17. Topographical relationship of vertebral segments—spinal cord segments.

The spinal cord is suspended in the dural canal by the **denticulate ligaments.** In each segment these ligaments are attached to the dura by "teeth" and to the pia by a reticular mantle of collagen fibers. The pia-arachnoid invests the ligament (Figs. 5-11, 5-12, and 5-13).

A strand of connective tissue fibers of the pia-arachnoid mater running along the ventromedian line is known as **linea splendens.**

Lengthening and Shortening of the Vertebral Canal

In ventral flexion the vertebral canal elongates and tenses the posterior longitudinal ligament and, even more, the ligamenta flava.

In dorsal flexion the vertebral canal shortens and the ligamenta flava slacken.

The common but mistaken view of the past held that the spinal cord and dura move up and down the canal with flexions and extensions of the spine. In reality,

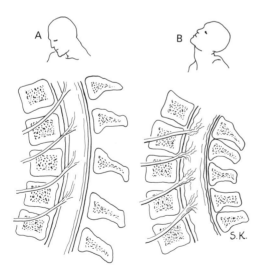

Fig. 5-18. Lengthening (A) and shortening (B) of the vertebral canal.

however, the cord, dura, and nerves are stretched in ventral flexion, whereas in dorsal flexion they slacken (Fig. 5-18).

The two spinal cord regions with the most extreme stretching and slackening are C6 to T2 and L4 to S5, respectively, due to the higher mobility of the corresponding vertebral regions.

Internal View of the Spinal Cord

A cross section of the spinal cord displays in its center the central canal and an H-shaped mass of gray matter surrounded by white matter (Fig. 5-19).

The **white matter** consists mostly of fibers. Its white color results from the abundance of myelin.

The **gray matter** contains neurons with their processes and glia, but it consists first and foremost of cell bodies and dendrites.

The cells of the gray matter originate from the four walls of the neural tube. The two anterior walls are called **basal plates** and the two posterior walls **alar plates.** They give rise to the anterior and posterior extensions of the gray matter, respectively. The junction between the alar and basal plates is known as **sulcus limitans** (Fig. 5-19C).

The two posterior extensions of the gray matter are the **posterior horns,** and their two anterior extensions are the **anterior horns.**

Much smaller than the anterior and posterior horns are the **lateral horns,** consisting of visceral motor neurons and situated bilaterally from T1 down to L2. The term horn is appropriate in reference to the spinal cross-sectional view, but when reference is made to these structures in their three-dimensional shape, the terms **posterior, anterior,** and **lateral gray columns** are used (Fig. 5-20).

Many of the neurons composing the

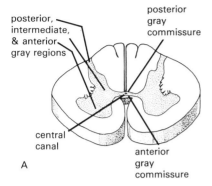

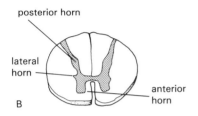

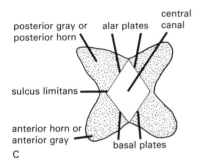

Fig. 5-19. Cross-section of spinal cord. (A) Cervical level; (B) thoracic level; (C) cell growth from neural tube.

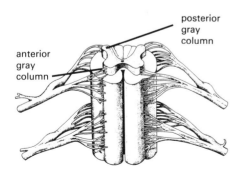

Fig. 5-20. Two spinal cord segments.

posterior horn region are picking up the impulses transmitted to them by the sensory roots. The posterior horn, or posterior gray column, is considered a sensory region.

The anterior horn region contains distinct motor neurons, whose axons form the motor roots. The anterior horn, or anterior gray column, is considered a motor region.

The region between the anterior and posterior horns is called **intermediate zone, intermediate region,** or **intermediate gray region.**

A **commissure** (L. *committere* to join together) is a region of union between two parts. The two thin bands of gray matter anterior and posterior to the central canal are the **anterior** and **posterior spinal gray commissures.**

Spinal Cord Nuclei

A histological analysis of the gray matter in each segment shows that some neurons are grouped together forming nuclei (Fig. 5-21). Some of the spinal nuclei are listed below:

1. The **posteromarginal nucleus** is situated at the margin of the posterior horn.
2. The **substantia gelatinosa (of Rolando)** occupies the posterior portion of the posterior horn. It has several components, four of which are
   A. the endings of small sensory fibers of the sensory root;
   B. many small neurons intrinsic to the substantia gelatinosa;
   C. dendrites of neurons whose cell bodies are situated in the center of the posterior horn; and
   D. the endings of some fibers that come from the brain.

The substantia gelatinosa exerts a modulating influence on the link primary afferents and spinal cord. For instance, some endings of small sensory fibers carrying nociceptive signals synapse in dendrites within the substantia gelatinosa. The small gelatinous neurons may amplify or inhibit such relays depending on their activity.

3. The **nucleus proprius,** also called the **chief, proper,** or **main sensory nucleus,** occupies the center of the posterior horn.

The dual role of this nucleus is to intervene in spinal reflexes and to transmit sensory information to other centers. These actions are regulated by the cerebral cortex.

The nucleus proprius contains

A. collateral endings of medium and large sensory fibers transmitting sensory modalities other than pain and temperature;

B. endings from the cerebral cortex; and

C. medium and small intrinsic neurons whose dendrites protrude in the substantia gelatinosa and whose axons synapse in motor neurons or travel in the white matter toward other centers.

4. The **dorsal nucleus (of Clarke)** is found in each segment from T1 down to L2 to L3. Its position is anteromedial to the nucleus proprius, and it is characterized by large neurons, whose axons are sent through the white matter upward, reaching the cerebellum. Sensory root fibers end in the nucleus and transmit proprioceptive information. All nuclei of Clarke together form the **column of Clarke.**

5. The **intermediolateral nucleus** occupies the small lateral horn, which, as was mentioned above, extends from T1 down to L2. The **intermediomedial nucleus** is located medially. Both the intermediolateral and the intermediomedial nuclei receive sensory visceral input and send (efferent visceral) axons through the motor roots toward the viscera.

It has been claimed that the intermediomedial nuclei are mainly related to the viscera of the trunk and the intermediolateral nuclei to the trunk wall and extremities. Each of the sacral segments 2, 3, and 4 has, instead of intermediomedial and intermediolateral nuclei, only one intermediate nucleus.

6. The **somatic motor neurons** are grouped in several motor nuclei for different muscle groups, all located in the anterior horn.

One distinguishes between the **medial** and **lateral groups of motor nuclei.** The medial group, which is present along all the segments of the spinal cord, innervates the muscles of the trunk. The lateral group innervates the muscles of the upper and lower limbs and is therefore prominent only in the segments C4 to T1 and L2 to S3.

Two main populations of neurons form these nuclei: the large **alpha** (α) **motor neurons** (for striated muscle fibers) and the smaller **gamma** (γ) **motor neurons** (for spindle muscle fibers).

The input to these nuclei may come directly or, most frequently, indirectly through other interneurons from posterior roots, cerebral cortex, and other centers, e.g., the brain stem.

The **phrenic motor nucleus,** whose fibers form the phrenic nerve and innervate the diaphragm muscle, belongs to the medial group of motor nuclei in segments C3 through C5. It receives to some extent afferents from the cerebral cortex but mostly from the brain stem respiratory center.

7. Situated on the lateral surface of the gray matter is the **spinal reticular nucleus.**

Laminae of Rexed

Rexed published the results of his studies on the structure of spinal cord gray matter of cats in 1952. He had found a

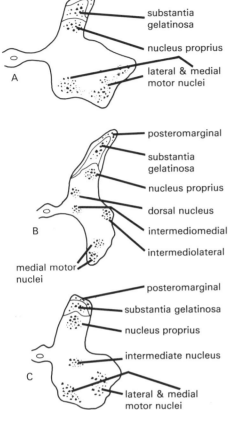

Fig. 5-21. Spinal cord cross-sections. (A) Cervical; (B) thoracic; (C) sacral.

4. lamina IX (which, by the way, is not laminated) corresponds to the motor nuclei; and
5. lamina X corresponds to the region around the central canal (Fig. 5-22).

The literature does not yet present consistent agreement concerning laminae V to VIII versus older nuclear terms.

structural laminar arrangement of this matter, which he labeled from I to X. The terminology has won scientific acceptance owing to its advantages when compared to the nuclear terminology, which addresses itself only to discrete regions of the cord.

When studying old and new findings in this area, it is wise to exercise caution. Currently, it is commonly agreed that

1. lamina I is a very thin layer at the tip of the posterior horn;
2. lamina II corresponds to the substantia gelatinosa;
3. laminae III and IV correspond to the main sensory nucleus;

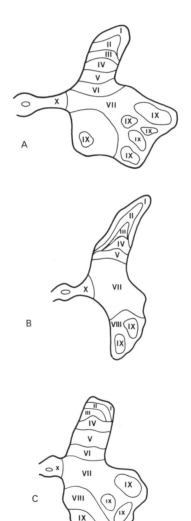

Fig. 5-22. Laminae of Rexed. (A) Cervical; (B) thoracic; (C) sacral.

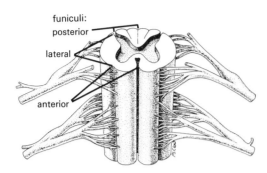

Fig. 5-23. Spinal cord white matter. Funiculi.

White Matter—Funiculi

The white matter of the spinal cord is arranged in three **funiculi** (L. little cords), i.e.,

1. the **anterior funiculus,** between the anteromedian fissure and the anterior gray column;
2. the **lateral funiculus,** between the anterior and posterior gray columns; and
3. the **posterior funiculus,** between the posterior gray column and the posterior median septum (which is a projection of the pia and the glia toward the posterior gray commissure from the posterior median sulcus). The posterior median septum separates the **left** and **right posterior funiculi** (Fig. 5-23).

The three pairs of spinal funiculi are also called the **anterior, lateral,** and **posterior spinal white columns.** They are composed mostly of vertically positioned ascending and descending fibers, whose origins are the following three: (1) the posterior roots mostly in the posterior funiculi; (2) the spinal gray matter, which sends ascending, and also some descending, fibers in the lateral, posterior, and anterior funiculi; and (3) descending fibers from the cerebrum and the brain stem mostly in the lateral and anterior funiculi.

Additional Terms Related to the Spinal Cord White Matter

There are other terms in the literature related to regions of the spinal cord white matter, e.g.,

anterolateral funiculus—the anterior portion of the lateral funiculus (Fig. 5-24)
posterolateral funiculus—the posterior portion of the lateral funiculus
anterolateral white column—the anterior region of the spinal cord white matter
posterolateral white column—the posterior region of the spinal cord white matter.

White Matter—Tracts

As a neuroanatomical term, a **tract** is defined as a group of fibers which travel together and have the same type of origin, course, and termination as well as function. It is convenient to qualify the meaning of "the same type" with some examples.

An ascending spinal tract is formed by contributions of fibers from the same region of many or all segments, which ascend (course) together and end higher up in a nucleus.

The name of a tract is composed by its origin and its termination, e.g., spinothalamic tract. In cases where two tracts have similar origin and termination, they

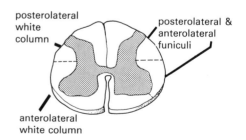

Fig. 5-24. Spinal cord white matter.

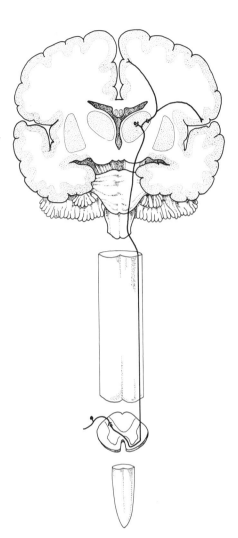

Fig. 5-25. Anterolateral spinothalamic tract.

the same origin, function, or termination. Although new data reveal greater complexity than reported in the past, the usage nevertheless still remains profitable.

The cells whose axons form part of the ascending paths are called **tract cells.**

White Matter—Fasciculi

When a bundle of fibers in the central nervous system (CNS) does not have the characteristics of a tract, it is called a **fasciculus.** The fibers of a fasciculus have different functions, origins, and/or terminations. The following are four of the fasciculi in the spinal cord:

1. The **fasciculus spinospinalis (propriospinalis)** interconnects spinal cord segments. It originates and ends in the spinal cord gray matter. The fasciculus contains ascending and descending fibers and participates in intersegmental spinal reflexes. Its position is immediately adjacent to the gray matter. This is the largest fasciculus (Fig. 5-26).
2. The **fasciculus posterolateralis,** also called the **posterolateral zone,** the **fasciculus dorsolateralis,** the **dorsolateral zone,** or **Lissauer's zone,** is a discrete

are distinguished by an additional term, which describes their topographical course, like anterior, lateral, or posterior, e.g., anterior spinothalamic, lateral spinothalamic, meaning that these tracts ascend in the anterior and lateral funiculi, respectively. These two tracts are frequently cited in the literature as one, namely, the anterolateral spinothalamic tract (Fig. 5-25).

The information collected particularly in the last decade furnishes grounds to question the validity of the term tract as it has been defined, because in many cases the fibers composing a tract may not have

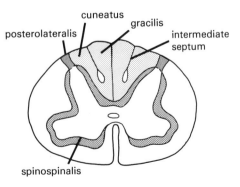

Fig. 5-26. Fasciculi.

bundle of small fibers at the tip of the posterior horns. Two main fiber groups make up this fasciculus:

  A. Small primary afferent fibers in their proximity to the posterior horn give off short branches ascending and descending one or two segments away (i.e., up or down).

  B. Small fibers from the posterior horn cells, e.g., substantia gelatinosa cells, enter the Lissauer's zone and give off short branches ascending and descending one or two segments away.

These two fiber types end in the posterior horns of neighboring segments.

3. The **fasciculus gracilis** makes up nearly all of the posterior funiculus in the lower half of the cord, from T7 down, and the medial portion of the posterior funiculus in the upper half, from T6 up to the medulla oblongata. The fibers of this fasciculus come from the sensory roots (T7 to coccyx) and carry tactile information to the brain from the lower half of the body. Its ascending fibers terminate in the nucleus gracilis, which is located in the inferior portion of the medulla, posteromedially.

4. The **fasciculus cuneatus** forms the lateral portion of the posterior funiculus in the upper half of the cord, from T6 up to the medulla oblongata. The fibers composing this fasciculus come from sensory roots C1 to T6. Its ascending fibers terminate in the nucleus cuneatus and accessory nucleus cuneatus, which are lateral to the nucleus gracilis. They carry tactile and proprioceptive information from the upper half of the body to the brain (through the nucleus cuneatus) and to the cerebellum (through the accessory nucleus cuneatus).

In the upper half of the cord the **intermediate septum** separates the fasciculi gracilis and cuneatus.

Endings of Sensory Root Fibers in the Spinal Cord and the Medulla Oblongata

The sensory root fibers, at their entrance to the spinal cord, rearrange into two bundles, i.e.,

1. the **medial bundle** or **division,** characterized by fibers of large diameters, which ascend, forming part of the posterior funiculus, and terminate in nucleus gracilis or cuneatus; and

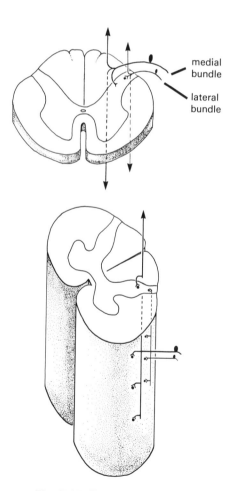

medial bundle

lateral bundle

Fig. 5-27. Spinal cord input.

2. the **lateral bundle** or **division,** characterized by fibers of small diameter,
which penetrate into the spinal gray
matter through the tip of the posterior
horn and terminate in the cord gray
matter (Fig. 5-27).

Apart from this rearrangement of the
fibers into medial and lateral bundles, one
must recall that all the sensory fibers, as
they approach their spinal level, divide
into a fork with ascending and descending
branches, from which horizontal branches
are given off (Fig. 5-27).

Some of the descending branches of the
primary afferent fibers gather into two distinct fasciculi, the **septomarginal** (lower
half of cord) and the **interfascicular** (upper half) **fasciculi** (Fig. 5-26).

Ascending Fibers of Posterior Versus Anterior and Lateral Funiculi

The following are the respective basic
patterns for two distinct groups of ascending pathways:

1. Some sensory root fibers enter the posterior funiculus, ascend in it, terminate
in the medulla oblongata and transmit
through the nuclei gracilis and cuneatus discriminative tactile and proprioceptive information to the cerebrum, where it becomes conscious
information (Fig. 5-28).
2. The ascending fibers of the anterior
and lateral funiculi come from neurons
of the cord gray matter, called second
sensory neurons, which receive information from primary sensory neurons,
whose cell bodies are in the spinal ganglia. Only 10 percent of these ascending
fibers of the anterior and lateral funic-

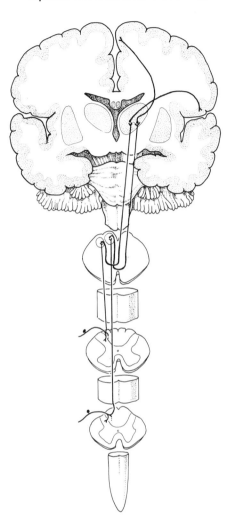

Fig. 5-28. Discriminative ascending path.

uli ultimately reach the cerebrum to relay signals at a conscious level. The
transmitted information is less discriminating than the information ascending
through the posterior funiculus, but
the potential for nociceptive (pain) information is strong. The bulk of the ascending anterior and lateral fibers ends
in the brain stem and contributes to unconscious circuitry.

General View of the Spinal Cord Circuitry

1. The spinal cord is engaged in its own ongoing activity carried out by neurons within each segment and between segments.
2. The spinal cord receives inputs from the body through the sensory roots and from the cerebrum and brain stem through descending tracts mostly in the anterior and lateral funiculi (Fig. 5-29).
3. The spinal cord sends information to the cerebrum and brain stem and an output to the body through the motor neurons.

These three activities are interdependent.

Spinal Cord Lesions

The information given until now about the spinal cord allows us to conclude a number of things, for instance, that (1) cutting the posterior funiculi will hinder discriminative tactile and proprioceptive conscious sensation; (2) cutting the anterior and lateral funiculi will abolish voluntary movements and perception of pain; and (3) cutting the motor roots or destroying the motor neurons will paralyse muscles of the body.

Identification of Spinal Cord Cross-Sections

If one quantifies with X the number of ascending fibers in the white matter toward the brain stem and cerebrum that each segment sends (upward), one finds 6X at the level of S1; 23X at T1; and 31X at C1.

If one again prescribes X for the number of descending fibers from the brain and the brain stem toward each cord segment (downward), one finds 31X at C1; 23X at T1; and 6X at S1. One can thus conclude that white matter increases from the sacral to the cervical segment. There is some disproportion at the **cervical** (C4 to T1) and **lumbar** (L2 to S3) **enlargements,** owing to the abundance of intrinsic (local) fibers, i.e., the **spinospinal fasciculus,** in the white matter of these segments. To identify the level of cross section this dis-

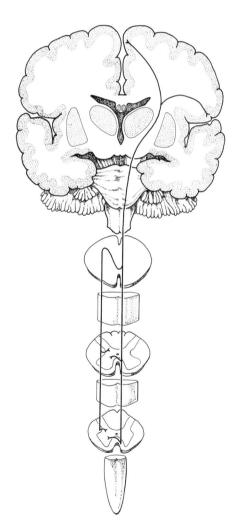

Fig. 5-29. Descending path: corticospinal.

proportion of white matter should be considered as well as the following facts:

1. The anterior median fissure is the only fissure of prominence.
2. The posterior intermediate septum is present only in cervical and upper thoracic segments.
3. The anterior horn becomes broader at C4 to T1 and L2 to S3, due to the presence of the lateral group of motor nuclei.
4. The lateral horn is present only at T1 to L2–3 (Fig. 5-30).

Somatotopic Representation in the Spinal Cord

Somatotopic representation relates to body regions. The spinal cord is organized in the same pattern as the regions of the body, and one speaks hence of a somatotopic organization of the nervous system. Examples of this arrangement at the spinal cord level are found in the anterior horns and in the funiculi (Fig. 5-31).

To understand the laminar arrange-

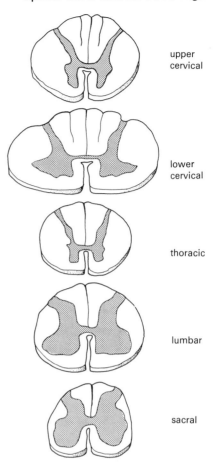

upper cervical

lower cervical

thoracic

lumbar

sacral

Fig. 5-30. Spinal cord cross-sections.

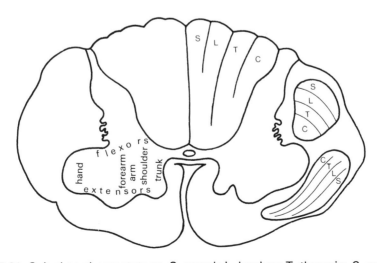

Fig. 5-31. Spinal cord somatotopy. S, sacral; L, lumbar; T, thoracic; C, cervical.

ment in the funiculi (Fig. 5-32) one must remember the origins of the fibers and their orientation. This pattern has developed to impede the waste of "wiring," which a mess of criss-crossing fibers would have made inevitable.

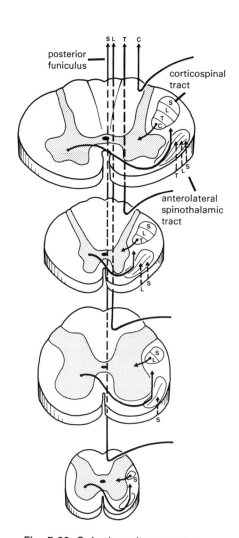

Fig. 5-32. Spinal cord somatotopy.

Suggested Readings

Barson AJ: The vertebral level of termination of the spinal cord during normal and abnormal development, J Anat 106:489–497, 1970.

Bennett GJ, Hayashi H, Abdelmoumene M, Dubner R: Physiological properties of stalked cells of the substantia gelatinosa intracellularly stained with horseradish peroxidase, Brain Res 164:285–289, 1979.

Brown AG: Organization in the Spinal Cord: The Anatomy and Physiology of Identified Neurons, Springer-Verlag, New York, 1981.

Carpenter MB: Human Neuroanatomy. Seventh Edition. Williams and Wilkins, Baltimore, pp. 213–237, 1970.

DeMyer W: Anatomy and clinical neurology of the spinal cord. In Baker AB, Baker LH, Eds. Clinical Neurology, Vol. 3. Harper and Row, Philadelphia, Chapter 31, 1981.

Fishman RA: Cerebrospinal Fluid in Diseases of the Nervous System, WB Saunders, Philadelphia, 1980.

Haughton VM, Ed.: Computed Tomography of the Spine, Churchill Livingstone, New York, 1983.

Matsushita M, Ikeda M, Hosoya Y: The location of spinal neurons with long descending axons (long descending propriospinal tract neurons) in the cat: a study with the horseradish perioxidase technique, J Comp Neurol 184:63–80, 1979.

Williams PL, Warwick R: Functional Neuroanatomy of Man, WB Saunders, Philadelphia, pp. 806–840, 1975.

Willis WD, Coggeshall RE: Sensory Mechanism of the Spinal Cord, Plenum Press, New York, 1978.

6

Brain Stem

Main Features of the Brain Stem

To understand the structural shape and the function of the **brain stem** it is important to be familiar with five main features of this region.

Structures Concerned with Equilibrium and Movement

The **cerebellum** and other structures are specialized in the automatic control of equilibrium and movement.

Fiber Paths

Situated between the cerebrum and the spinal cord, the brain stem contains not only **fibers (paths)** which connect its intrinsic structures among themselves but also fibers connecting (Fig. 6-1A):

1. the brain stem with the cerebrum and vice versa;
2. the spinal cord with the brain stem and vice versa; and
3. the spinal cord to the cerebrum and vice versa.

Interneurons—Tegmentum

The number of **interneurons** connecting sensory with motor neurons is larger in the brain stem than in the spinal cord to manage the complex circuitry implicit in the association and coordination of many vital functions, e.g., respiration, blood circulation, and sleep, as well as locomotion and instinctual reflexes. This mass of interneuronal tissue makes up most of the brain stem. The most complex arrangement of the interneurons is situated in a region called the **tegmentum** (Fig. 6-1B).

Cranial Nerves

The **cranial nerves** are more complex than the spinal nerves. In the spinal cord it is easy to recognize general patterns for the 31 pairs of spinal nerves (sensory-motor, posterior-anterior, ganglia, nuclei, etc.).

By contrast, however, each cranial nerve is unique. Some cranial nerves are sensory only, others are motor only, and yet others are mixed (sensory and motor) as in the spinal cord. A cranial nerve has none, one, or two sensory ganglia. It has one, two, or even four types of nuclei.

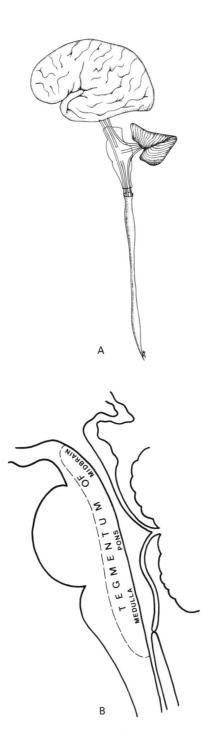

A

B

Fig. 6-1. (A) Brain stem connections; (B) tegmental region.

Rhombic Configuration

The bent neural tube of the embryonic stage unbends in its fetal stage in the region of the brain stem. This results in the **rhombic configuration (rhomboid fossa)** of the dorsal pons and the medulla oblongata, much resembling the bend of a hollow cane.

To acquire a more detailed conception of what these general features outline, it is necessary to explore the inside of the brain stem in cross-sections and surface projections of the medulla, pons, and midbrain.

Cross-Section at the Medullary Level

Structures Concerned with Equilibrium and Movement

The **inferior olivary nucleus** (Fig. 6-2) produces the oval bulge known as the **inferior olive** on the ventral surface of the medulla. The function of the inferior olivary nucleus is to encode body movements and to transmit this information to the cerebellum. For this purpose the message comes from the spinal cord through the spino-olivary tract and is transmitted to the cerebellum through the olivocerebellar tract.

Fiber Pathways

The pair of **nuclei gracilis** and **cuneatus** (Fig. 6-2) can be noted on the posterior surface of the medulla as four bulging masses. These nuclei are relay stations on the path transmitting sensory signals from the body to the cerebrum, where they become conscious information.

The long route along which the signals travel is called the **discriminative conscious path** (Fig. 5-28). It is formed by a "chain" of three neurons.

The first neurons are **primary sensory**

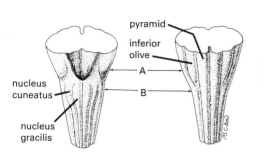

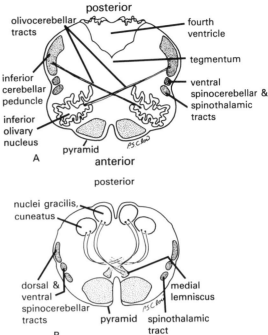

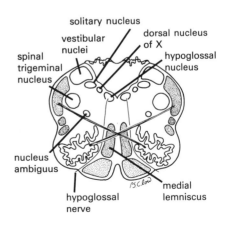

Fig. 6-2. Medulla oblongata. (A) Upper cross-section; (B) lower cross-section.

neurons. As we already know, their neuronal cell bodies are located in the spinal ganglia. Their processes start as sensory receptors in the periphery, continue in the posterior roots, ascend in the posterior funiculi, and reach the nucleus gracilis or cuneatus. The cells making up these nuclei send their axons anteriorly and toward the opposite side (decussation of the medial lemniscus) where they continue upward as a narrow band of fibers close to the medial line and finally reach the thalamus. This band of fibers is the **medial lemniscus** (L. fillet or narrow band) (Fig. 6-2B; Fig. 6-3).

The neurons and their axons of the nuclei gracilis and cuneatus are called the **second** or **secondary sensory neurons,** which together make up the medial lemniscus path. The primary and second sensory neuronal path is known as the **posterior (white) column—medial lemniscus path** and also as the **posterior funiculus—medial lemniscus path.**

The **third neurons** of the path are

found in the thalamus. They send their axons to the cerebral (thalamocortical) cortex (Fig. 5-28). Another important fiber path is made up by the **left** and **right corticospinal tracts,** which are seen anteromedially in a medullary cross-section. These tracts form anterior surface bulges called the **pyramids** (Fig. 6-2).

Fig. 6-3. Cross-section of medulla.

Coming from the lateral funiculus of the spinal cord and ending in the cerebellum are the **anterior** and **posterior spinocerebellar tracts** (Figs. 6-2 and 6-3). The anterior tract continues to ascend and enters the cerebellum through the superior cerebellar peduncle; the posterior tract enters the cerebellum through the inferior cerebellar peduncles.

The **spinothalamic** and **spinotectal tracts,** together called the **spinal lemniscus,** ascend posteriorly to the inferior olivary nucleus toward the thalamus and the tectum of the midbrain (Figs. 5-25 and 6-3).

Medullary Tegmentum

A distinct light gray region is observed occupying the posteromedial region of the medulla. Apart from the numerous neuronal cell bodies, there are also many fibers here, some of which make up a very intricate mesh. This region is the **tegmentum** (L. lower roof or ceiling) **of the medulla** (Fig. 6-2). It consists of interneurons concerned with the regulation of vital functions. Within this interneural medullary tegmentum one can identify components such as a reticular meshwork with Golgi type I axons. These axons spread throughout the whole nervous system and participate in the control of vital functions.

Cranial Nerve Nuclei

Discrete patches of dark gray are seen within the tegmental region. These are typical nuclei with well-packed neuron cell bodies. These nuclei are the points of origin (motor) or of arrival (sensory) of the fibers composing the medullary cranial nerves (Fig. 6-3).

Several cross-sections of the medulla contain nuclei of cranial nerves V, VIII, IX, X, XI, and XII.

Cranial Nerve V

The **cranial nerve V,** i.e., the **trigeminal nerve,** is not seen surfacing on the medulla oblongata, but at this level there are a nucleus and a tract corresponding to this nerve, namely, the **spinal trigeminal tract** and **nucleus** (Figs. 6-3 and 6-4).

Cranial Nerve VIII

The **cranial nerve VIII,** i.e., the **vestibulocochlear** or **statoacoustic nerve,** has two distinct branches, the **static** and the **acoustic.** Both branches are sensory. Its sensory ganglia are the vestibular and spiral ganglia. Laterally, it surfaces on the upper border of the medulla. It picks up stimuli from two distinct sensory organs (Fig. 6-5), i.e.,

1. the **vestibule** and **semicircular canal,** transmitting signals which are basic to

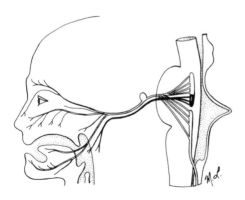

Fig. 6-4. Trigeminal nerve.

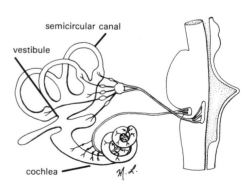

Fig. 6-5. Vestibulocochlear nerve.

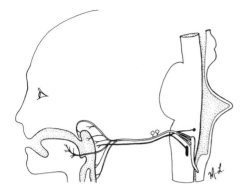

Fig. 6-6. Glossopharyngeal nerve.

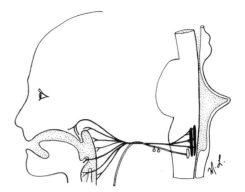

Fig. 6-7. Vagus nerve.

the related functions of static equilibrium, orientation, dynamic equilibrium or, in other words, posture and movement; and

2. the **cochlea,** a spirally shaped "tube," transmitting signals related to sound and hearing.

The nuclei of these two components of the cranial nerve VIII are the **vestibular nuclei** (four) (Fig. 6-3) and the **cochlear nuclei** (two).

Cranial Nerve IX

The **cranial nerve IX,** the **glossopharyngeal nerve** (Fig. 6-6), is sensory and motor. It has two sensory ganglia, namely, the superior and inferior ganglia. It surfaces laterally on the upper portion of the medulla. It carries sensory information of several kinds; taste from the posterior one-third of the tongue and tactile information from the pharynx and the posterior one-third of the tongue. It carries special information from baroreceptor and chemoreceptor organs. Motor fibers innervate the stylopharyngeus muscle, which is involved in swallowing.

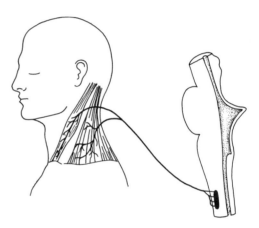

Fig. 6-8. Spinal accessory nerve.

The main nuclei of this nerve are: the **solitary, inferior salivatory,** and **ambiguus nucleus** (Fig. 6-3).

The afferent fibers of the solitary nucleus form the **solitary tract** or fasciculus.

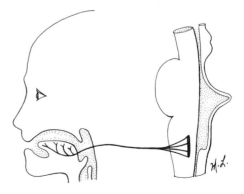

Fig. 6-9. Hypoglossal nerve.

Cranial Nerve X

The **cranial nerve X,** the **vagus nerve** (Fig. 6-7), is sensory and motor. It has two sensory ganglia, i.e., the superior and inferior ganglia. It surfaces below the glossopharyngeal nerve and carries sensory information from the pharynx, larynx, baroceptor, and chemoreceptor organs, and viscera from the neck, thorax, and abdomen. It innervates the muscles involved in swallowing and phonation as well as the muscles of thoracic and abdominal viscera.

The main nuclei of this nerve are the **solitary, ambiguus,** and **dorsal vagal nucleus** (Fig. 6-3).

Cranial Nerve XI

The **cranial nerve XI,** the **spinal accessory nerve** (Fig. 6-8), is only motor. This nerve surfaces below the vagus nerve. It innervates the sternomastoid and trapezius muscles, two muscles involved in head, neck, and shoulder movements.

The main nucleus of this nerve is the **spinal accessory nucleus.**

Cranial Nerve XII

The **cranial nerve XII,** the **hypoglossal nerve** (Fig. 6-9), is motor only. It surfaces between the inferior olive and pyramid and innervates the muscles of the tongue.

The main nucleus of this nerve is the **hypoglossal nucleus** (Fig. 6-3).

Cross-Section at the Pontine Level

Structures Concerned with Equilibrium and Movement

In the ventral portion of the cross-section the numerous so-called **pontine nuclei** (Fig. 6-10) create the belt-like appearance of the ventral pons. The neurons composing these nuclei receive information of the movements which the brain cortex is demanding to have executed. The information becomes recorded as well as transmitted to the cerebellum.

The paths are **corticopontine** (afferent to the nuclei) and **pontocerebellar** (efferent from the nuclei) (Fig. 6-10).

Fiber Pathways

1. The **medial lemniscus** (Fig. 6-10) continues upward and toward the sides, diverting from its medial position.
2. The **lateral lemniscus** is an ascending band of fibers, forming a link of the auditory pathway. This pathway starts in the inner ear apparatus. The auditory signals, through a chain of neurons at medullary levels, reach the lateral lemniscus. The lateral lemniscus is lateral to the medial lemniscus at the level of the pons (Fig. 6-10).
3. The **corticospinal tracts** that are seen forming the pyramids are diffused in smaller bundles between the pontine nuclei. Other fiber bundles ending in pontine nuclei form the descending corticopontine tract and the horizontally arranged pontocerebellar tract (see above).
4. The **anterior spinocerebellar tract** continues ascending in its lateral position and reaches the cerebellum through the superior cerebellar peduncle, a portion of which is seen in the upper pons region (Fig. 6-10).

    The **posterior spinocerebellar tract** is not seen in the pons, because it reaches the cerebellum through the inferior cerebellar peduncle.
5. The **spinothalamic** and **spinotectal tracts (spinal lemniscus)** continue ascending dorsolaterally (Fig. 6-11).

Pontine Tegmentum

A tegmental region, similar to the one observed in the medullary cross-section, is

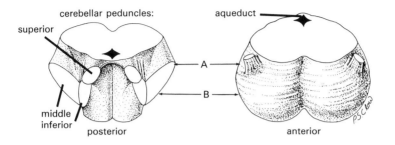

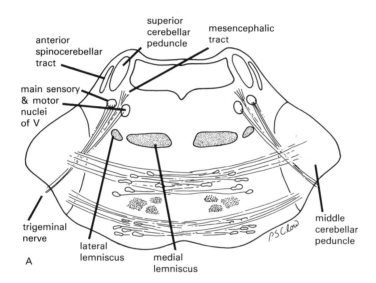

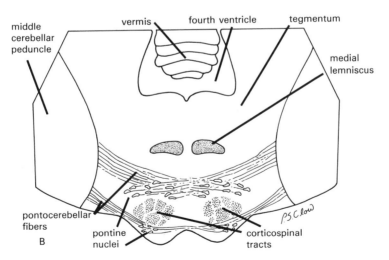

Fig. 6-10. Pons. (A) Upper cross-section; (B) lower cross-section.

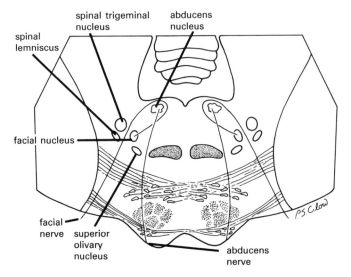

Fig. 6-11. Cross-section of pons.

seen at the pontine level. This is the **tegmentum of the pons.**

Cranial Nerve Nuclei

The **cranial nerve nuclei** seen in the tegmentum of the pons belong to cranial nerves V, VI, and VII.

Cranial Nerve V

The **cranial nerve V,** the **trigeminal nerve** (Fig. 6-4), has three branches. It surfaces laterally on the basal pons. First and foremost it carries sensory information of different types (tactile, pain, and proprioception) from most of the head. Its sensory ganglion is the **trigeminal semilunar** or **gasserian ganglion.** It also carries motor fibers to the muscles of mastication and other small muscles.

The main nuclei of this nerve are: the **mesencephalic, chief sensory, trigeminospinal,** and **masticatory nuclei** (Figs. 6-10 and 6-11).

Cranial Nerve VI

The **cranial nerve VI,** the **abducens nerve** (Fig. 6-12), is motor only. It surfaces medially on the lower border of the pons.

It innervates a muscle of the eye.

The main nucleus of this nerve is the **abducens nucleus** (Fig. 6-11).

Cranial Nerve VII

The **cranial nerve VII,** the **facial nerve** (Fig. 6-13), is sensory and motor. Its sensory ganglion is the **geniculate ganglion.** It surfaces laterally on the lower border of the pons. It carries sensory signals from the salivary and lacrimal glands; taste from the anterior two-thirds of the tongue; and cutaneous signals from the external ear. Motor fibers travel to the muscles of facial expression and efferents to salivary and lacrimal glands.

The main nuclei of this nerve are the

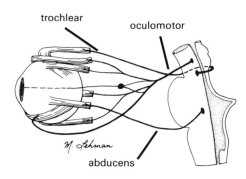

Fig. 6-12. Cranial nerves III, IV, and VII.

solitary, facial, lacrimal, and **superior salivatory nuclei.**

Cross-Section at the Midbrain Level

Structures Concerned with Equilibrium and Movement

Quadrigeminal Bodies

The **quadrigeminal** (L. four identical) **bodies** (Fig. 6-14), formed by the **superior**

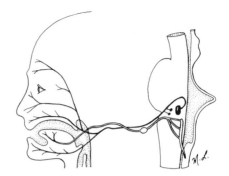

Fig. 6-13. Facial nerve.

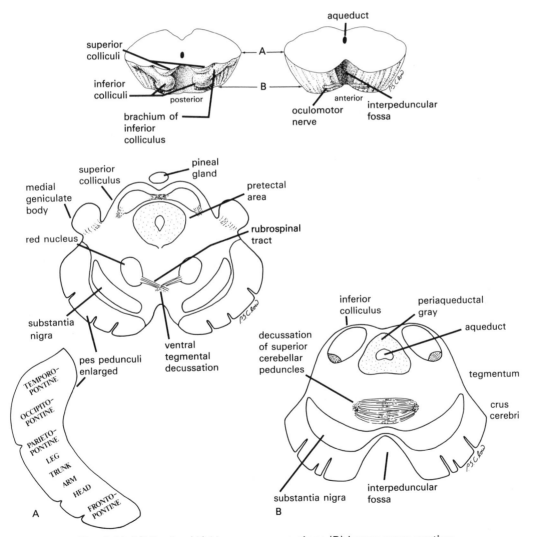

Fig. 6-14. Midbrain. (A) Upper cross-section; (B) lower cross-section.

and **inferior colliculi,** are seen protruding in the dorsum of the midbrain, thus constituting the bulging part of the **tectum** (L. upper roof) **of the midbrain.**

The tectum of the midbrain is the region of the midbrain dorsal to the aqueduct. The colliculi have very well-organized sets of neurons, which are arranged in layers.

The region just anterior to the superior colliculus is called the **pretectal area.**

Signals come to the colliculi from (1) the body, through the spinotectal tract; (2) the ear, through the auditory path, which is identified as the lateral lemniscus; (3) the eye, through the visual path; and (4) the cortex.

Output fibers from the tectum reach a number of structures, e.g., cranial nerve nuclei, the pretectal area, the reticular formation, the pontine nuclei, and the cervical spinal cord, in the last example forming the **tectospinal tract.** These connections permit the execution of patterned reflex movements involved in the orientation of the eyes and head to the source of the signal. The colliculi may be considered as centers for sound and visual localization and orientation reactions.

Red Nucleus

The **red nucleus** (Fig. 6-14) is an oval structure of the size of a colliculus. It is situated in the center of the mesencephalon close to the midline.

The red nucleus is concerned with excitation of flexor muscles and inhibition of extensor muscles. It receives afferents from various regions like the cerebellum, tectum, and cerebral cortex. It has output to several regions, like the cerebellum, inferior olive, reticular formation, and the spinal cord; this last path is the **rubrospinal tract.**

Substantia Nigra

Anterolateral to the red nucleus is the **substantia nigra** (Fig. 6-14), a distinct mass

abundant in melanin, which makes it appear black. It is a modulator of patterns of movements through inhibitory discharges. It has input and output with regions involved in the patterning of movements. A massive discharge of substantia nigra neurons abolishes striate muscle tone.

Note: L. *crus* (pl. *crura*) leg, stalk, or peduncle. The term **crus cerebri** is synonymous with cerebral peduncle. These terms refer to the whole midbrain region except the tectum, i.e., tegmentum, substantia nigra, and ventral white tracts.

Another term for the ventral white tracts is **pes pedunculi.** The substantia nigra and ventral tracts together constitute the **basis pedunculi.**

Pathways

The pathways of the midbrain are (1) the ones just mentioned above, i.e., the tectospinal and rubrospinal tracts; and (2) motor tracts descending from the brain cortex. They are positioned ventral to the substantia nigra and form the pes pedunculi (Figs. 6-14 and 6-15). The tracts course from a medial to a lateral position, i.e.,

the **frontopontine tract:** from the cortex of the frontal lobe to the pontine nuclei;

the **corticobulbar tract:** from the frontal and parietal cortex to motor nuclei of the cranial nerves;

the **corticospinal tract:** from the frontal and parietal cortex to the spinal cord; and

the **parieto-, occipito-,** and **temporopontine tracts:** from the parietal, occipital, and temporai cortex to the pontine nuclei.

(3) The ascending sensory paths from the spinal cord and brain stem toward the thalamus are the three lemnisci mentioned at the level of the pons in addition to the fibers of the trigeminal nuclei coursing toward the thalamus. The anteroposterior arrangement of the lemnisci is medial, tri-

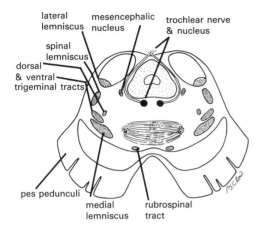

Fig. 6-15. Cross-section of midbrain.

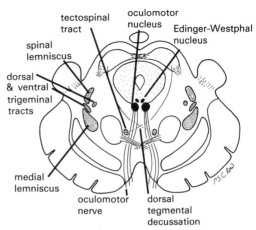

Fig. 6-16. Cross-section of midbrain.

geminal, spinal, and lateral.

The lateral lemniscus ends in the inferior colliculus. Past this level the spinal and trigeminal lemnisci are reduced in size, because many of the fibers that carry noxious signals or alarm signals end in the superior colliculus or the reticular formation.

Efferent fibers from the cerebellum toward the diencephalon travel within the superior cerebellar peduncle and, at the level of the inferior colliculus, cross the midline, continue to ascend and end in the thalamus. This is called the **decussation of brachium conjunctivum** or the **decussation of the superior cerebellar peduncle** (Fig. 6-14B).

Midbrain Tegmentum

The **midbrain tegmentum** (Fig. 6-14), which contains several nuclei, is a region at midbrain level similar to the tegmenta described in the medulla and pons. The region around the aqueduct is known as the **periaqueductal gray.**

Cranial Nerve Nuclei

The **cranial nerve nuclei** at the midbrain level belong to cranial nerves III, IV, and V.

Cranial Nerve III

The **cranial nerve III,** the **oculomotor nerve** (Fig. 6-12), is motor only. It surfaces medially on the interpeduncular fossa and innervates muscles of the eye.

The main nuclei of this nerve are the **oculomotor** and the **Edinger-Westphal nuclei** (Fig. 6-16).

Cranial Nerve IV

The **cranial nerve IV,** the **trochlear nerve** (Fig. 6-12), is motor only. It surfaces medially below the inferior colliculi and innervates a muscle of the eye.

The main nucleus of this nerve is the **trochlear nucleus** (Fig. 6-15).

Cranial Nerve V

The **cranial nerve V** is not seen surfacing on the midbrain. However, at this level there is a nucleus whose cell fibers travel with the V nerve, i.e., the **mesencephalic nucleus** (Fig. 6-15) of the trigeminal nerve.

Now that some of the components of the three levels of the brain stem have been introduced, a detailed account of the individual cranial nerve nuclei follows.

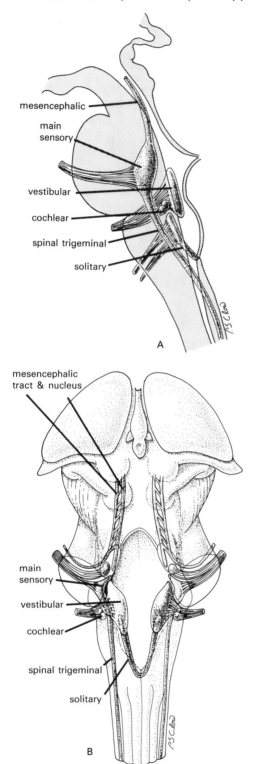

mesencephalic

main
sensory

vestibular

cochlear

spinal trigeminal

solitary

A

mesencephalic
tract & nucleus

main
sensory

vestibular

cochlear

spinal trigeminal

solitary

B

Fig. 6-17. Lateral (A) and posterior (B) views of brain stem. Sensory nuclei.

Cranial Nerve Nuclei—Sensory

There are six cranial nerve sensory nuclei in the brain stem. Five of these consist of secondary sensory neurons which receive a stimulus through the primary sensory neurons. The cell bodies of the primary sensory neurons form the cranial ganglia, except for the **mesencephalic nucleus,** where they form the very nucleus.

Mesencephalic Nucleus

The **mesencephalic nucleus** (Fig. 6-17) is a slender nucleus situated lateral in the mesencephalon. Its function concerns proprioception. The axons of the cell bodies have two branches: one coming from sensory proprioceptive endings in muscles of mastication as well as other muscles of head, pharynx, and larynx; and the other synapsing with a motor nucleus, i.e., the **masticatory nucleus,** which is a key component in a circuit for reflexes (Fig. 6-18).

Chief Sensory Nucleus

The **chief sensory nucleus** (Fig. 6-17), also called the **principal sensory nucleus,** is located laterally in the pons. It is characterized by large neurons. Its function concerns discriminative touch and pressure from most of the head. It sends fibers to the thalamus ipsilaterally **(dorsal trigeminothalamic tract)** and contralaterally **(ventral trigeminothalamic tract).**

Trigeminospinal Nucleus

The **trigeminospinal nucleus** (Fig. 6-17) is a slender nucleus situated laterally and extending from the chief sensory nucleus to the substantia gelatinosa of cervical segment 1. It is characterized by small neurons. Its function concerns nociceptive and light touch signals from most of the pharynx and larynx. It sends fibers to cranial nerve motor nuclei for reflexes and as-

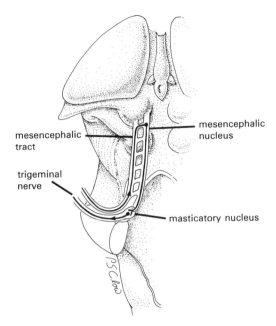

Fig. 6-18. Masticatory reflex path.

cending fibers to the thalamus, mostly contralaterally, forming part of the **ventral trigeminothalamic tracts.**

The fibers coming into the nucleus arrange themselves as the **spinal trigeminal (trigeminospinal) tract.** The trigeminospinal tract and the trigeminospinal nucleus correlate in structure and function with the dorsolateral fasciculus and the substantia gelatinosa, respectively.

Dorsal and Ventral Cochlear Nuclei

Laterally, in the rostral end of the medulla, are the **dorsal** and **ventral cochlear nuclei** (Fig. 6-17). Their function concerns hearing signals. The fibers ascend toward the inferior colliculus, forming the **lateral lemniscus.** The inferior colliculus sends fibers to the brain stem nuclei which permit auditory reflexes. The main output is directed toward the thalamus and travels from there to the brain cortex, forming part of the **conscious auditory path** (Fig. 6-19).

Vestibular Nuclear Complex

The **vestibular nuclear complex** (Fig. 6-17) is placed laterally mainly in the rostral area of the medulla. Its function concerns equilibrium and posture. It consists of the **lateral, superior, medial,** and **inferior vestibular nuclei** (Figs. 6-17 and 6-20).

These nuclei receive input from the vestibular nerve. They have a feed-back loop with the cerebellum through the inferior cerebellar peduncle. In addition to this feed-back loop with the cerebellum, they have three outputs:

1. The **lateral vestibulospinal tract** (Fig. 6-20) courses from the lateral vestibular nucleus (i.e., nucleus of Deiter) to the spinal cord. It excites neurons innervating extensor muscles mainly of the trunk and inhibits neurons of flexor muscles.
2. The **medial longitudinal fasciculus (MLF)** originates in the four vestibular nuclei. Its fibers travel toward the midline, where they branch out in ascending and descending fibers.

   Two related functions are handled by the MLF. One is by ascending fibers to interconnect motor nuclei, especially

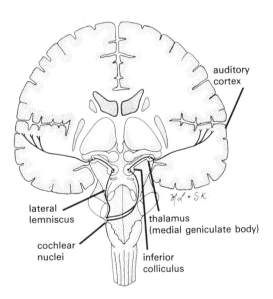

Fig. 6-19. Auditory path.

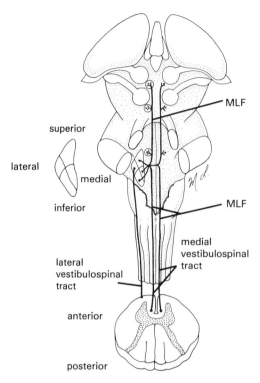

Fig. 6-20. Vestibular paths. Posterior view.

the ones concerned with eye movement, and the other to coordinate neck muscles by descending fibers which reach the cervical segments of the spinal cord. These descending fibers are specifically known as the **medial vestibulospinal tract.** Movement of the eyes, head, and neck are very important in equilibrium.

3. In the **vestibulothalamocortical path,** fibers from the vestibular nuclei ascend contralaterally with the medial lemniscus to end in the thalamus, which sends the impulses to the cortex.

Solitary Nucleus

The **solitary nucleus** (Fig. 6-17) is situated dorsally along the length of the medulla. It is involved in (1) taste signals coming from the tongue; (2) baroceptor signals and chemical signals (oxygen tension, CO_2) from baroceptor and chemoreceptor organs; and (3) sensory visceral signals from thoracic and abdominal viscera.

As the afferent fibers approach the solitary nucleus they form the **solitary tract.**

Summary of Cranial Nerve Sensory Nuclei

The connections between the fibers arriving to the nuclei and the cranial nerve of origin are presented in Table 6-1.

Cranial Nerve Nuclei—Motor

There are 13 cranial nerve nuclei (Fig. 6-21). Eight are true motor nuclei; their

Table 6-1. Cranial Nerve Sensory Fibers; Their Origin, Route, Signal Type and Destination

Nucleus	Cranial Nerve	Type of Signal	Region
Mesencephalic	V	Proprioception	
Chief	V	Discriminative Touch and pressure	Most of the head
Trigeminospinal	V	Nondiscriminative Touch, pain, temperature	
Solitary	VII, IX, X	Taste, visceral, baroceptor, chemoreceptor	Viscera
Vestibular	VIII	Equilibrium	Vestibular organ
Cochlear	VIII	Hearing	Cochlear organ

Note: The mesencephalic, chief, and trigeminospinal nuclei receive inputs also from cranial nerves other than V.

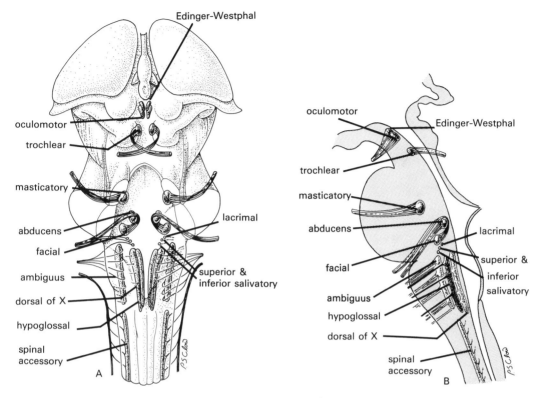

Fig. 6-21. Posterior (A) and lateral (B) views of brain stem. Motor nuclei.

neurons innervate muscle fibers directly. The other five send efferent fibers ending in visceral motor ganglia of the peripheral nervous system (PNS). These five nuclei are marked below with an asterisk (*) to distinguish them from the true motor nuclei.

1. The **oculomotor nucleus** is located ventral to the aqueduct in the rostral portion of the midbrain. Its fibers form the oculomotor nerve (III).
2. The ***Edinger-Westphal nucleus** is situated beside the oculomotor nucleus. Its fibers contribute to the oculomotor nerve (III).
3. The **trochlear nucleus** is located immediately caudal to the oculomotor nucleus in the midbrain. Its fibers form the trochlear nerve (IV).
4. The **abducens nucleus** is placed medi-

ally on the floor of the fourth ventricle in the pons. Its fibers form the abducens nerve (VI).

The four nuclei above innervate muscles of the eye.

5. The **trigeminal motor nucleus** is located medial to the chief sensory nucleus in the pons. Its fibers form part of the trigeminal nerve (V). It innervates muscles of mastication.
6. The **facial motor nucleus,** situated ventrolaterally in the pons, innervates muscles of facial expression. Its fibers form the facial nerve (VII).
7. The ***lacrimal nucleus** is located medial to the facial motor nucleus. It is a link in the innervation of the lacrimal gland and the nasal mucosa. Its fibers contribute to the facial nerve (VII).
8. The ***superior salivatory nucleus** is found beside the facial motor nucleus.

It is a link in the innervation of the salivary glands. Its fibers contribute to the facial nerve (VII).

9. The *inferior salivatory nucleus is situated below the superior salivatory nucleus at the medullary level. It is a link in the innervation of one salivary gland. Its fibers contribute to the glossopharyngeal nerve (IX).

10. The nucleus ambiguus, located laterally, dorsal to the inferior olivary nucleus, innervates muscles of the soft palate, pharynx, and larynx. Its fibers contribute to the glossopharyngeal (IX) and vagus (X) nerves.

11. The *dorsal nucleus of vagus is found along the medulla, dorsally, beside the central canal and in the caudal region of the floor of the fourth ventricle. It is a link in the innervation of the viscera of the thorax and abdomen. Its fibers contribute to the vagus nerve (X).

12. The hypoglossal nucleus is located between the dorsal nucleus of the vagus and the midline. It innervates muscles of the tongue. Its fibers form the hypoglossal nerve (XII).

13. The spinal accessory nucleus is found in cervical spinal cord segments C1 to C6 in the lateral region of the anterior gray horn. It innervates the trapezius and sternomastoid muscles. Its fibers exit as rootlets along the side of the cord and form the spinal accessory nerve (XI).

Interneurons—Reticular Formation

Most of the central nervous system (CNS) consists of different interneurons, e.g., the inferior olives, pontine nuclei, substantia nigra, and colliculi. In the brain stem there are other interneurons that have a number of characteristics in common with each other. They are together known as the reticular formation.

Since many regions of the CNS, other than the brain stem, can be described as reticular networks, it is generally agreed that the term reticular formation be restricted to the neuron cell bodies of the brain stem and their meshwork formed by the cell processes which not only permeate the brain stem but also reach higher and lower CNS structures. In various other re-

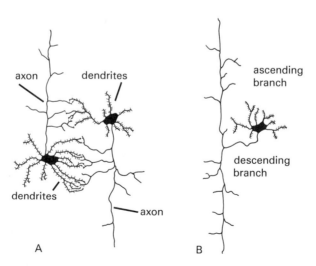

Fig. 6-22. Reticular neurons. (A) Synaptic interaction; (B) axonal branching.

gions of the CNS other reticular networks with their neuron cell bodies are distinguished, e.g., the reticular nucleus of thalamus.

Structure of the Reticular Formation

The reticular neurons have prolific dendritic processes and long axons (Golgi type I) with abundant collaterals. Due to these processes the aggregates of reticular neurons form nuclei which are not as easily identifiable as other neuronal nuclei.

The orientation of the dendritic processes is perpendicular to the long axis of the brain stem. The orientation of the axons is parallel to the long axis of the brain stem (Fig. 6-22).

Some more rostrally located nuclei project their axons caudally, descending, and others, located more caudally, send their axons rostrally, ascending. This overlapping arrangement permits interactive linkage between the two projections (Fig. 6-22).

Reinforcing this coordinated activity of the reticular formation are reticular neurons whose axons branch out in a rostral and caudal direction (Fig. 6-22).

Two regions of the reticular formation can be defined, i.e., the **lateral** and the **medial areas.** The lateral area, which occupies one-third of the reticular formation, receives several types of stimuli and acts upon the medial area, which comprises the remaining two-thirds (Fig. 6-23).

Afferents and Efferents of the Reticular Formation—Connectivity

The reticular formation receives information of all sensory modalities from spinal cord and cranial nerve nuclei as well as from the cerebral cortex, the septal area, and the diencephalon. The efferents of the reticular formation reach, apart from brain stem structures, the diencephalon, the septal area, and the spinal cord (reticulospinal tract).

Function of the Reticular Formation

The reticular formation influences almost all functions controlled by the nervous system, somatic and visceral, sensory and motor. It serves as an important substrate of integrative CNS functions, influencing the mind and behavioral states in the broadest range from awakening, alerting, and attentiveness to disruption of functions, drowsiness, and sleepiness.

To understand how the functions of the reticular formation can be so disparate in their consequences (sleep or wakefulness, alertness or drowsiness) one must not consider the isolated types of inputs but all the inputs and their modes of integration.

Most anesthetics block synaptic transmission, affecting very efficiently the polysynaptic paths. The reticular formation is

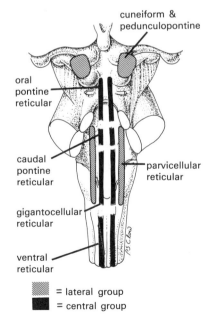

cuneiform &
pedunculopontine

oral
pontine
reticular

caudal
pontine
reticular

parvicellular
reticular

gigantocellular
reticular

ventral
reticular

= lateral group
= central group

Fig. 6-23. Central and lateral reticular nuclei.

greatly affected because of its well-developed polysynaptic structure.

Serious damage to the reticular formation produces a state of coma. Because of its role in regulating visceral vital functions, inhalation, expiration, blood circulation, etc., lesions to the brain stem may be life threatening.

Raphe Nuclei

Setting aside other differences, the structural arrangement of the raphe nuclei (Fig. 6-24) is a characteristic intrinsic also to the reticular formation. This likeness motivates some scientists to include the raphe nuclei as part of the reticular formation, while others regard them as a group of their own.

The raphe nuclei are positioned in the midline, forming a continuous column. They send fibers to the cerebral hemispheres, the diencephalon, the brain stem, and the spinal cord.

One of the raphe nuclei, the **raphe magnus** (Fig. 6-24), sends a synaptic fiber path to the spinal cord dorsal horns. This path releases **serotonin,** which activates interneurons that release **enkephalin,** a peptide similar to morphine, which blocks nocicep-

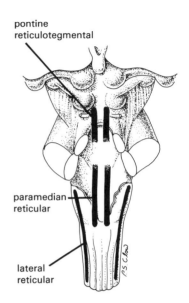

Fig. 6-25. Precerebellar reticular nuclei.

tive signals with ensuing loss of pain sensations.

Precerebellar Nuclei

The term **precerebellar nuclei** includes all the nuclei that send many of their efferent fibers to the cerebellum. The most important ones are the pontine nuclei, the inferior olives, red nucleus, and three reticular nuclei (Fig. 6-25), which are considered a group of their own.

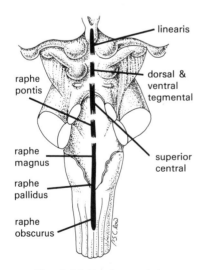

Fig. 6-24. Raphe nuclei.

A Simple Model of Motor Activity

Using only the aforementioned components, one can describe the structure and function of the cerebellum and brain stem in a simplified manner as a black box with

1. a **middle cerebellar peduncular inlet** from the cortex through the pontine nuclei to the cerebellum for voluntary automatic adjustments;
2. a **superior cerebellar peduncular inlet-outlet** for complex flexion and exten-

sion functions; and

3. an **inferior cerebellar peduncular inlet-outlet** for extensor functions.

The vestibular nucleus and the vestibulospinal tract excite extensor muscles. The red nucleus and the rubrospinal tract excite flexor muscles.

The reticular formation has inhibitory and excitatory inputs and modulates extensor and flexor muscles through the reticulospinal tracts. A section at any level between the superior inlet-outlet of the cerebellum or red nucleus, down to (but above) the inferior inlet-outlet of the cerecellum or vestibular nucleus, produces pronounced extensor rigidity.

A Model of Cranial Nerve Reflex Circuitry

A simple model of cranial nerve reflex circuitry could be exemplified as follows: a person eating too fast, bites her/his lip. A strong nociceptive stimulus travels through the trigeminal nerve and passes the Gasserian ganglion, the trigeminospinal tract, and nucleus. From there, connections are established with

1. the facial motor nucleus, which responds with a mass discharge through the facial nerve and contracts the muscles of facial expression in pain;
2. the lacrimal nucleus, which also through the facial nerve reaches the lacrimal gland and stimulates the secretion of tears; and
3. the thalamus, through the trigeminal lemniscus, where at conscious levels it informs of the pain and warns to proceed more cautiously.

Suggested Readings

Abrahams VC, Rose PK: Projections of extraocular, neck muscle, and retinal afferents to superior colliculus in the cat: their connections to cells of origin of tectospinal tract, J Neurophysiol 38:10–18, 1975.

Adams JC: Ascending projections to the inferior colliculus, J Comp Neurol 183:519–538, 1979.

Allen GI, Oshima T, Toyama K: The mode of synaptic linkage in the cerebro-ponto-cerebellar pathway investigated with intracellular recording from pontine nuclei cells of the cat, Exp Brain Res 29:123–136, 1977.

Arvidsson J, Grant G: Further observations on transganglionic degeneration in trigeminal primary sensory neurons, Brain Res 162:1–12, 1979.

Barr ML, Kiernan JA: The Human Nervous System. Fourth Edition. Harper and Row, Philadelphia, pp. 81–156, 1983.

Bentivoglio M, Macchi G, Rossini P, Tempesta E: Brain stem neurons projecting to neocortex: a HRP study in the cat, Exp Brain Res 31:489–498, 1978.

Bertrand F, Hugelin A, Vibert JF: Quantitative study of anatomical distribution of respiration related neurons in the pons, Exp Brain Res 16:383–399, 1973.

Blomquist A, Fink R, Bowsher D, Griph S, Westman J: Tectal and thalamic projections of dorsal column and lateral cervical nuclei: a quantitative study in the cat, Brain Res 141:335–341, 1978.

Bobillier P, Seguin S, Petijean F, Salbert D, Touret M, Jouvet M: The raphe nuclei of the cat brain stem: a topographical atlas of their efferent projections as revealed by autoradiography, Brain Res 113:449–486, 1976.

Carpenter MB: Human Neuroanatomy. Seventh Edition. Williams and Wilkins, Baltimore, pp. 285–398, 1976.

Fields HL, Basbaum AJ: Brainstem control of spinal pain-transmission neurons, Ann Rev Physiol 40:217–248, 1978.

Partlow GD, Colonnier M, Szabo J: Thalamic projections of the superior colliculus in the rhesus monkey, Macaca mulatta. A light and electron microscopic study, J Comp Neurol 171:285–378, 1977.

Pasquier DA, Reinoso-Suarez F: Differential efferent connections of the brain stem to the hippocampus in the cat, Brain Res 120:540–548, 1977.

Pompeiano O: Reticular formation. In Iggo A, Ed.: Handbook of Sensory Physiology, Vol.

II: Somatosensory System, Springer-Verlag, Berlin, pp. 381–488, 1973.

Scheibel AB: The brainstem reticular core and sensory function. In Darian-Smith I, Ed.: American Handbook of Physiology, Vol. 2. Second Edition. American Physiological Society, Washington, DC, 1980.

Sjölund B, Björklund A, Eds.: Brain Stem Control of Spinal Mechanisms. Fernström Foundation Series, 1, Elsevier Excerpta Medica, Elsevier Science Publishers, New York, 1982.

Snell RS: Clinical Neuroanatomy for Medical Students, Little, Brown and Co., Boston, pp. 169–220, 1980.

7

Diencephalon

Components and Function of the Diencephalon

The **diencephalon,** which makes up the core of the cerebrum, is less than 1/40 of the size of the cerebral hemispheres. In spite of its unimpressive size, however, it manages to be a link between the spinal cord and the hemispheres, the brain stem and the hemispheres, and different regions within each hemisphere.

Four diencephalic regions are recognized: the **thalamus, subthalamus, hypothalamus,** and **epithalamus.**

Three categories of functions are identified: **somatic sensory, somatic motor,** and **visceral functions.**

The correlations of regions and functions are shown in Table 7-1.

It is important that the conceptual classification presented in Table 7-1 be interpreted in the light of the following facts:

1. The correlation region–function merely aims at attracting attention to dominant roles, while in fact none of

Table 7-1. Correlation of Regions and Functions

Region	Function
Thalamus	Multiple sensibilities
Subthalamus	Motor link
Hypothalamus ⎱	Neuroendocrine
Epithalamus ⎰	Homeostatic

the cited functions are exclusive to a region.
2. No neurons of the diencephalon are directly linked with muscles or other peripheral tissue. Hence, all the neurons here are, in reality, interneurons.
3. A neuronal network permeates the four regions and establishes interactions and modulations within and between them.

Position and Configuration of the Diencephalon

It would be very difficult, if not impossible, to build a correct mental image of the shape and position of the diencephalon

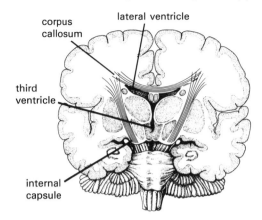

Fig. 7-1. Coronal section of the brain.

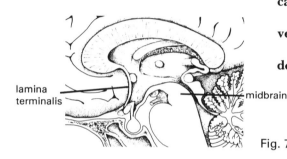

Fig. 7-2. Midsagittal section of diencephalon.

furnished on the description of the details of its boundaries alone. Additional facts and concepts are needed for such an image as well as for the correct interpretation of two dimensional illustrations of the diencephalon.

Boundaries of the Diencephalon

The following are the basic limits of the diencephalon:

medial limit: the third ventricle (Fig. 7-1)
rostral (anterior) limit: lamina terminalis (Fig. 7-2)
caudal (posteroinferior) limit: the midbrain (Fig. 7-2)
ventral limit: protrudes on the ventral (inferior) surface of the brain (Fig. 7-3)
dorsal limit: mostly the floor of the bodies

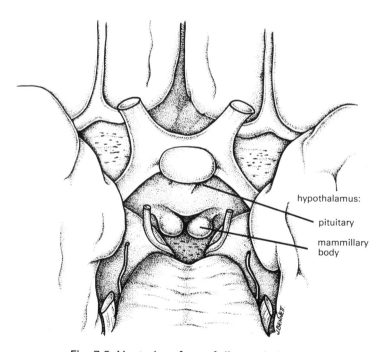

Fig. 7-3. Ventral surface of diencephalon.

of the lateral ventricles (Fig. 7-1)

lateral limit: in each side a posterior portion of the so-called **internal capsule,** which is white matter (Fig. 7-1)

Topographical Planes of Reference of the Diencephalon

The bundles of fibers that symmetrically link the left and right structures are called **commissures** (L. *committere* to join to-

gether). In a midsagittal section of the brain one can easily identify two of them, the **anterior** and **posterior commissures.** Joining the two is the **anterior commissure-posterior commissure (AC–PC) line,** which has an average length of 25 mm in an adult human (Fig. 7-4).

In the midsagittal plane of the brain, showing the AC–PC line, a **horizontal plane** can be traced that also shows the line that is perpendicular to the midsagittal plane. Both planes are the coordinates of the brain most commonly used as points of reference in neurosurgery.

A plane, which is perpendicular to the

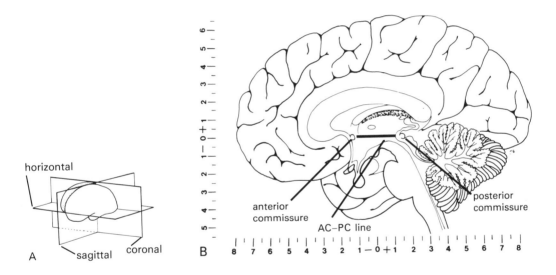

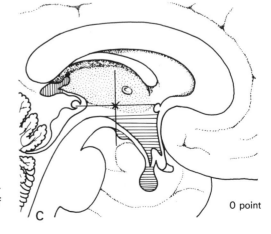

Fig. 7-4. Topography of diencephalon. (A) Coordinate planes; (B) AC–PC line; (C) 0 point of coordinates.

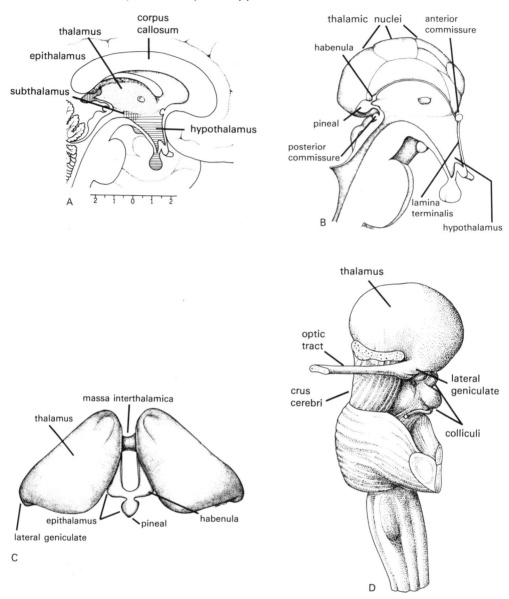

Fig. 7-5. Different views of diencephalon. (A) Left midsagittal surface; (B) midsagittal surface dissected to expose dorsal surface of thalamus; (C) dorsal view of thalamus; (D) lateral view of brain stem and diencephalon.

midsagittal and horizontal, is the **transverse plane,** also known as the **coronal** and **verticofrontal plane.**

The midsagittal point of the AC–PC line (12.5 mm from each commissure) defines the 0 (zero) point of the coordinates in the midsagittal, horizontal, and coronal planes.

Size and Position of Diencephalic Regions

The following are approximate weights of diencephalic regions:

thalamus	19 g
hypothalamus	4 g

subthalamus   1 to 2 g
epithalamus   1 g

The hypothalamus and subthalamus are situated ventral (inferior) and the thalamus and epithalamus are situated dorsal to the AC–PC line. The zero coronal (vertical) plane section cuts through the thalamus, hypothalamus, and subthalamus. Successive caudal planes to the zero coronal first cut only the thalamus and subthalamus and later the thalamus and epithalamus. Successive rostral planes to the zero coronal cut only the thalamus and hypothalamus (Fig. 7-5).

Some other important facts regarding the topographical orientation are that (1) the zero coronal plane passes through the posterior portion of the mammillary bodies and (2) the subthalamus is continuous caudally with the midbrain tegmentum.

By looking at the surface projection of the hypothalamus in the midsagittal plane, one receives the impression that it covers approximately as large an area as the thalamus. Nevertheless, the thalamus is almost five times the size of the hypothalamus. The deceiving appearance is explained by the following facts:

1. The hypothalamus is narrower than the thalamus in horizontal and coronal planes.
2. In a midsagittal section of the brain, the dorsum of the thalamus is hidden from view by other structures.
3. The posterior region of the thalamus bulges posteriorly (beyond the posterior commissure), laterally, and then caudally.

A horizontal section of the brain cutting through the red nucleus (of the midbrain) displays also posterolaterally the lateroposteroinferior tip of the thalamus. The lateral surfaces of the thalamus, delineated by the posterior portion of the internal capsule, are oriented posterolaterally (Fig. 7-5D).

The epithalamus is partly seen with its pineal gland in the posterior union of the

medial, dorsal, and caudal surfaces of the thalamus (Fig. 7-5C).

The Thalamus

The thalamus is composed of a large number of nuclei. The reader must be aware that the literature on the thalamus presents many classifications of the thalamic nuclei. These classifications are as yet arbitrary. What is essential is to become familiar with their positions and connectivities. In this text they are classified into five

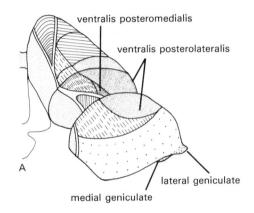

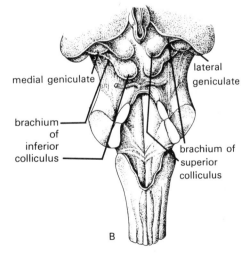

Fig. 7-6. (A) Specific thalamic nuclei; (B) colliculi and geniculate bodies.

main groups: (1) **specific relay nuclei,** (2) **sensory association nuclei,** (3) **proprioceptive-motor association nuclei,** (4) **integrative nuclei,** and (5) **nondiscriminative nuclei.**

Specific Relay Nuclei

The following are descriptions of **specific relay nuclei,** which receive specific sensory data.

The **medial geniculate nucleus** (or **body**) is concerned with hearing signals coming through the **brachium** (L. arm) of the **inferior colliculus** (Figs. 7-6 to 7-8).

The **lateral geniculate nucleus** (or **body**) is concerned with visual signals from the eye (Figs. 7-6 to 7-8).

The **ventralis posterior nucleus** handles mainly exteroceptive and proprioceptive somatosensory signals (Figs. 7-6 and 7-8). The nucleus is subdivided into (1) the **ventralis posterolateralis,** which receives signals from the spinal cord (body), and (2) the **ventralis posteromedialis,** which receives signals from the brain stem (head).

The somatosensory pathways from the spinal cord to the ventralis posterolateralis are the **spinal** and **medial lemnisci.**

The **trigeminothalamic tracts** constitute a somatosensory pathway from the brain stem to the ventralis posteromedialis.

The three specific relay nuclei send fibers to the cerebral cortex (Fig. 7-8):

1. medial geniculate (hearing) to temporal lobe;
2. lateral geniculate (vision) to occipital lobe; and
3. ventralis posterior (somatosensory) to parietal lobe.

The aforementioned sensory signals can be classified as exteroceptive—visual, auditory, tactile—and proprioceptive—from **joints, muscles, tendons.**

Sensory Association Nuclei

The **pulvinar nucleus (PN)** is the largest nucleus of the thalamus. It receives fibers from the lateral geniculate (visual), from the medial geniculate (auditory), and the ventralis posterior (somatosensory). It associates the signals and sends fibers to the cerebral sensory association cortex, a broad region, consisting of the parietal, occipital, and temporal lobes (Fig. 7-9).

The **lateral posterior nucleus (LP)** and the **lateral dorsal nucleus (LD)** have input-output similar to those of the pulvinar (Fig. 7-9).

Proprioceptive-Motor Association Nuclei

The thalamus houses two nuclei to associate proprioceptive-motor signals of different types and sources.

The **ventralis lateralis nucleus (VL)** receives fibers from the ventralis posterior concerned with proprioception and associates their signals with others coming from the cerebellum through the cerebellotha-

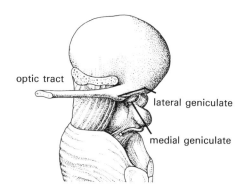

optic tract

lateral geniculate

medial geniculate

Fig. 7-7. Ending of optic tract in lateral geniculate nucleus of thalamus.

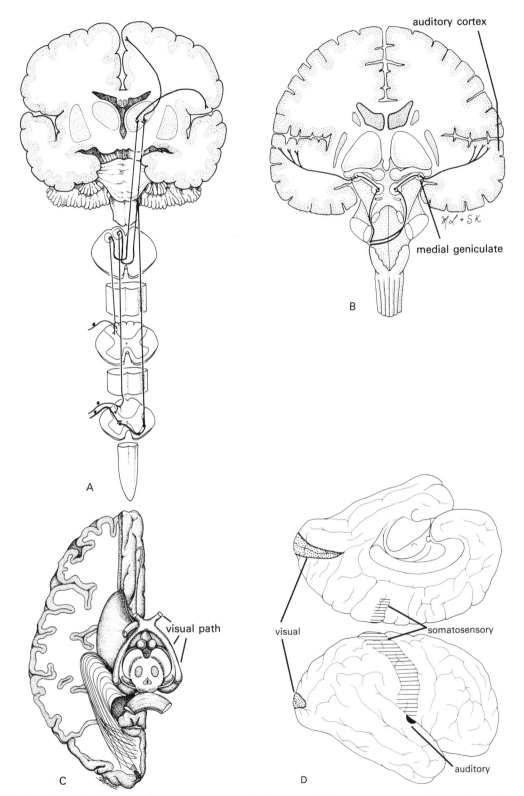

Fig. 7-8. Specific signal pathways to the cerebral cortex. (A) Somatosensory; (B) auditory; (C) visual; (D) cortical areas.

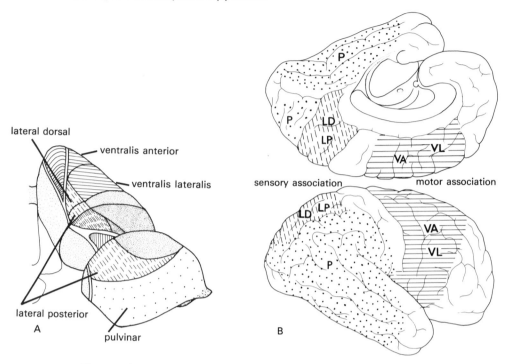

Fig. 7-9. (A) Association thalamic nuclei; (B) cortical areas.

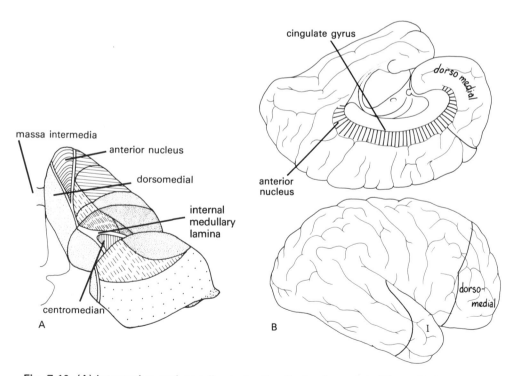

Fig. 7-10. (A) Integrative and nondiscriminative thalamic nuclei; (B) cortical areas.

lamic tract. It sends fibers to the frontal lobe, to mostly motor areas.

The **ventralis anterior nucleus (VA)** receives proprioceptive fibers also from the ventralis posterior and associates the signals with the motor ones coming from a subcortical nucleus, the so-called **globus pallidus.** This path is the **pallidothalamic tract.** The ventralis anterior sends fibers to the frontal lobe, to mostly premotor areas.

Integrative Nuclei

Had mention been made only of the sets of nuclei described above, it would appear as if the thalamus and cerebral cortex were split in the processing of sensory and proprioceptive-motor signals. In reality, however, the thalamus harbors other sets of nuclei that act in support of its integrative function. Integration is a higher level of association.

The **dorsomedial nucleus (DM)** receives fibers from all the thalamic nuclei and picks up their signals integrated with the inputs from nondiscriminative nuclei and others of visceral nature coming from the hypothalamus.

The dorsomedial nucleus sends fibers to the frontal lobe and the **septal area,** a region anterior to the lamina terminalis. The septal area appears to be the most intriguing region of the brain. The connections of the dorsomedial nucleus establish an important substrate for all brain functions of an integrative nature (Fig. 7-10).

The **anterior nucleus (A)** communicates with the mammillary bodies through the mammillothalamic tract and makes an important connection with the cortex of the **cingulate gyrus** (Fig. 7-10).

The **nucleus reticularis thalami** covers the thalamus dorsolaterally. Strategically situated, it plays a major interactive role with signals coming into or out of the thalamus, activating or inhibiting them.

The nucleus reticularis thalami is separated from the lateral border of the thalamus by a narrow band of fibers, the so-called **external medullary lamina (EML).**

Nondiscriminative Nuclei

In the context of thalamic nuclei, the term "nondiscriminative" merely implies that the nuclei process sensory signals of nondiscriminative nature.

Within the group of nondiscriminative thalamic nuclei there are two subgroups.

Intralaminar Nuclei

The intralaminar nuclei (I) correspond to nuclei found within a layer of fibers called the **internal medullary lamina (IML).** The IML courses between the dorsomedian nucleus (medially) and the other thalamic nuclei (Fig. 7-10). Rostrally, this lamina forks out, embracing the anterior nucleus.

The intralaminar nuclei establish connections with subcortical and other thalamic nuclei and the reticular formation as well as with the cortex of the temporal lobe. The largest intralaminar nucleus is the **centromedian nucleus.**

The **posterior nuclear complex (PO)** of the internal medullary lamina contains a number of ill-defined nuclei.

Midline Nuclei

It has been found that in approximately 70 percent of human brains, the **midline nuclei,** facing the wall of the third ventricle, establish connections with the corresponding nuclei of the opposite side, crossing the third ventricle as the **massa interthalamica,** also called the **massa intermedia, adhesio interthalamica,** or **middle commissure.**

Rostrally, the midline nuclei establish association through the internal and external medullary laminae with the anterior nucleus and subcortical nuclei. In their favorable location, they interact with the dorsomedial nucleus and hypothalamus.

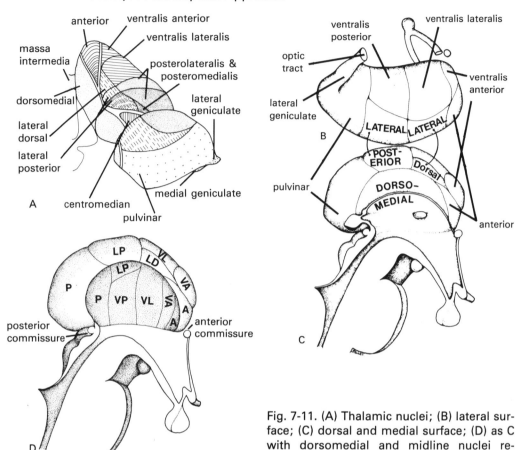

Fig. 7-11. (A) Thalamic nuclei; (B) lateral surface; (C) dorsal and medial surface; (D) as C with dorsomedial and midline nuclei removed.

These two subgroups of nuclei play a significant role in modulating the activity of other diencephalic and brain stem regions (reticular formation).

Given their position, function, and connections, the nondiscriminative nuclei play a critical part in any identifiable general function and state of the cerebrum (consciousness, emotions, alertness, sleepiness, memory).

Terminology of Thalamic Nuclei

The names given to the thalamic nuclei allude to their topographical position. In order to reinforce this terminology a re-

view of the nuclei is presented (Fig. 7-11):

medial nuclei—dorsomedial and midline nuclei

lateral nuclei—lateral dorsal and lateral posterior nuclei

ventral nuclei—ventralis posterior ventralis lateralis, and ventralis anterior

anterior nucleus

pulvinar (L. a cushioned seat)—the lower and posterior mass below which are two other rounded nuclei, i.e., the medial and lateral geniculate bodies

metathalamus—a term sometimes used to indicate the medial and lateral geniculate bodies

internal medullary lamina with a number of intralaminar nuclei, e.g., centromedian nucleus and nuclei of posterior complex

external medullary lamina, a lamina of fibers on the lateral surface of the thalamus

The **reticular thalamic nucleus** has a reticular cellular arrangement similar to that of the reticular formation.

Thalamic Circuitry

A number of inputs or outputs of thalamic nuclei have already been mentioned. Add to the picture of the circuitry the fact that all those connections have feed-back paths that establish loops between the connected structures. The thalamic nuclei hence have many interconnecting loops between themselves as well as with nuclei of other central nervous system (CNS) regions, especially the brain cortex.

The fiber connections of the thalamus with the cortex is called **thalamic radiation** because of its radiated arrangement.

Visual Paths—Conscious

Axons from a type of neuronal cells composing the retina of the eyes exit the eyeballs posteriorly, forming the two thick **optic nerves.** Some fibers decussate, forming the **optic chiasm** (Fig. 7-12).

The optic chiasm indents the anterior wall of the third ventricle, thus forming the **optic (supraoptic, preoptic, chiasmatic) recess,** separating it from the infundibular recess (Fig. 7-13). Posterior to the optic chiasm, the **optic tract,** i.e., fibers from the same optic nerve, and (decussated) fibers from the other optic nerve, continue posteriorly. The optic tract diverges to embrace the hypothalamus and reaches the lateral geniculate bodies, where its fibers synapse. Fibers from the lateral geniculate nucleus are projected to the visual cortex.

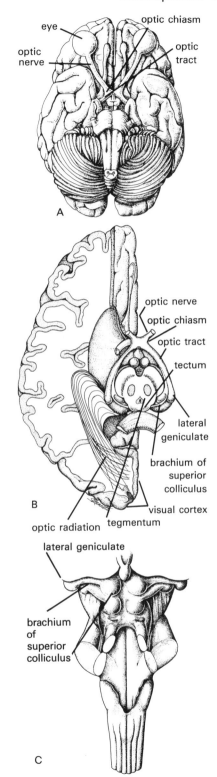

Fig. 7-12. Visual paths. (A) Basal view of brain; (B) as A dissected to show visual path; (C) geniculotectal path.

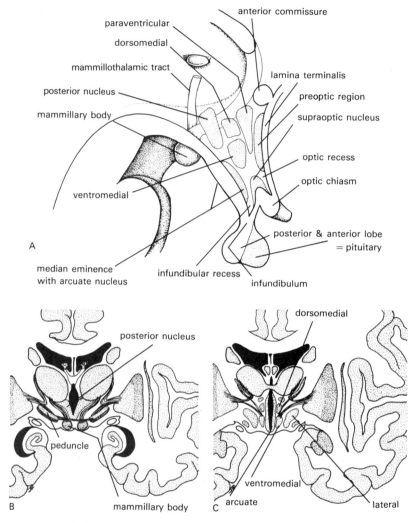

Fig. 7-13. Hypothalamus. (A) Medial view; (B) coronal view; (C) coronal view.

The path thus described is considered as the path for conscious visual information.

Reflex Visual Path

Some of the fibers of the optic tract bypass the lateral geniculate body, continue toward the midbrain through the brachium of the superior colliculus, and synapse in tectal, pretectal, and tegmental neurons to trigger visual reflexes.

Hypothalamus

The hypothalamus is essentially concerned with the control of the optimal conditions of the interior of the body, or **homeostasis.** This includes, for instance, body temperature, quantity of body water, hunger, visceral and hormonal activities, and dependent trophic and reproductive functions. It is awe-inspiring to conceive that the 4 g of tissue that constitute the hypothalamus possess powers so complex that we have only just begun to understand them.

Boundaries of the Hypothalamus

Four important landmarks to the hypothalamus (Fig. 7-13) are

rostrally—the anterior commissure, preoptic region, lamina terminalis, and optic chiasm
caudally—the subthalamic region and midbrain; the anatomical caudal limit is the posterior edge of the mammillary bodies
laterally—bordering on the optic tracts (Fig. 7-12)
ventrally—protruding on the ventral surface of the brain

Divisions of the Hypothalamus

In the hypothalamus there are a **lateral zone** and a **medial zone.** The lateral zone contains the **lateral nucleus** and the **medial zone** is divided into three regions, i.e., the **anterior, middle,** and **posterior regions.**

Anterior Region

Anteriorly (rostrally), above (dorsal to) the chiasm, lies the **anterior** or **suprachiasmatic region.** Two nuclei of this region are the **supraoptic** and the **paraventricular.**

Middle Region

Behind the anterior region is the **middle region,** which is also called the **tuberal region.** It contains in the upper portion the **dorsomedial** and **ventromedial nuclei.** In the lower portion, bulging at the base, there is a thickening of the wall of the third ventricle. This portion is the **tuber cinereum** (L. ash-colored swelling).

The **arcuate (infundibular) nucleus** is a well-defined nucleus in the tuber cinereum. This nucleus produces on the third

ventricle a bulge, known specifically as the **median eminence.**

The tuber cinereum continues with the **infundibulum** or **infundibular stalk** or **stem** and the **pituitary gland** or **hypophysis.** This gland has an **anterior (adenohypophysis)** and a **posterior (neurohypophysis) lobe** with a small intermediate region.

Posterior Region

Behind the middle region lies the **mammillary** or **posterior region,** which contains the mammillary body and the **posterior nucleus.**

Note: The reader must be aware that the literature on the hypothalamus describes many other nuclei and presents other classifications and divisions of this region. The three regions and groups of nuclei described here are widely accepted.

Subependymal Gray

To serve the purpose of accurate conceptualization, it is convenient at this point to introduce the **subependymal gray,** a region of gray matter. It includes the gray immediately below the ependyma of the whole ventricular system. This region is identified at different levels, i.e., the periventricular gray of the thalamus, the hypothalamus, the mesencephalon (periaqueductal gray), and the central canal (substantia gelatinosa centralis).

These levels of the ependymal gray have a number of characteristics in common:

1. They interact as a system.
2. They are related to visceral, homeostatic functions.
3. They are directly, through discrete specialized regions, or indirectly affected by the chemical composition of the cerebrospinal fluid (CSF).
4. They have connections with the reticular formation of the brain stem.

In studying the hypothalamus it is important to appreciate that a major link between it and other CNS regions is formed through this subependymal gray.

Non-Neural Inputs to the Hypothalamus

The hypothalamus is under the influence of the physical and chemical characteristics of the blood and the CSF, e.g., their temperature, osmolar values, and hormonal levels, affecting each particular nucleus in a manner responsive to the nature of the homeostatic imbalance.

Neural Connections of the Hypothalamus

The periventricular gray of the hypothalamus establishes reciprocal connections with

1. the midline nuclei of the thalamus;
2. the midbrain, through the periaqueductal gray and the dorsal longitudinal fasciculus, which are linked with the reticular formation; and
3. the cerebral hemispheres, especially the frontal lobe, through the preoptic region, a region with nuclei outgrowing

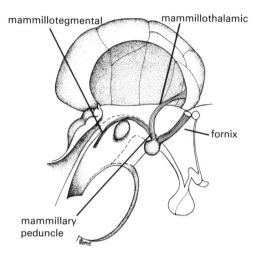

Fig. 7-14. Mammillary peduncle.

from the lamina terminalis and situated in front of the hypothalamus.

The projections of fibers of the mammillary bodies form the **mammillary peduncle** (Fig. 7-14), which splits into two fasciculi. One of them, the **mammillothalamic fasciculus (bundle of Vic d'Azyr)**, establishes connections with the anterior nucleus of the thalamus and the other, the **mammillotegmental fasciculus,** bends

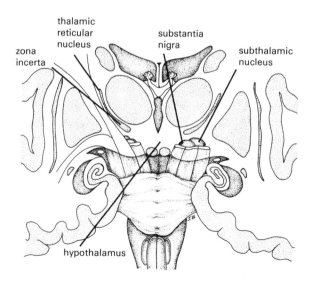

Fig. 7-15. Subthalamic region.

dorsocaudally and establishes connections with the tegmentum of the midbrain.

Subthalamus

The **subthalamic region** or **subthalamus** is an ill-defined area limited by the midbrain, thalamus, hypothalamus, internal capsule, and third ventricle (Fig. 7-15). It contains fasciculi and tracts, the **zona incerta,** and the **subthalamic nucleus of Luys.**

Fasciculi and Tracts

Among the fiber paths are

1. the **medial** and **spinal lemnisci** and the **trigeminal tracts** coursing toward the thalamus (Fig. 7-16);
2. a fascicle of fibers coursing from the cerebellum toward the ventral lateral nucleus of thalamus;
3. the reticular bundle of fibers connecting the brain stem and diencephalon

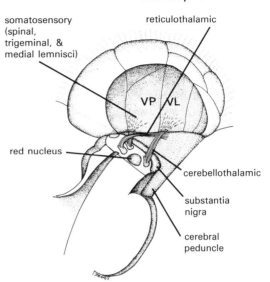

Fig. 7-16. Subthalamic region fasciculi.

(Fig. 7-16); and
4. two fasciculi, the ansa lenticularis and lenticular fasciculus, coursing from a subcortical nucleus, the globus pallidus, across and around the internal capsule toward the thalamus (Fig. 7-17).

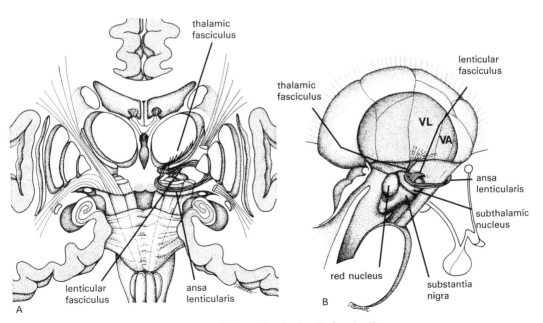

Fig. 7-17. Subcorticothalamic fasciculi.

Zona Incerta

Limited by fascicles, the **zona incerta** is a continuation of the nucleus reticularis thalami (Fig. 7-15).

Subthalamic Nucleus

The **subthalamic nucleus** (Fig. 7-17), also known as the **nucleus of Luys,** is well-defined and rests on the internal capsule. It appears as a rostral extension of the substantia nigra.

The subthalamic nucleus has reciprocal connections with the globus pallidus, across the internal capsule, through the subthalamic fasciculus. The nucleus receives corticosubthalamic fibers from the frontal cortex via the internal capsule.

Function of the Subthalamic Region or Subthalamus

Generally speaking, the subthalamus is associated with somatic motor functions. More specifically, however, as its role is complex, it is wise to be aware of a number of facts:

This miniscule region contains different types of fiber paths. Some are identified as sensory, others come from subcortical nuclei, like the globus pallidus, and course toward the thalamus.

In the subthalamus there are reticular structures of extremely complex functions.

The effects of localized lesions within this region are difficult to assess and interpret.

Hence, this region contains structures involved in a variety of functions. Clinical and experimental data clearly indicate that alterations in this region play an important role in motor disorders. More will be said on this subject in the context of studying the cerebral hemispheres in depth.

Epithalamus

The **epithalamus** consists of the **pineal gland** and the **habenular nuclei** with their connections.

Pineal Gland

The **pineal gland** or **body** (Fig. 7-18), also called **epiphysis,** is shaped like a pine cone. Ontogenetically, it originated as an outgrowth of the ependyma and is composed of secretory cells, which produce hormones. The gland is highly vascularized and is influenced by a number of blood constants and the CSF. The hormones produced by the gland are taken up by the vessels.

In a posterior view, the pineal gland can be seen hanging from above between the superior colliculi. The gland is attached anteriorly by a thin stalk to the posterior commissure ventrally and to the habenular

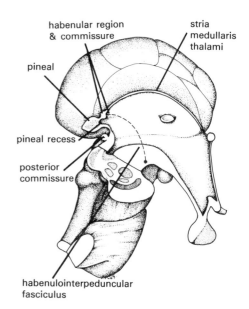

Fig. 7-18. Epithalamic region.

commissure dorsally. Between the two commissures is the **pineal recess.**

Habenula

The **habenula** is a set of very small nuclei above the posterior commissure. Its three connections form the **habenular trigone.**

One arm of the habenular trigone, the **stria medullaris thalami,** serves the input to the habenular nuclei. It is composed of a bundle of fibers coming from different regions, especially the septal area. The fibers travel along the border created by the dorsal and medial surfaces of the thalamus.

Note: Along the stria medullaris thalami there is a line of attachment of the choroid plexus where a thin membrane (the ependyma) merges with the substance of the brain. This line of attachment is called **tenia thalami** (L. from Gr. *tainia* band or tape).

Some fibers end in the habenular nuclei. Other fibers bypass it and end in the opposite habenular nuclei. These fibers, together with the ones from the opposite side, form the second arm of the trigone, the **habenular commissure.**

The third arm of the trigone, the **habenulointerpeduncular fasciculus,** is formed by the fiber output of the nuclei. It is sent caudally toward the interpeduncular nucleus in the mesencephalic tegmentum. From the interpeduncular nucleus, connections are established with the reticular formation, influencing visceral activities among others. The habenular nuclei are links between the septal area, other hemispheric diencephalic regions, and the brain stem.

Suggested Readings

Barr ML, Kiernan JA: The Human Nervous System. Fourth Edition. Harper and Row, Philadelphia, pp. 176–203, 1983.

Carpenter MB: Human Neuroanatomy. Seventh Edition. Williams and Wilkins, Baltimore, pp. 435–495, 1976.

Hensel H: Thermoreception and Temperature Regulation, Monographs of the Physiological Society, No. 38, Academic Press, London, 1981.

Jones EG, Leavitt RY: Retrograde axonal transport and the demonstration of non-specific projections to the cerebral cortex and striatum from thalamic intralaminar nuclei in the rat, cat and monkey, J Comp Neurol 154:349–378, 1975.

Macchi, G, Rustioni A, Spreafico R, Eds.: Somatosensory Integration in the Thalamus, Elsevier Excerpta Medica, Elsevier Science Publishers, New York, 1983.

Morgane PJ, Panksepp J, Eds.: Anatomy of the Hypothalamus, Marcel Dekker, New York, 1979.

Reichlin S, Baldessarini RJ, Martin JB, Eds.: The Hypothalamus, Ass Res Nerv Dis Res Publ, Vol. 56, Raven Press, New York, 1978.

Smith CG: Basic Neuroanatomy. Second Edition. University of Toronto Press, Toronto, pp. 59–99, 1971.

Valverde F: Aspects of cortical organization related to the geometry of neurons with intracortical axons, J Neurocytol 5:509–529, 1976.

Williams PL, Warwick R: Functional Neuroanatomy of Man, WB Saunders, Philadelphia, pp. 891–921, 1975.

8

Cerebral Hemispheres

Surface of Cerebral Hemispheres

In relation to the cerebral hemispheres a number of terms were introduced in Chapter 2: longitudinal (sagittal) fissure; central sulcus or sulcus of Rolando; post-central and precentral gyri; lateral fissure or fissure of Sylvius; frontal, parietal, occipital, and temporal lobes. The following comments are intended to reinforce and expand the understanding of these terms and add new ones.

The **longitudinal fissure** contains the **falx cerebri** and ends posteriorly in the **transverse fissure** (Fig. 8-1).

The **transverse fissure** separates the posterior portion of the cerebral hemispheres from the cerebellum and the colliculi. It is limited anteriorly by the dorsum of the thalamus and the corpus callosum. This fissure contains the **tentorium cerebelli.**

The **central sulcus** forms the boundary between the frontal and parietal lobes (Fig. 8-2).

The **lateral fissure** separates the **frontal** and **parietal lobes** from the **temporal lobe.**

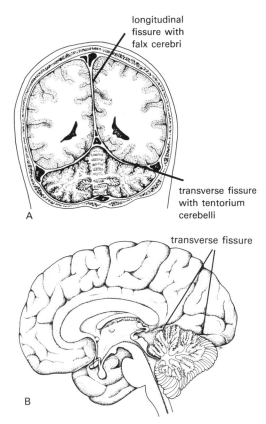

Fig. 8-1. (A) Coronal section of the head; (B) medial surface of right hemisphere.

127

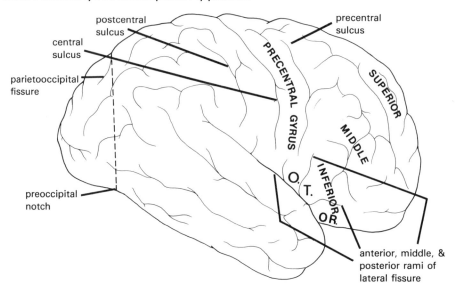

Fig. 8-2. Lateral surface of right hemishere. O, opercular; T, triangular; OR, orbital portions.

An indentation in the inferior border of the lateral surface of the hemisphere, the **preoccipital notch,** is regarded as a point of reference to mark the **occipital cortex.** An imaginary line traced between the parietooccipital sulcus and the notch delineates the anterior boundary of the occipital lobe.

The part of the frontal cortex anterior to the precentral gyrus and precentral sulcus is imperfectly divided into three gyri, the **superior, middle,** and **inferior frontal gyri,** by two sulci, the **superior** and **inferior frontal sulci.**

In the stem of the lateral fissure one can observe three arms, the **anterior, middle,**

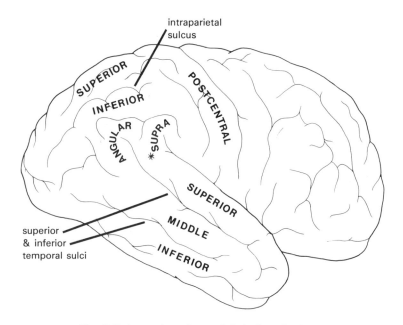

Fig. 8-3. Lateral surface of right hemisphere.

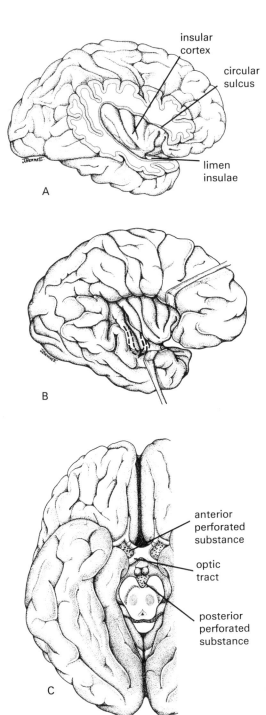

insular
cortex

circular
sulcus

limen
insulae

A

B

anterior
perforated
substance

optic
tract

posterior
perforated
substance

C

Fig. 8-4. (A) Insula exposed to view; (B) Heschl's convolutions; (C) inferior basal surface of hemisphere.

and **posterior rami** (L. *ramus* branch). The projection of the anterior and middle rami into the inferior frontal gyrus divides it into the **opercular, triangular,** and **orbital portions.**

The part of the parietal cortex that is posterior to the postcentral sulcus is divided into the **superior** and **inferior parietal lobules** by the **intraparietal sulcus** (Fig. 8-3).

The ends of the posterior ramus of the lateral fissure and the superior temporal sulcus stretching into the inferior parietal lobule demarcate the **supramarginal gyrus** and the **angular gyrus,** respectively.

The temporal lobe is divided into three gyri, the **superior, middle,** and **inferior temporal gyri,** by two sulci, the **superior** and **inferior temporal sulci.**

Hidden by the **opercula** (L. lips) of the lateral fissure lies more of the cortical area, i.e., the so-called **insula, insular lobe,** or **island of Reil,** composed of short and long gyri. By removing what conceals the insula, the **frontal, parietal,** and **temporal opercula,** one can observe the insula encircled by the **circular sulcus** (Fig. 8-4).

The hidden surface of the superior temporal gyrus, forming the ventral wall of the lateral fissure, is marked by short, transverse gyri. They are known as the **transverse temporal gyri of Heschl (Heschl's convolutions)** (Fig. 8-4B).

Sandwiched between the inferior part of the insula and the **anterior perforated substance,** a region lateral to the optic tract, lies a small cortical region called the **limen insulae** (Fig. 8-4A).

Medial and Inferior Surfaces of the Hemispheres

The **cingulate gyrus** encircles the corpus callosum and is separated by the **callosal sulcus.** This gyrus is separated from

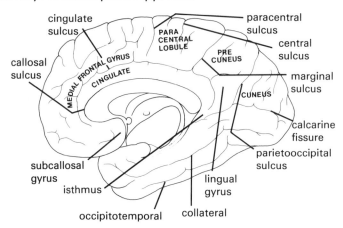

Fig. 8-5. Medial and inferior surfaces of right hemisphere.

the remaining cortex by the **cingulate sulcus** (Fig. 8-5).

Between the cingulate sulcus and the superior frontal gyrus lies the **medial frontal gyrus.**

The projection of the cingulate sulcus toward the termination of the postcentral sulcus in the medial surface is the **marginal sulcus.**

The **calcarine** and **parietooccipital sulci,** situated posteriorly, demarcate a region called the **cuneus.**

The **precuneus region** is located between the marginal, parietooccipital, and cingulate sulci.

The projection of the precentral sulcus in the medial surface to the point where it joins the cingulate sulcus is called the **paracentral sulcus.**

The region between the paracentral, marginal, and cingulate sulci is the **paracentral lobule.** It contains the medial projections of the precentral and postcentral gyri.

The cortex anterior to the paracentral sulcus and anterosuperior to the cingulate sulcus is part of the **superior frontal gyrus.**

Anterior to the lamina terminalis and inferior to the corpus callosum lies the **subcallosal gyrus.** The cortex anterior to this gyrus is known as the **subcallosal area.**

The inferomedial border of the frontal lobe is formed by the **gyrus rectus** or **straight gyrus** (Fig. 8-6).

The inferior surface of the frontal lobe, lateral to the straight gyrus, is formed by the **orbital gyri.** They are separated from the straight gyrus by the **olfactory sulcus.**

The medial border of the inferior surface of the temporal lobe is set apart from the diencephalon by the **choroidal fissure.** The inferior temporal cortex, lateral to this fissure, is the **parahippocampal gyrus,** limited laterally by the **collateral sulcus.**

Posterior to the parahippocampal gyrus and between the precuneus and cuneus lies the **lingual gyrus.**

The region embraced by the calcarine and collateral sulci is called the **medial occipitotemporal** or **fusiform gyrus.**

The narrowing portion of the cingulate gyrus, whose shape is affected by the calcarine sulcus, and which ends in the parahippocampal gyrus, is called the **isthmus** (of the cingulate gyrus).

To the side of the collateral sulcus lies the **lateral occipitotemporal gyrus,** separated laterally from the inferior temporal gyrus by the **occipitotemporal sulcus.**

Anterolaterally, the parahippocampal gyrus is limited by the short **rhinal sulcus** (Fig. 8-6), which sometimes is continuous with the collateral sulcus.

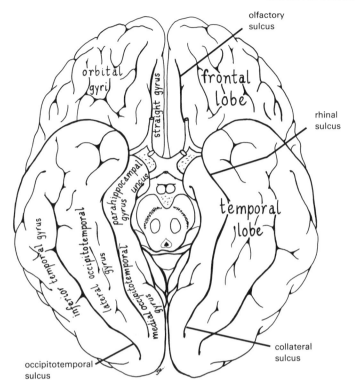

Fig. 8-6. Inferior surface of cerebral hemispheres.

The anterior portion of the parahippocampal gyrus bends, forming the **uncus** (L. hook).

The total surface area of the brain is approximately 1,600 cm². A great many terms relate to this surface.

The described mapping of the cerebral cortex is a method based on its convolutions, gyri, and sulci. (**Note:** The student must be aware of the great variability of gyri and sulci; each brain has its own unique pattern.)

Other methods of mapping are based on the cytoarchitectonics of the cortex.

The cerebral cortex does not have a uniform structure throughout the hemispheres. It varies from region to region in thickness, cellular content, and pattern of laminar arrangement.

Founded on such differences, several maps have been contrived. The one most widely accepted is the classification developed by Brodmann. He divided the cerebral cortex into areas and labeled 47 of them with numbers. The selection of the numbers is based on the sequence of the ontogenetic maturation of the respective cortical areas.

Olfactory Path

The **olfactory mucosa,** in the roof of each nasal cavity, contains the **olfactory cells.** Their axons, which are unmyelinated, enter the cranium through the cribiform plate of the ethmoid bone and end in the **olfactory bulb.** Axons of cells from the olfactory bulb form the olfactory tract, which travels posteriorly with an orientation similar to that of the **olfactory sulcus,**

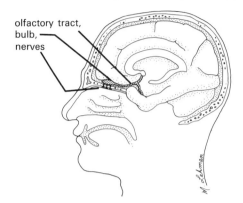

Fig. 8-7. Olfactory path.

until it reaches the level of the **anterior perforated substance.** There it bifurcates into two striae, the **lateral** and **medial olfactory striae** (Figs. 8-7 and 8-8).

The three-pronged formation consisting of the olfactory tract and striae is called the **olfactory trigone.**

The lateral olfactory stria has connections with (1) the cortex of the uncus; (2) the amygdala, a nucleus within the uncus; (3) the anterior region of the parahippocampal gyrus, which is called the **entorhinal area** (Gr. *ento* inner; **rhinos** nose); and (4) the anterolateral portion of the limen insulae.

The lateral olfactory stria, uncus, limen insulae, and entorhinal area are large in lower vertebrates, bulging into a pear-shaped formation called the **pyriform lobe** (L. *pirum* pear). These structures, the uncus, limen insulae, entorhinal area, and part of the amygdala, form the **lateral olfactory area.** In man, by comparison, the pyriform lobe is decidedly inconspicuous with regard to size and shape to the point where its name clearly is but a carry-over from a more primitive phylogenetic stage.

The medial olfactory stria ends in the **anterior olfactory nucleus.**

Some fibers from the olfactory trigone penetrate the anterior perforated substance. Small in number in man, these fibers are the remnants of an **intermediate olfactory stria.** The aforementioned cortical areas receiving olfactory signals are known as the **rhinencephalon** (Gr. nose-brain).

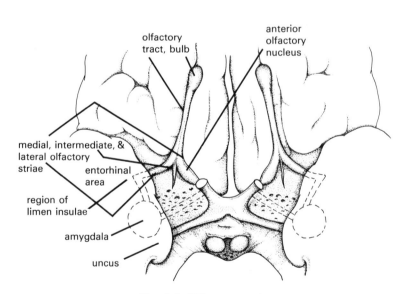

Fig. 8-8. Olfactory path.

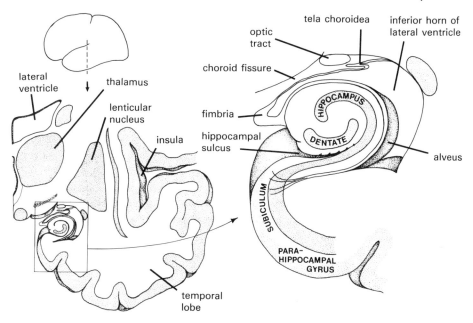

Fig. 8-9. Hippocampal formation of left hemisphere.

Hippocampal Formation

The medial edge of the parahippocampal cortex grows in the shape of a coil (Fig. 8-9). The inner, medial region of this coiled gray is called the **dentate gyrus,** and its outer region is known as the **hippocampal gyrus, hippocampus,** or **Ammon's horn.**

The region curving from the parahippocampal cortex to the hippocampus is a transition region called the **subiculum** (L. small strip). The subiculum, hippocampus, and dentate gyrus together constitute the **hippocampal formation** (Fig. 8-10).

Through the choroidal fissure the temporal horn receives a plexus of vessels, the **anterior choroid plexus.** Between the dentate gyrus and subiculum is the **hippocampal sulcus** (Fig. 8-9). The hippocampus is located on the floor of the temporal horn of the lateral ventricle.

Myelinated fibers coming out from the

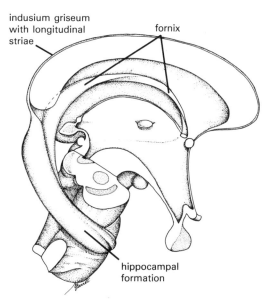

Fig. 8-10. Hippocampal formation of right hemisphere.

subiculum bend and cover the dorsal (upper) surface of the hippocampus, imparting a whitish appearance. This is the **alveus,** whose fibers form a ridge medially.

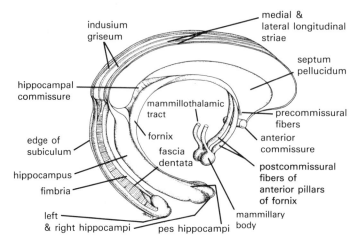

Fig. 8-11. Fornical loop.

This ridge is the **fimbria,** which becomes progressively thicker posteriorly as more fibers are added and turn posteriorly in their orientation (Figs. 8-9 and 8-11).

In Figure 8-11 the two hippocampal convolutions are represented isolated (subiculum and parahippocampal gyrus are removed). The left convolution displays its inferior surface, i.e., the dentate gyrus surface bordering on the hippocampal sulcus. This surface of the dentate gyrus displays teeth-like components, from which it derives its name **fascia dentata.** The right convolution displays its superior surface, which is the dorsum of the hippocampus bordering on the inferior horn of the lateral ventricle.

Below the most posterior and inferior part of the corpus callosum, the hippocampus and a strip of the dentate gyrus **(fasciolar gyrus)** curve over the corpus callosum, becoming the **indusium griseum** or **supracallosal gyrus,** which is very thin and difficult to detect. It contains the medial and lateral longitudinal striae.

The striae follow the contour of the callosum and reach the septal area from the hippocampal formation.

The parahippocampal gyrus continues posterosuperiorly with the isthmus of the cingulate gyrus.

The fimbria curves under the corpus callosum, becoming the **fornix.**

Fornix–Fornical Loop

The **fornix** (Fig. 8-11) is situated under the corpus callosum. Three regions are identified in the fornix: the **posterior pillars** or **crura of fornix,** the **body,** and the **anterior pillars.**

The fornix, which is a continuation of the fimbria, provides the connection between the hippocampus and the mammillary bodies.

A few fibers from the posterior pillars cross from one to the other, forming the

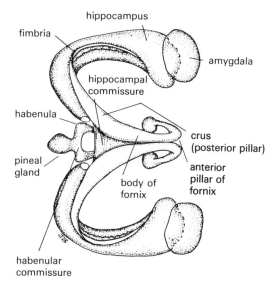

Fig. 8-12. Hippocampal commissure.

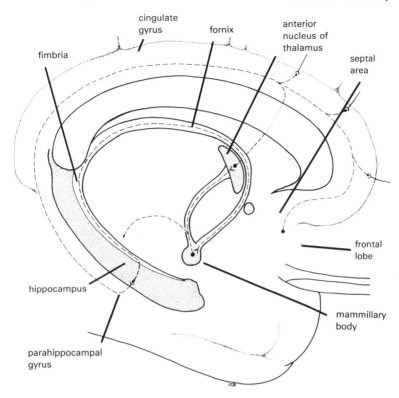

Fig. 8-13. Connections of fornical loop.

hippocampal commissure (Figs. 8-11 and 8-12).

Stretching from the body of the fornix to the lower surface of the corpus callosum is the **septum pellucidum** (Fig. 8-11), which forms the medial walls of the body and the anterior horns of the lateral ventricles.

The body of the fornix becomes the anterior pillars, each one curving ventrally in front of the interventricular foramen and dorsal to the anterior commissure. Some fibers of the fornix are connected with the septal area. These compose the **precommissural fibers** of the anterior pillar of the fornix. The remaining fibers of the anterior pillar are the **postcommissural fibers,** which continue their course to the mammillary bodies, passing between the medial and lateral hypothalamic nuclei.

The mammillary bodies are connected with the anterior nucleus of the thalamus via the mammillothalamic tract.

The anterior nucleus of the thalamus is connected with the cingulate gyrus. In turn, this gyrus is joined through the isthmus to the parahippocampal gyrus, which is linked to the hippocampal formation (Fig. 8-13).

The described loops and connections of the hippocampal formation are considered fundamental substrates in the patterning process of memory imprinting storage and retrieval.

Subcortical Nuclei

There are five major **subcortical nuclei,** namely, the **amygdala (amygdaloid complex), the **claustrum,** the **caudate,** the **putamen,** and the **pallidum.**

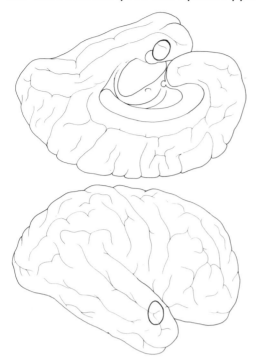

Fig. 8-14. Surface projection of amygdala.

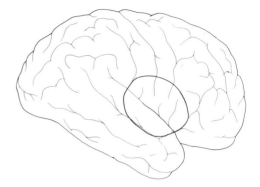

Fig. 8-15. Surface projection of claustrum.

its role in visceral activities, influencing emotional and behavioral states.

Claustrum

The **claustrum** (Fig. 8-15) is a thin, curved lamina of the size of the insula, thickening somewhat at the base. Its function is debated. Its involvement in the processing of complex sensory visceral signals has been suggested.

Amygdala or Amygdaloid Body

Amygdala in Greek means "almond," which describes its shape. Its topographical surface projection is depicted in Figure 8-14. Also, due to its phylogenetically very early development, it is known as **archistriatum.**

Among the functions of the amygdala is

Caudate Nucleus

The **caudate** (L. *cauda* tail) is attached to the wall of the lateral ventricle, which it follows. It has a **head,** a **body,** and a long **tail.** The head is apposed to the anterior horn of the ventricle, the body to the body of the ventricle, and the tail to the inferior horn.

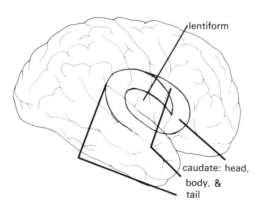

lentiform

caudate: head, body, & tail

Fig. 8-16. Surface projection of caudate and lentiform.

The topographical surface projection of the caudate nucleus is depicted in Figure 8-16.

Putamen and Pallidum (or Globus Pallidus)

The **putamen** and **pallidum** are packed together, appearing like a single nucleus, and therefore are conceived as one structure. It resembles a lentil or lens and is interchangeably called **lenticular** or **lentiform nucleus** (Fig. 8-17). Its surface projection is shown in Figure 8-16.

Related Terminology

The caudate, putamen, and pallidum are together known as the **corpus striatum.**

In respect to their phylogenetic development, the pallidum is older and is known as the **paleostriatum.** The caudate and putamen are known as the **neostriatum** or, simply, **striatum.**

The basal region of the head of the caudate is united with the rostral region of the putamen. The remainder of the caudate and putamen maintains only striated connections (Fig. 8-17).

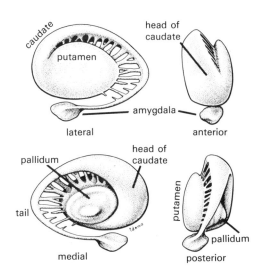

Fig. 8-17. Four views of left corpus striatum and amygdala.

The Term Basal Ganglia

The ill-defined and misleading term **basal ganglia** should be abandoned (see page 26). Nevertheless, in order to understand the literature, one must be aware that through the times it has referred to a varying selection of components which have included structures of the diencephalon, subcortical nuclei, substantia nigra, and red nucleus.

Topographical Maps of Cerebral Structures

Following the same coordinate system as described in the previous chapter, a coronal map and a horizontal map, each with 12 planes, are illustrated in Figures 8-18 to 8-41. They are of use for this chapter and beyond. Sound knowledge of brain topography is a must by the end of Chapter 9.

Coronal Planes

The five subcortical nuclei are enclosed within the −20 and +36 planes.

The **+36 coronal plane** marks the most anterior regions of the head of the caudate; the claustrum; the insular cortex; and the anterior horn of the lateral ventricle. The temporal lobe is not cut in this plane.

The **+20 coronal plane** cuts through the most anterior portion of the putamen. The striated gray between the head of the caudate and putamen is very pronounced.

The **+12 coronal plane** shows the anterior commissure and the border of the union of the temporal lobe to the core of the brain. The lentiform nucleus (putamen and pallidum) is thick in this plane.

The amygdala is situated between the +12 and 0 planes.

The bending of the parahippocampal

(Text continues on p. 141.)

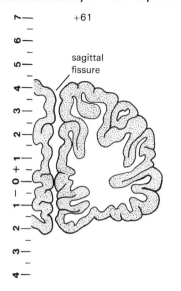

Fig. 8-18. Coronal plane +61.

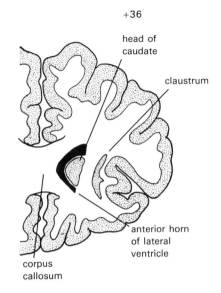

Fig. 8-19. Coronal plane +36.

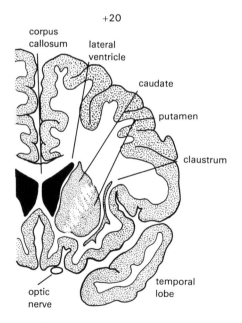

Fig. 8-20. Coronal plane +20.

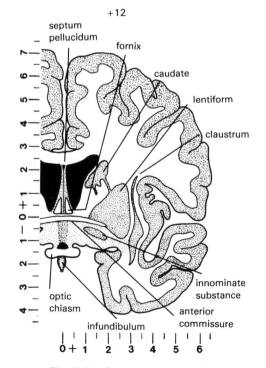

Fig. 8-21. Coronal plane +12.

+9

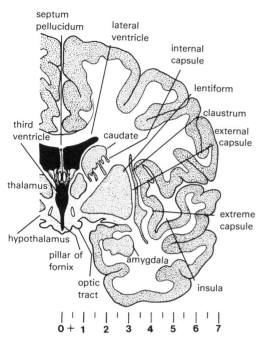

septum pellucidum

lateral ventricle

internal capsule

lentiform

claustrum

third ventricle

caudate

external capsule

thalamus

extreme capsule

hypothalamus

pillar of fornix

amygdala

optic tract

insula

| | | | | | | | | | | | | |
0 + 1 2 3 4 5 6 7

Fig. 8-22. Coronal plane +9.

+5

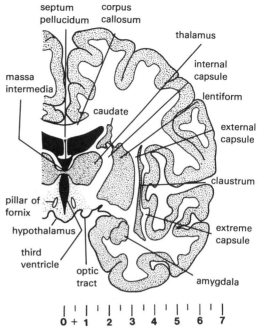

septum pellucidum

corpus callosum

thalamus

massa intermedia

internal capsule

caudate

lentiform

external capsule

claustrum

pillar of fornix

hypothalamus

third ventricle

optic tract

extreme capsule

amygdala

| | | | | | | | | | | | | |
0 + 1 2 3 4 5 6 7

Fig. 8-23. Coronal plane +5.

0

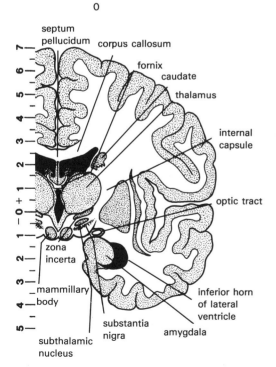

septum pellucidum

corpus callosum

fornix

caudate

thalamus

internal capsule

optic tract

zona incerta

mammillary body

substantia nigra

inferior horn of lateral ventricle

amygdala

subthalamic nucleus

Fig. 8-24. Coronal plane 0.

−6

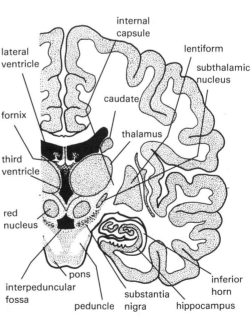

internal capsule

lateral ventricle

lentiform

subthalamic nucleus

fornix

caudate

thalamus

third ventricle

red nucleus

pons

interpeduncular fossa

peduncle

substantia nigra

inferior horn

hippocampus

Fig. 8-25. Coronal plane −6.

−12

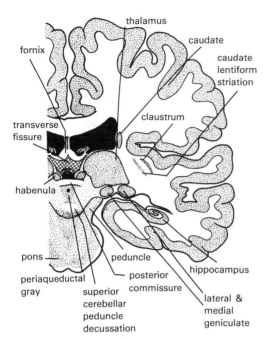

Fig. 8-26. Coronal plane −12.

−20

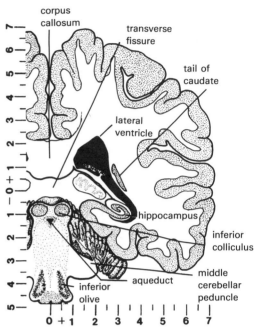

Fig. 8-27. Coronal plane −20.

−30

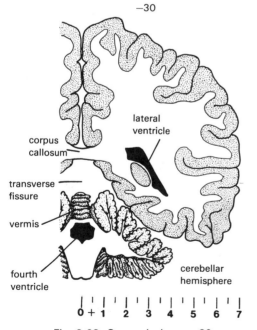

Fig. 8-28. Coronal plane −30.

−60

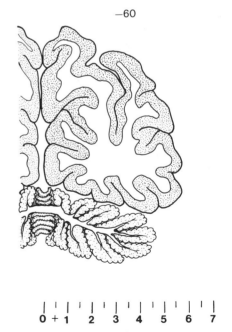

Fig. 8-29. Coronal plane −60.

gyrus into the uncus occurs between the same planes that reveal the amygdala, i.e., +12 and 0.

The **0 coronal plane** cuts through the thalamus, hypothalamus, and subthalamus as well as the five subcortical nuclei.

The **−12 coronal plane** marks the posterior limits of the insular cortex. The claustrum and putamen also end in this plane or slightly beyond it. The pallidum ends somewhat more anterior to this plane, which passes through the posterior commissure.

The **−20 coronal plane** cuts through the curved portion of the caudate—the transition of the body to the tail. It also cuts through the atrium of the lateral ventricle.

The tail of the caudate and the inferior horn of the lateral ventricle extend from −20 to +4.

Horizontal Planes

The **+40 horizontal plane** displays cortical gray and white matter.

The **+25 horizontal plane** shows the cortex and the white matter (particularly the corpus callosum); the upper portion of the body of the lateral ventricles; and the body of the caudate nucleus.

The **+20 horizontal plane** reveals the body of the lateral ventricles with the beginning of its anterior horn extension, which is covered by the callosum. It also displays a portion of the head and body of the caudate.

The **+15 horizontal plane** reveals two portions of the corpus callosum; the anterior horn and body of the lateral ventricle; the head and tail of the caudate; and minor portions of the insular cortex, the thalamus, and the fornix.

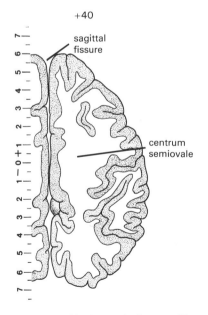

Fig. 8-30. Horizontal plane +40.

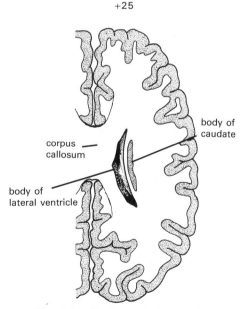

Fig. 8-31. Horizontal plane +25.

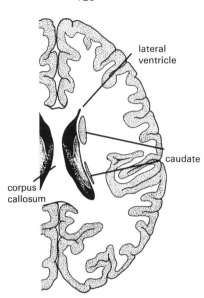

Fig. 8-32. Horizontal plane +20.

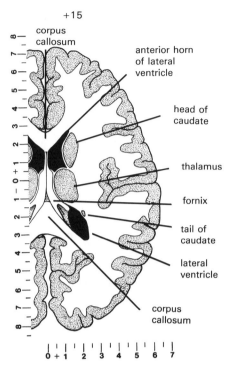

Fig. 8-33. Horizontal plane +15.

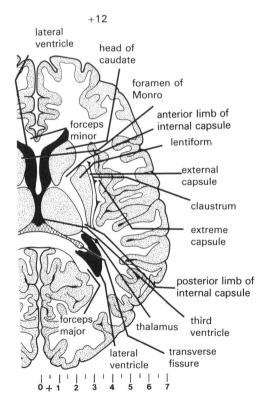

Fig. 8-34. Horizontal plane +12.

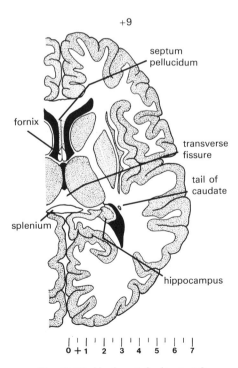

Fig. 8-35. Horizontal plane +9.

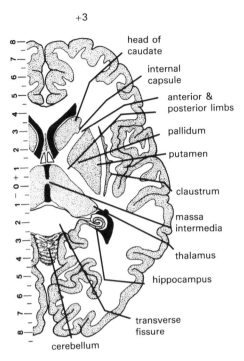

Fig. 8-36. Horizontal plane +3.

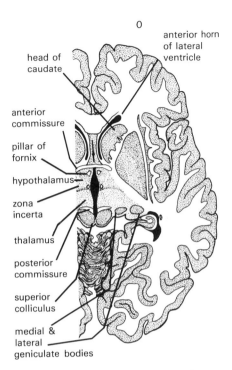

Fig. 8-37. Horizontal plane 0.

The **+12 horizontal plane** displays the anterior horn and the atrium of the lateral ventricle; the head and tail of the caudate; the insular cortex; the claustrum; and the lentiform nucleus.

The **+3 horizontal plane** shows the anterior and inferior horns; the head and tail of the caudate; the insular cortex; the claustrum; and the lentiform nucleus.

The **0 horizontal plane** displays the anterior and inferior horns of the lateral ventricles; the head and tail of the caudate; the insular cortex; the claustrum; and the lentiform nucleus. The striae uniting the head of the caudate and the putamen are seen in this plane and are larger than in

the upper planes. The 0 horizontal plane cuts the anterior and posterior commissures.

The **−6 horizontal plane** reveals the inferior ending of the anterior horn of the lateral ventricle; the inferior horn of the lateral ventricle; the insular cortex; the claustrum (thicker than in previous planes); the caudate and putamen, which are nearly united; the tail of the caudate; and the inferior horn of the lateral ventricle.

The **−9 horizontal plane** displays the insular cortex; a small portion of the claustrum with some thickness; a rounded mass of gray composed of the nucleus accum-

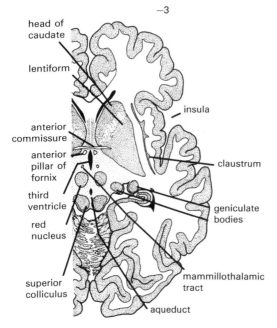

Fig. 8-38. Horizontal plane −3.

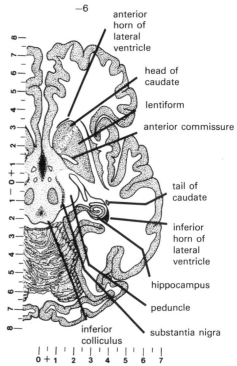

Fig. 8-39. Horizontal plane −6.

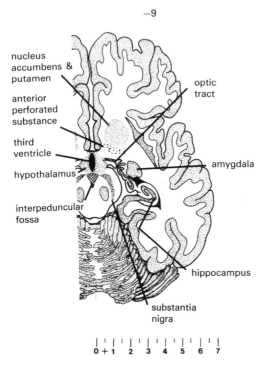

Fig. 8-40. Horizontal plane −9.

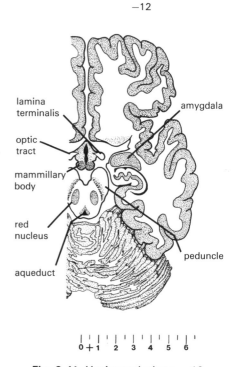

Fig. 8-41. Horizontal plane −12.

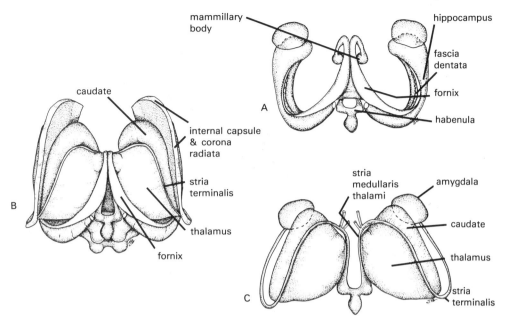

Fig. 8-42. (A) Topography of fornix; (B) stria terminalis; (C) stria medullaris.

bens and the putamen; the amygdala; the inferior horn of the lateral ventricle; and the tip of the tail of the caudate.

Note: The **tenia choroidea,** a line of attachment with the choroid plexus, runs along the thalamus and stria terminalis.

Main Connections of the Subcortical Nuclei

Amygdala

The amygdala has connections with the primary olfactory cortex (the pyriform lobe) and other cortical regions, the claustrum, the septal area, the thalamus, hypothalamus, epithalamus, and the reticular formation.

A well-defined bundle of fibers of the amygdala is the **stria terminalis,** which follows the contours of the caudate nucleus, until it reaches the interventricular foramen region, where it turns toward the septal area and the anterior hypothalamic region. Some fibers of the stria terminalis join the stria medullaris (Fig. 8-42).

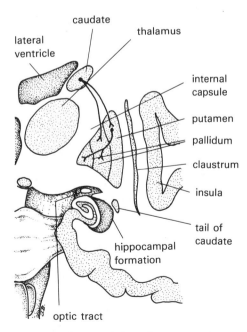

Fig. 8-43. Connectivity of corpus striatum.

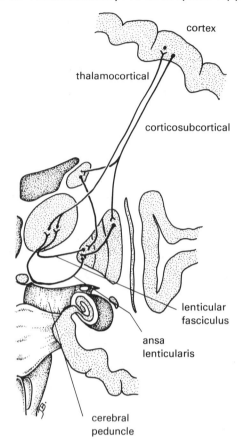

Fig. 8-44. Corticosubcorticocortical loop.

Claustrum

The connections of the claustrum are debated. Three of the alleged connections are the cerebral cortex, the intralaminar nuclei of the thalamus, and the amygdala.

Corpus Striatum

The three nuclei of the corpus striatum are viewed as acting in cascade: **caudate—putamen—pallidum** (Fig. 8-43), where its final output ends in the ventralis lateralis and ventralis anterior nuclei of the thalamus. The corpus striatum receives input from the cerebral cortex, the thalamus, the subthalamus, and the substantia nigra. A schematic diagram of the circuitry of the corpus striatum is presented in Figure 8-44.

It is important to recognize that the corpus striatum is a link from cortex to thalamus. With this connection a continuous loop is established: **sensory systems input—thalamus—cortex—corpus striatum—thalamus—cortex.** This loop influences not only motor activity but also other dimensions of behavior.

Suggested Readings

Astruc J: Corticofugal connections of area 8 (frontal eye field) in Macaca mulatta, Brain Res 33:241–256, 1971.

Jones EG, Powell TPS: Anatomical organization of the somatosensory cortex. In Iggo A, Ed.: Handbook of Sensory Physiology, Vol. 2. Somatosensory System, Springer-Verlag, Berlin, pp. 279–620, 1973.

Lassen NA, Ingvar DH, Skinhöj E: Brain function and blood flow, Sci Amer 239(4):62–71, 1978.

Mehler WR: The basal ganglia—circa 1982. A review and commentary. In Gildenberg AL, Ed.: Applied Neurophysiology, Karger, Basel, pp. 261–290, 1982.

O'Keefe J, Nadel L: The Hippocampus as a Cognitive Map, Oxford University Press, Oxford, 1978.

Stephens RB, Stilwell DL: Arteries and Veins of the Human Brain, Charles C Thomas, Springfield, 1969.

Swanson LW: The anatomical organization of septo-hippocampal projections. In Functions of the Septo-Hippocampal System, CIBA Foundation Symposium 58 (new series), Elsevier Excerpta Medica, Amsterdam, pp. 25–43, 1978.

Van Hoesen GW: The parahippocampal gyrus: new observations regarding its cortical connections in the monkey, Trends in Neuroscience 5(10):345–350, 1982.

Williams PL, Warwick R: Functional Neuroanatomy of Man, WB Saunders, Philadelphia, pp. 921–984, 1975.

Zarzecki P, Shinoda Y, Asanuma H: Projection from area 3a to the motor cortex by neurons activated from group I muscle afferents, Exp Brain Res 33:269–282, 1978.

9

Cerebral Hemispheres— Connections

White Matter

The **white matter** can be classified into three types: **commissural, association,** and **projection fibers.**

Commissural Fibers

The **commissural fibers** are nerve fibers that cross the midline and interconnect similar regions in the two cerebral hemispheres.

Corpus Callosum

The **corpus callosum** (Fig. 9-1) is made up of fibers that radiate to interconnect the left and right homologeous regions of the frontal, parietal, temporal, and occipital lobes.

The following terminology relates to the different regions of the corpus callosum:

splenium—the rounded posterior extremity

genu—the rounded anterior extremity

body—the region between the splenium and the genu

rostrum (L. beak)—the ventral tapering portion from the genu to the lamina terminalis

The genu projects most of the fibers to the frontal lobes in a formation resembling a pair of forceps. This is appropriately called the **forceps minor.** The **forceps major** is a similar arrangement from the splenium to the occipital poles.

The **body** radiates to the temporal and parietal lobes.

Fibers of the corpus callosum spread and form a thin sheath, called **tapetum,** over the inferior horn of the lateral ventricle.

Anterior and Posterior Commissural Fibers

The bundle of fibers composing the **anterior commissure** connects primarily the temporal poles but also the frontal lobes (+ olfactory circuitry) (Fig. 9-2). The **pos-**

terior commissure consists mostly of fibers internally interconnecting the left and the right sides of the tectum and the tegmentum of the midbrain. The **habenular commissure** consists of fibers interconnecting the left and right habenular nuclei.

Hippocampal Commissural Fibers

The **hippocampal** (also known as **fornical**) **commissural fibers** (very few in man)

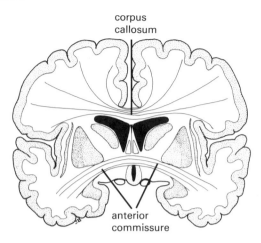

Fig. 9-2. Commissural fibers.

(Fig. 8-12) are those which pass from one fornix to the other.

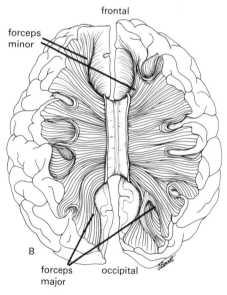

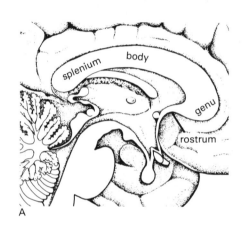

Fig. 9-1. Corpus callosum. (A) Midsagittal plane; (B) dorsal view of dissected corpus.

Association Fibers

Association fibers (Fig. 9-3) are nerve fibers that interconnect cortical regions of the same cerebral hemisphere. They are classified into **short** and **long.**

Short Association Fibers

The **short association** (or **arcuate**) **fibers** interconnect adjacent convolutions.

Long Association Fibers

The **long association fibers** interconnect cortical regions of different lobes within the same hemispheres. Five main bundles are identified:

1. The **cingulum,** buried primarily in the subcallosal, cingulate, and parahippocampal gyri, interconnects these regions as well as other lobes.
2. The **uncinate fasciculus** interconnects the frontal with the temporal lobe.
3. The **inferior occipitofrontal fasciculus**

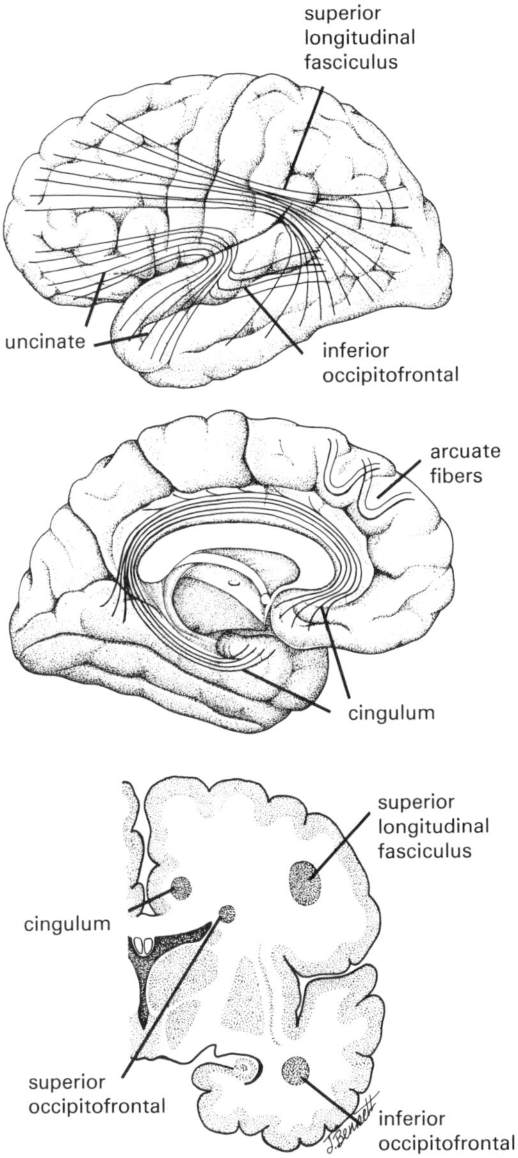

superior
longitudinal
fasciculus

uncinate

inferior
occipitofrontal

arcuate
fibers

cingulum

superior
longitudinal
fasciculus

cingulum

superior
occipitofrontal

inferior
occipitofrontal

Fig. 9-3. Bundle of association fibers.

Projection Fibers

The **projection fibers** (Fig. 9-4) project from the diencephalon to the cerebral hemispheres and from the hemispheres to the diencephalon, the brain stem, and the spinal cord. The internal capsule, which handles the input-output of the hemispheres, contains projection fibers.

Other Terms Related to White Matter

A number of terms aim to define regions of the white matter.

The **internal capsule** is the white matter medial to the lentiform nucleus and lateral to the diencephalon and the caudate nucleus.

The **corona radiata** (Fig. 9-4) is seen spreading from the upper limit of the internal capsule, i.e., between the caudate nucleus and the upper portion of the putamen. It consists of the fibers of the internal capsule which fan out like a crown to and from the cortex.

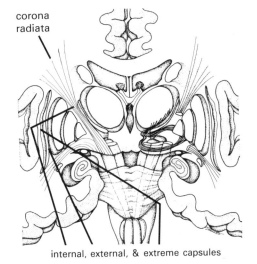

corona
radiata

internal, external, & extreme capsules

Fig. 9-4. White matter capsules and corona radiata.

interconnects the frontal and the occipital lobes.

4. The **superior longitudinal** (or **arcuate**) **fasciculus** interconnects the four lobes.
5. The **superior occipitofrontal** (or **subcallosal**) **fasciculus** interconnects the frontal and the occipital lobes.

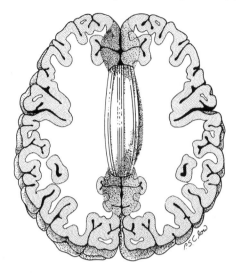

Fig. 9-5. Centrum of white matter.

The **external capsule** is the layer of white matter lateral to the lentiform nucleus and medial to the claustrum.

The **extreme capsule** is the layer of white matter between the claustrum and the insular cortex.

The extreme and external capsules are composed of association fibers.

The **centrum semiovale** (Fig. 9-5) is the semiovally shaped white matter observable in horizontal sections above the corpus callosum.

Primary, Association, and Integration Cortical Areas

A **primary cortical area** is a region of the cortex receiving (sensory) or projecting (motor) a first level of signal information. For example, the **primary visual cortex** is the area of cortex that receives first and principally visual signals.

Association cortex refers to areas of the cortex receiving (associating) more complex levels of signal information.

The particular modality invested in the

signals which are received normally lends its name to the adjective describing the term, e.g., **visual association cortex.** If the signals received and associated by an area of cortex belong to more than one sensory modality, the area may be called by different names, e.g., by a name composed by the modalities involved or by the uncommitted term **complex association cortex** or simply **sensory association cortex.**

An area of the cortex that receives signals from many complex association areas is called **integration cortical area.**

Input to Primary Cortical Areas

Thalamic Path to Primary Somatosensory Cortex

Fibers from the ventralis posterior nucleus of the thalamus ascend, forming part of the posterior limb of the internal capsule, reach the postcentral gyrus or the **primary somatosensory cortex** (areas 1, 2, and 3 of Brodmann). This thalamocortical projection has two main features:

1. It follows the somatotopic plan. It has been mapped by electrical recordings

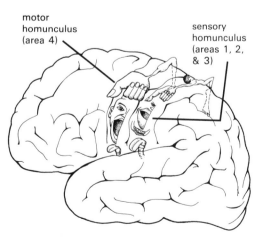

Fig. 9-6. Cortical representation.

of body stimuli and its schematic representation displays what is called a **homunculus** (L. little man or dwarf) (Fig. 9-6).

2. There is a disproportion between individual body areas and their respective representation in the cortical area. For instance, the legs are shown as dwarfed, whereas the fingers and lips take up proportionately much larger areas.

Thalamic Path to Primary Visceral Sensory Cortex

In the thalamic path to the primary visceral sensory cortex there are two projections. One small group of fibers follows the same pattern as the thalamic path to the primary somatosensory cortex, i.e., from the ventralis posterior nucleus. Another group of fibers projects from the intralaminar nuclei to the upper lip (parietal operculum) of the lateral fissure and the anterior pole of the temporal lobe.

Thalamic Path to Primary Visual Cortex

In the thalamic path to the primary visual cortex, fibers from the lateral geniculate nucleus of the thalamus form part of the **retrolenticular limb** of the internal

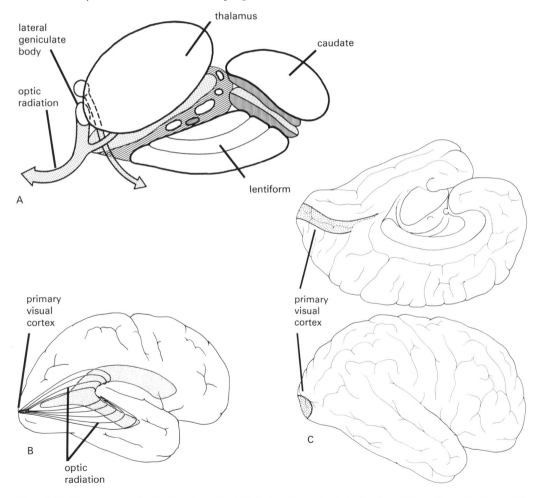

Fig. 9-7. Thalamocortical visual path. (A) Lateral geniculate body; (B) optic radiation; (C) primary visual cortex.

capsule and reach the **calcarine region** of the occipital lobe, or primary visual cortex (area 17 of Brodmann). This fiber path is the **geniculocalcarine tract.** It is worth mentioning that this tract makes a sharp bend in its course because of the presence of the confluence of the horns of the lateral ventricle. Once the tract can proceed posteriorly, the fibers fan out and embrace the posterior horn of the lateral ventricle to reach the **calcarine cortex.** The radiated portion of the tract is called the **optic radiation** (Fig. 9-7).

The cortex of area 17 is also known as **striate cortex** or **area** because of its cross-sectional macroscopic stripe first described by Gennari.

Thalamic Path to Primary Auditory Cortex

As part of the **auditory path,** fibers travel from the medial geniculate nucleus of the thalamus, forming part of the **sublenticular limb** of the internal capsule, and reach the **auditory region** of the tem-

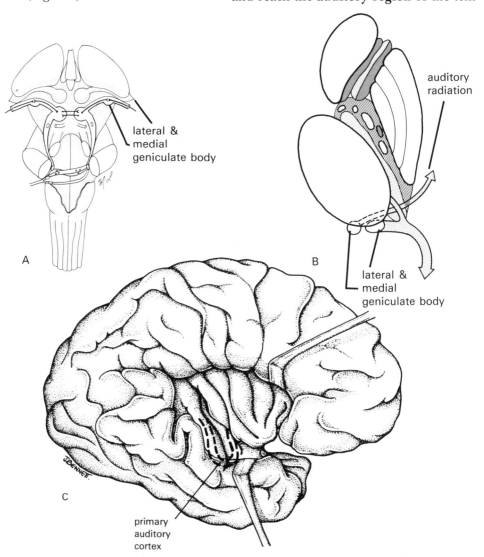

Fig. 9-8. Thalamocortical auditory path. (A) Brain stem; (B) medial geniculate body; (C) primary auditory cortex.

poral lobe, or primary auditory cortex (area 41 of Brodmann). This **geniculotemporal tract,** once it is out from under the lentiform nucleus, fans out and reaches the auditory cortex. The radiated portion is known as the **auditory radiation** (Fig. 9-8).

When the specific sensory signals have reached the specific sensory cortical areas, an enormous amount of association and communication processes follows (Fig. 9-9).

Cortical Association Areas

There are **simple** and **very complex** cortical association areas.

The **simple cortical association areas** have connections with the corresponding primary area, specific thalamic nucleus, and associative thalamic nuclei.

The **simple somatosensory association area,** i.e., **area 5 of Brodmann** (Fig. 9-10), has connections with areas 1, 2, and 3; the ventralis posterior nucleus of the thalamus; and the sensory association nuclei of the thalamus.

The **simple visceral association area** (the **insular cortex**) has connections with the cortex of the parietal opercula, the ventralis posterior, and the intralaminar nuclei of the thalamus.

The **simple visual association area (secondary visual area** or **parastriate area),** i.e., **area 18 of Brodmann,** has connections with area 17, the lateral geniculate body, and the sensory association nuclei of the thalamus.

The **simple auditory association area (secondary auditory area),** i.e., **area 42 of Brodmann,** has connections with area 41, the medial geniculate body, and the sensory association nuclei of the thalamus.

The **very complex cortical association areas** mature in a sequence of stages. First, simple cortical association areas associate in pairs, for instance, the somatosensory

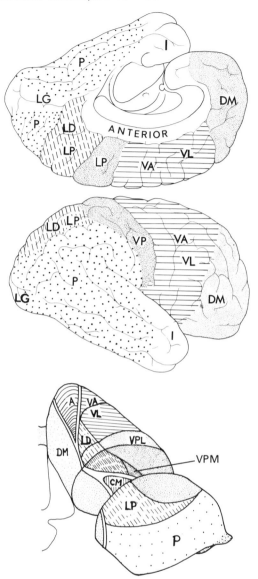

Fig. 9-9. Thalamocortical connections.

cortex and visual cortex in area 9 and area 19 **(peristrate area);** and the visual and auditory cortex in areas 19 and 20. Subsequently, more complex associations are executed in areas 21, 22, 37, and 38 of Brodmann. These areas have connections also with the sensory association nuclei and the intralaminar nuclei. Areas 39 and 40 associate multiple sensibilities by establishing

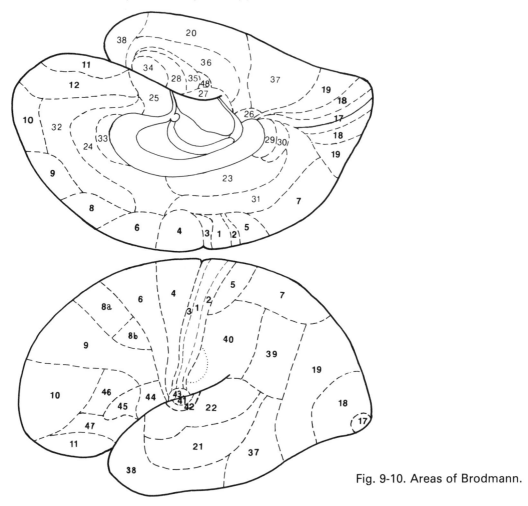

Fig. 9-10. Areas of Brodmann.

connections with all the surrounding areas and with an integrative nucleus of the thalamus (the dorsomedial nucleus).

Other Cortical Connections

More or less in parallel with this process of maturation of sensory associative circuits, three other circuit maturation processes occur.

1. One such process is the channeling of cerebral activities through the hippo-

campus, ending via the fornical path and the thalamus in the cingulate gyrus (Fig. 8-13). This gyrus also establishes direct connections with the four lobes.

2. Another process is the maturation of commissural paths interconnecting symmetrical regions of the hemispheres. This process triggers what is called **secondary sensory areas,** where sensory information from both hemispheric regions is recorded. These areas are poorly known in humans. Best known is one called the **secondary sensory area II (SS II)** (Fig. 9-11), situated in the upper bank of the lateral fissure.

3. A third such maturation process is the

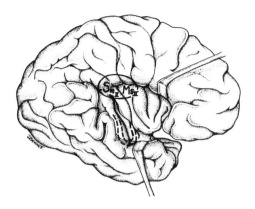

Fig. 9-11. Secondary sensory area = secondary somesthetic area = Sm II and secondary motor area = Ms II.

connections of the frontal lobe with the other three lobes.

Cortical Motor Areas

The term cortical motor area at one time referred exclusively to cortical area 4 of Brodmann. It was then believed that the corticospinal (pyramidal) path originated only in that area.

The concepts regarding cortical motor areas have since changed and a number of related terms has consequently followed.

The **primary somatic sensorimotor area** or **cortex** (abbreviated **primary S-M**) includes areas 1, 2, 3, 4, and 6 of Brodmann,

which all contribute fibers to the corticospinal tract.

To distinguish between the areas 1, 2, and 3, which are mainly sensory, and areas 4 and 6, which are mainly motor, two other terms are in use:

Primary somesthetic area, or **S-m I,** emphasizes the involvement of the sensory areas 1, 2, and 3 in motor functions.

The **primary motor area,** or **M-s I,** stresses the motor functions of the somatic area 4.

The secondary sensory area, or the **secondary somesthetic area,** also expressed as **S-m II,** defines an area in the upper bank of the fissure of Sylvius. It is chiefly sensory and has bilateral representation of the body.

The **secondary motor area,** or **M-s II,** overlaps the S-m II area. Stimulation of the M-s II area produces bilateral contraction of muscles.

The **supplementary motor area,** also expressed as **supplementary s-M,** defines an area corresponding to the portion of area 6 of Brodmann in the medial surface of the cerebral hemisphere above the cingulate gyrus. This area has bilateral representation of the body (Fig. 9-12).

The **premotor area** is the portion of area 6 of Brodmann in the lateral surface of the cerebral hemisphere.

Frontal cortical eye fields (Fig. 9-10) refer to a portion of area 8 of Brodmann, which appears to be involved in the control of eye movements. When the area is lesioned, the eyes become deviated toward the same side as the lesion.

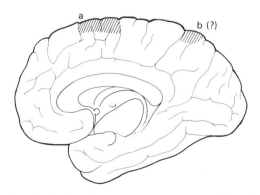

Fig. 9-12. Supplementary motor area (a) and supplementary sensory area (b).

Details Regarding Area 4 of Brodmann

Area 4 of Brodmann, or area M-s I, has a somatotopic organization similar to that of areas 1, 2, and 3, as evidenced in the mapped homunculus (Fig. 9-6).

Area 4 has cortical connections mainly with areas 1, 2, 3, and 6. It also establishes connections with the corpus striatum and the thalamus (ventralis lateralis and ventralis anterior), forming a subcortical loop. Proprioceptive signals from other neural regions are channeled through this loop principally toward areas 4 and 6.

Area 4, acting as the main distributor, contributes approximately 50 percent of the fibers from the cortex toward the spinal cord.

Details Regarding the Premotor Area

The **premotor area** supplies approximately 15 percent of the fibers coursing from the cortex toward the spinal cord. It appears that the premotor area contributes to a repository of pattern movements of muscle groups, chiefly channeled through area 4. It manifests many similarities with area 4, with which it has important connections. Its main differences as compared to area 4 are noted below:

1. There is no simple somatotopic arrangement as in area 4. Each small region affects many groups of muscles.
2. The premotor area has more connections with the anterior frontal cortex than does area 4.
3. It does not have a type of cells typical of the primary somatomotor cortex, i.e., the **giant pyramidal cells of Betz.**

Integration of Cortical Functions

The brain matures cortical areas in the anterior frontal cortex, where sensory and motor information are integrated. This is done in sequential stages, as the information becomes available in its ontogenetically progressive complexity.

Areas 9 to 12 of Brodmann in the anterior frontal cortex integrate sensory and motor cortex information by establishing connections with the precentral regions and with the parietal, occipital, and temporal lobes.

Area 43 matures its sensory connections coming through the thalamus from the pharynx, larynx, mouth, and tongue and surrounding sensory and motor cortical areas, especially area 44.

Area 44, which is known as the **motor speech area** or the **motor speech center (Broca's area),** matures its dual connections from motor and sensory areas concerned with the control of the muscles involved in speech. As an infant matures, area 44 starts receiving more complex input from **area 46,** where a higher order of integration of multiple types of signals (sound, touch, vision, etc.) is executed.

Area 45 has a portion invested with a similar function as that of area 44 and included in the motor speech area. The remaining portion of area 45 is also concerned with written language and has connections similar to those of area 44.

It is in the second year of life that areas 43 to 46 come to maturity.

Apart from its connections with other cortical areas, the integrating frontal cortex has other important connections with the region of the lamina terminalis, which is another telencephalic integrating region.

The dorsomedial nucleus of the thalamus connects with the cerebral cortex, in particular the region of the lamina terminalis.

Cortical Projection Fibers

Direct Corticospinal Projection Fibers

Direct corticospinal projection fibers originate mainly from areas 1, 2, and 3 of Brodmann; the fibers end mostly in laminae IV and V of Rexed and control the sensory input to the posterior horn;

areas 4 and 6 of Brodmann, ending mostly in laminae VI and VII and controlling the motor activity of the anterior horn.

Decussations of the Direct Corticospinal Tract

At the limit between the spinal cord and brain stem, the majority of the corticospinal fibers of each side changes position. Eighty-five to 90 percent of the fibers from

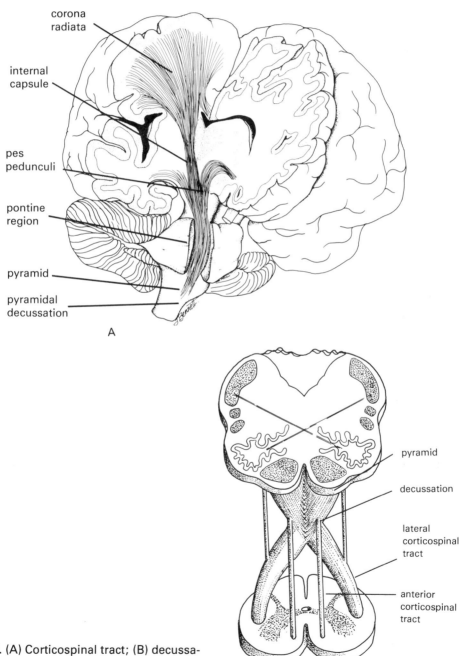

Fig. 9-13. (A) Corticospinal tract; (B) decussation of corticospinal tract.

the left hemisphere turn to the right, descending in the lateral funiculus of the spinal cord to establish connections with the right gray matter of the spinal cord, while 85 to 90 percent of the fibers coming from the right hemisphere do the opposite (Fig. 9-13). The remaining 10 to 15 percent from each hemisphere stay on their course and descend ipsilaterally in the corresponding anterior and lateral funiculi. However, most of the fibers descending in the anterior funiculus, at the level where they establish connections with the gray of the spinal cord, shift and innervate the opposite gray matter.

The direct corticospinal fiber path descending in the lateral funiculus forms the **lateral corticospinal tract,** while the fibers descending in the anterior funiculus form the **anterior corticospinal tract.**

Course of the Direct Corticospinal Tract

The uninterrupted direct corticospinal tract forms part of a number of anatomical regions through its downward course: the corona radiata, the internal capsule, the peduncular region, the pontine region, the pyramids, the pyramidal decussation, and the lateral and anterior corticospinal tracts (Fig. 9-13).

Indirect Corticospinal Tracts

From the primary somatic sensorimotor cortex a number of fibers also forms two large indirect corticospinal tracts, namely, the **corticorubrospinal** and the **corticoreticulospinal tracts,** and one minor indirect corticospinal tract, namely, the **corticotectospinal tract** (Fig. 9-14). These indirect routes make the bundles of fibers separate from the direct corticospinal tract on the upper portion of the mesencephalon to reach the tectum, the red nucleus, and the brain stem reticular formation.

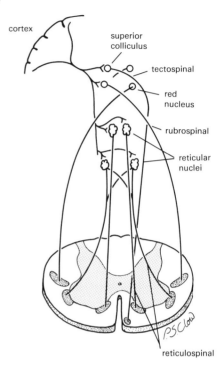

Fig. 9-14. Indirect corticospinal paths.

Neurons from these three structures project to the spinal cord.

Cortical Projection Fibers to Cranial Nerve Nuclei

Fiber bundles that originate in the primary somatic sensorimotor cortex first travel together with the corticospinal tract. At the appropriate brain stem levels, fibers separate to innervate the corresponding cranial nerve motor nuclei (e.g., oculomotor, facial, hypoglossal) or interneurons near the sensory and motor nuclei, controlling the activity of sensory and motor cranial nerve nuclei. Also indirect routes through the red nucleus, reticular formation, and tectum are established. These connections are known as the **corticobulbar tract.**

Cortical Projection Fibers to Pontine Nuclei

A massive amount of fibers from the four lobes of a cerebral hemisphere descends through the internal capsule and cerebral peduncle to end in the pontine nuclei of the same side. Fibers of these pontine nuclei cross to the opposite side to reach the opposite cerebellar hemisphere through the middle cerebellar peduncle. Fibers from that cerebellar hemisphere travel through the superior cerebellar peduncle, cross to the opposite side, and reach the ventralis lateralis and ventralis anterior nuclei of the thalamus. Fibers from these nuclei reach the somatic sensorimotor cortex. This complex circuit, the **corticopontocerebellothalamocortical loop,** is an important presetting loop of motor activity (Fig. 9-15).

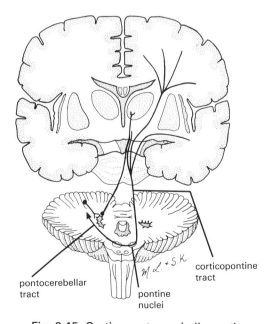

Fig. 9-15. Corticopontocerebellar path.

pontocerebellar tract

pontine nuclei

corticopontine tract

Other Cortical Projections

There are conceivably direct fiber tracts from the cortex to practically all the regions of the brain stem, except for the lateral vestibular nucleus (the nucleus of Deiter).

Note: An important topographical difference between cortical descending fibers beyond the internal capsule and the ascending fibers coursing from the spinal cord, the brain stem and the cerebellum toward the diencephalon, is that the descending fibers travel in the ventral region of the midbrain and the ascending fibers travel in the tegmental region of the midbrain.

Review of the Cortical Connections with Subcortical and Thalamic Nuclei

In Chapters 7 and 8, emphasis was placed on the connections of the four cortical lobes with the corpus striatum and the thalamus, establishing a corticosubcorticothalamocortical loop; and the thalamocorticothalamic connections.

Functions of the Primary Somatic Sensorimotor Cortex

Electrical stimulation of any of the areas of the primary somatic sensorimotor cortex never elicits coordinated purposeful movement, only contraction of muscles or muscle groups. These areas alone cannot produce intelligent motor movement.

If a surgical lesion of the corticospinal tracts or primary somatic sensorimotor cortex is performed, abolition of movement results, especially those of rapid, skilled, intelligent, volitional nature, first and foremost with those of the hands.

One can state that in a functioning nervous system the primary sensorimotor cortex and its direct and indirect corticospinal tracts, in very close cooperation, control the performance of skilled movement mainly by modulating the activity of the spinal patterns of movement. The efficiency of such activity is dependent on proper activity in many other regions and pathways, e.g.:

1. the brain stem, the spinal cord, the thalamus, and the cortex, which furnish the route for ascending sensory information;
2. the corticopontocerebellothalamocortical loop; and
3. the corticosubcorticothalamocortical loop.

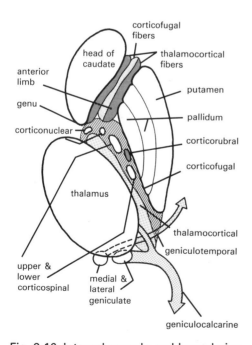

Fig. 9-16. Internal capsule and boundaries.

Overview of the Cerebral Cortex Connections Through the Internal Capsule

The understanding of the structure of the internal capsule is very important in the consolidation of a correct image of the cerebral topography. First of all, one must realize that the shape of the internal capsule is different at different plane levels. The two factors underlying this difference are the types of fibers composing the capsule, and their orientation.

Types of Fibers Composing the Internal Capsule

Composing the internal capsule are fibers constituting **thalamocortical** (i.e., thalamocortical and corticothalamic) **connections,** and fibers coursing from the cortex to other regions of the diencephalon, the corpus striatum, the brain stem, and the spinal cord.

Observations made in three planes are essential in acquiring an accurate image of the internal capsule.

Regions of the Internal Capsule

Three regions are distinguished in the internal capsule (Fig. 9-16): the **anterior limb** between the head of the caudate and lentiform nucleus, the **genu,** and the **posterior limb** between the thalamus and lentiform nucleus.

Views at Different Planes

The arrangement of the fibers from a ventromedial position to a dorsolateral is frontopontine, corticobulbar, corticospinal, parietopontine, occipitopontine, and temporopontine.

The corticopontine fibers constitute approximately half of the descending fibers.

The term **corticobulbar** or **corticonuclear fibers** refers to fibers coursing from the cortex to the nuclei of the brain stem with the exception of the ones coursing toward the pontine nuclei.

In the **horizontal plane −3** (Fig. 8-38), the anterior limb of the internal capsule is not yet clearly visible. The region is occupied mostly by the striations between the caudate and the putamen. The anterior limb appears above it, radiating to and from the frontal lobe.

The posterior limb of the internal capsule continues under the term **retrolenticular limb** behind the lentiform nucleus and gives off occipital and temporal radiations (Fig. 9-16).

Some fibers known as the **sublenticular limb** of the internal capsule course under the lentiform nucleus toward the temporal cortex.

The **horizontal plane +9** (Fig. 8-35) displays the anterior, posterior, and retrolenticular limbs and the genu of the internal

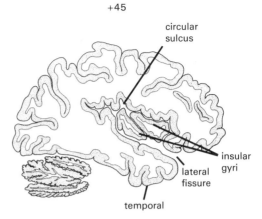

+45

Fig. 9-18. Sagittal plane +45.

circular sulcus

insular gyri

lateral fissure

temporal

capsule with its characteristic pattern of fiber distribution (Fig. 9-16).

Knowing that the central sulcus is inclined and that the inferior portion is more anterior (and the source of fibers of the head region), it is easy to understand their more ventral, anterior position in the internal capsule as compared to that of the fibers for the trunk and leg regions (Figs. 9-6 and 9-16).

Sagittal Planes of the Brain

To facilitate a three-dimensional image of the brain structures a map of eight sagittal brain sections is presented in Figures 9-17 to 9-24. The basis of the coordinate system is explained on page 111.

Dissection of the Cerebral Hemisphere

The two lateral views of dissected right hemispheres shown in Figure 9-25 display
(Text continues on p. 165.)

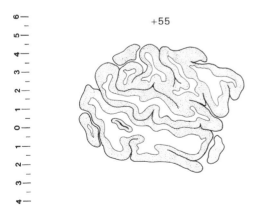

+55

Fig. 9-17. Sagittal plane +55.

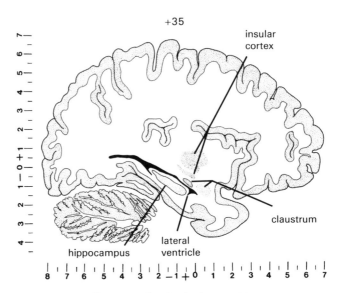

Fig. 9-19. Sagittal plane +35.

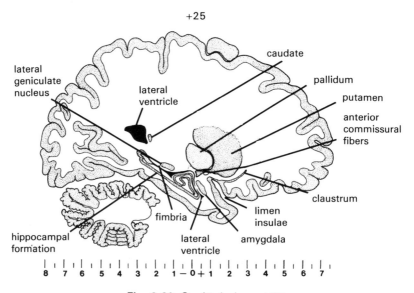

Fig. 9-20. Sagittal plane +25.

+20

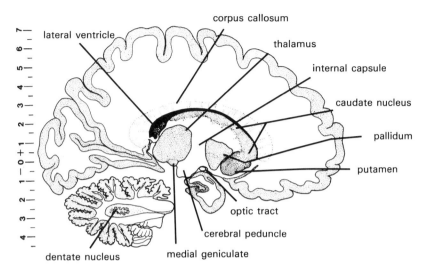

Fig. 9-21. Sagittal plane +20.

+15

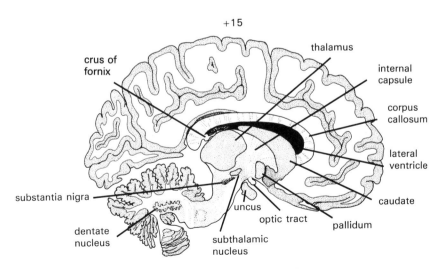

Fig. 9-22. Sagittal plane +15.

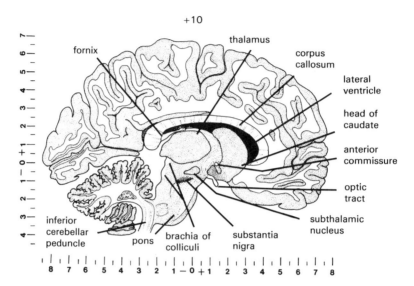

Fig. 9-23. Sagittal plane +10.

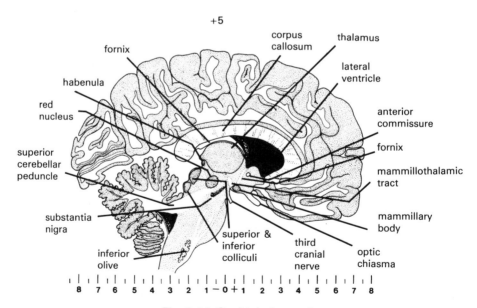

Fig. 9-24. Sagittal plane +5.

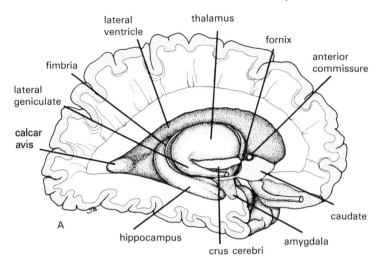

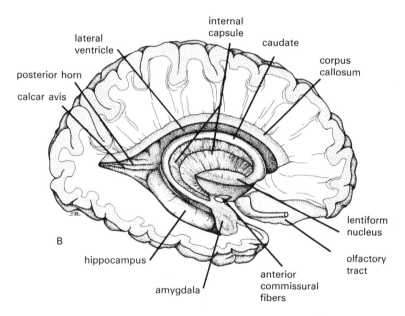

Fig. 9-25. (A) and (B); Lateral views of dissected right cerebral hemisphere.

a number of the structures mentioned in previous chapters.

A prominence produced by the indentation of the calcarine sulcus is observed in the medial wall of the posterior horn of the lateral ventricle. This prominence is called **calcar avis** (L. *calcar* spur; *avis* bird) in recognition of its shape.

Suggested Readings

Berke JJ: The claustrum, the external capsule and the extreme capsule of Macaca mulatta, J Comp Neurol 115:297–331, 1960.

Bindman L, Lippold O: The Neurophysiology of the Cerebral Cortex, University of Texas Press, Austin, pp. 3–60, 1981.

Brain, The: Sci Am 241(3), 1979.

Carpenter MB: Human Neuroanatomy. Seventh Edition. Williams and Wilkins, Baltimore, pp. 21–36, 1976.

Denny-Brown D, Kirke EJ, Yanagisawa N: The tract of Lissauer in relation to sensory transmission in the dorsal horn of spinal cord in the Macaque monkey, J Comp Neurol 151:175–200, 1973.

Eleftheriou BE, Ed.: The Neurobiology of the Amygdala, Plenum Press, New York, 1972.

Hornykiewicz O: Neurohumoral interactions and basal ganglia function and dysfunction. In Yahr MD, Ed.: The Basal Ganglia, Raven Press, New York, pp. 269–278, 1976.

Izquierdo I: The hippocampus and learning, Progr Neurobiol 5:37–75, 1975.

Coulter JD, Ewing L, Carter C: Origin of primary sensorimotor cortical projections to lumbar spinal cord of cat and monkey, Brain Res 103:366–372, 1976.

O'Keefe J, Nadel L: The Hippocampus as a Cognitive Map, Clarendon Press, Oxford, 1978.

Williams PL, Warwick R: Functional Neuroanatomy of Man, WB Saunders, Philadelphia, pp. 921–984, 1975.

Yahr MD, Ed.: The Basal Ganglia, Raven Press, New York, 1976.

III

Segmental Loops and Tracts

10

Autonomic Nervous System

The **visceral nervous system** is that part of the nervous system concerned with the innervation of the visceral body. This includes all the digestive, respiratory, cardiovascular, and glandular organs plus the erector pili muscles of the skin and other smooth muscles like the ones found in the eye and the orbit. It implies involvement in the regulation of digestion, respiration, blood circulation, body temperature, etc. All these functions together aim at maintaining an optimal stable internal body environment, the "milieu interieur."

As an example, the visceral nervous system regulates the heart beats, the blood supply to the heart, the blood pressure, the distribution of blood to different parts of the body, the O_2-CO_2 content of the blood, etc. The visceral nervous system accomplishes such complex tasks by automating all of them as much as possible within the peripheral nervous system.

The visceral nervous system is, of course, also an integral part of the whole nervous system and as such it is regulated by the brain. The brain regulates visceral functions at a subconscious level most of the time and through the conscious state of well-being.

It is unfortunate that the conscious state of well-being is very poorly developed in modern society as compared to other conscious states like those of pleasure or excitement. Indubitably, with the passage of time, our current food habits, for instance, will appear preposterous. For the present, however, it is sufficient to realize that the lack of care of the conscious state of well-being places the mechanisms of the visceral nervous system and consequently also the body organs at risk. This willful neglect of the conscious state of well-being is the basic cause of many disorders of modern times.

The visceral nervous system consists of afferent or sensory neurons, interneurons or intercalary neurons, and motor neurons.

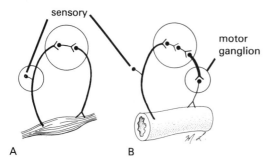

Fig. 10-1. (A) Somatic and (B) visceral loops.

Visceral Versus Somatic Nervous System

Knowing that the somatic nervous system is made up of the same three types of neurons as the visceral nervous system, it is convenient to compare the two of them.

The sensory component of the visceral nervous system is similar to that of the somatic sensory system, i.e., the sensory visceral afferent neuron cell body is found also in the spinal or cranial ganglia, and the axon proceeds from the periphery toward the central nervous system (CNS) through sensory posterior roots.

The interneuronal component of the visceral nervous system characteristically establishes mainly multisynaptic paths within the CNS.

The motor component of the visceral nervous system is strikingly different from the somatic motor output. Three principal differences (Fig. 10-1) are listed below.

The efferent visceral neuron cell bodies form specific nuclei in the CNS. The axons get out of the CNS but do not innervate muscles or organs. Instead they synapse into

a visceral motor neuron, whose cell bodies, found in the human body outside the

CNS, are grouped in clusters forming motor ganglia. The axons of these ganglion cell bodies reach the target organ (visceral smooth muscle, gland, etc.).

The third difference is one of terminology. All the visceral efferent and visceral motor neurons are described in the literature under the term **autonomic nervous system.**

One can easily deduct with what has been said that the autonomic nervous system is made up of a two neuron path. The first efferent neuron is called a **preganglionic neuron** or **first autonomic neuron.** Its axon is small and myelinated. The **preganglionic fiber** extends from its cell body in the CNS toward a ganglion outside the CNS, forming part of the peripheral nervous system (PNS).

The ganglion contains neurons that send their axons toward the effector organs. These neurons are called **visceral motor neurons, second autonomic neurons,** or (although it is a misnomer) **postganglionic neurons.** Their **postganglionic fibers** are unmyelinated and very small in diameter.

The ganglion also contains neurons that interact between preganglionic endings and postganglionic neurons. These **intrinsic ganglionic cells** are rich in dopamine (Fig. 10-2).

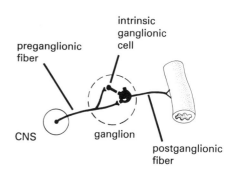

Fig. 10-2. Visceral ganglion.

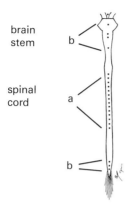

brain
stem

b

spinal
cord

a

b

Fig. 10-3. (Ortho)sympathetic (a) and parasympathetic (b).

spinal segments the cells are grouped together forming an intermediolateral and
an intermediomedial cell nucleus. All the
intermediolateral sympathetic nuclei, from
segment T1 through L2–3, form the **intermediolateral sympathetic cell column,**
or **thoracolumbar sympathetic column.** It
is convenient to be aware that the sympathetic preganglionic fibers are topographically confined to the thoracic and upper
lumbar segments of the spinal cord,
known as the **thoracolumbar division** of
the autonomic nervous system.

Motor Sympathetic Neurons

In difference to the limited number of
preganglionic cells and sympathetic nuclei
(which are 14 or 15 from T1 to L2–3) the
number of motor cells and sympathetic
ganglia is large. The sympathetic ganglia
are classified into two groups: **paravertebral ganglia** (also known by other names,
e.g., **sympathetic chain, sympathetic
trunk, vertebral ganglia**) and **abdominal
ganglia** (also known as **prevertebral ganglia**).

Paravertebral Ganglia

The paravertebral ganglia are found at
the sides of and close to the vertebrae. All
the paravertebral ganglia of one side are
joined together as a series of links forming
the sympathetic chain or trunk. There are
two such trunks, one on each side of the
vertebral column, extending from the cervical to the sacral region. The number of
ganglia in the sympathetic chain or trunk
(Fig. 10-4) is

cervical region—3
thoracic region—12
lumbar region—4 or 5
pelvic region—4 or 5
coccygeal region—1 (odd) ganglion common to the 2 sympathetic trunks

Division of the Visceral Efferent or Autonomic Nervous System

Two very distinct components of the autonomic nervous system (Fig. 10-3) can be
recognized: the **sympathetic** (or **ortho-
sympathetic**) **nervous system;** and the
parasympathetic nervous system.

Both of these are made up of a two neuron path, but the position, function, and
name of their neurons are different.

Sympathetic Nervous System

Preganglionic Sympathetic Neurons

Preganglionic sympathetic cells are
found in the 12 thoracic segments and the
first 2 or 3 lumbar segments of the spinal
cord. More specifically, in each of these

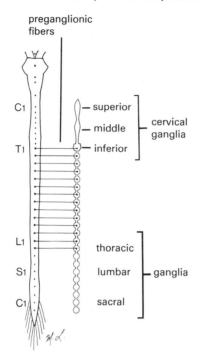

Fig. 10-4. Sympathetic chain.

The three cervical ganglia are called the **superior, middle,** and **inferior cervical ganglia.** The inferior cervical ganglion is sometimes fused with the first thoracic ganglion in a star shape. They are together called the **stellate ganglion.**

Input to the Sympathetic Trunk—White Rami

The preganglionic fibers from T1 to L2–3 travel with the corresponding ventral root. They then continue with the cor-

responding spinal nerve, leave it and reach the sympathetic trunk, where they synapse in motor neurons (Fig. 10-5). The path formed by these fibers between the spinal nerve and the sympathetic trunk is called the **white ramus communicans** on account of the whitish color of its fibers (myelinated fibers).

Output of Sympathetic Trunk—Gray Rami

Some of the postganglionic (nonmyelinated) fibers course out from the ganglion and re-enter a spinal nerve to reach and innervate an organ. The path between the ganglion and the spinal nerve is called a **gray ramus communicans** (Fig. 10-5).

Spread of Preganglionic Fibers Along the Sympathetic Trunk

The preganglionic fibers from T1–5 reach the ganglia of the upper portion of the sympathetic trunk (Fig. 10-6).

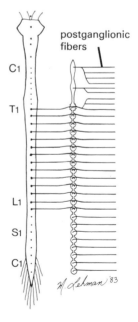

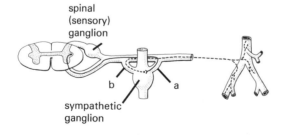

Fig. 10-5. White (a) and gray (b) rami communicantes.

Fig. 10-6. Postganglionic fibers.

The preganglionic fibers from T10 to L2–3 reach the ganglia of the lower portion of the sympathetic trunk.

This organization accounts for the existence of 14 to 15 white rami and 31 gray rami that reach the 31 spinal nerves.

Abdominal Sympathetic Ganglia

The **sympathetic abdominal ganglia** contain motor neurons and are found in the abdomen. They are also called **prevertebral ganglia,** as they are positioned in front of the vertebrae or, more precisely, at the base of the main arterial branches of the abdominal aorta (Fig. 10-7): the celiac artery with the **left** and the **right celiac ganglion;** the superior mesenteric artery with the **superior mesenteric ganglion;** the inferior mesenteric artery with the **in-**ferior **mesenteric ganglion;** the left and right renal arteries with the **left** and the **right renal ganglion;** and the left and right spermatic (or ovarian) arteries with the **left** and the **right spermatic** or **ovarian ganglion.**

The postganglionic fibers of the motor cells composing the ganglia egress in all directions, forming well-developed plexuses, which spread along the corresponding vessels. There are as many plexuses as the arteries mentioned above, and, in addition, the following can be mentioned:

The **aortic plexus,** along the abdominal aorta, continues further below as the **hypogastric plexus** along the hypogastric artery in the midline. The hypogastric plexus splits still further below into left and right extensions, reaches the pelvic region, and contributes to the formation of the **left** and **right pelvic plexuses,** positioned on the sides of the bladder and the rectum.

Another extension of the aortic plexus is the **iliac plexus** along the right and left iliac arteries.

All the aforementioned plexuses are reinforced not only with postganglionic sympathetic fibers coming from the sympathetic trunk ganglia of T5 down to the coccygeal ganglia but also with preganglionic fibers on their way to the abdominal ganglia.

Preganglionic Input to the Abdominal Ganglia

A number of preganglionic fibers from the spinal cord segments T5–6 to L2–3 travel without interruption toward the abdominal ganglia, where they make the synaptic contact. These long fibers form the **splanchnic nerves.**

Splanchnic Nerves

In the past, the term "splanchnic" (Gr. *splanchnikos* pertaining to the viscera) in its broadest sense has been used to name

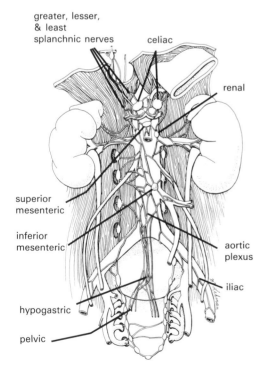

greater, lesser, & least splanchnic nerves

celiac

renal

superior mesenteric

inferior mesenteric

aortic plexus

iliac

hypogastric

pelvic

Fig. 10-7. Abdominal ganglia and plexuses.

many nerves innervating the viscera. However, the proper meaning is restricted to the nerves carrying preganglionic sympathetic fibers passing through sympathetic trunk ganglia without synapse and terminating in abdominal ganglia. The splanchnic nerves are the **greater, lesser,** and **least thoracic splanchnic nerves** and the **lumbar splanchnic nerves** (Fig. 10-8).

The greater splanchnic nerve originates from spinal cord segments T5–6 to T9–10; the lesser splanchnic nerve from spinal cord segments T9–10 to T11; the least splanchnic nerve from spinal cord segment T12; and the lumbar splanchnic nerve from spinal cord segments L1 to L2–3.

The greater, lesser, and least splanchnic nerves descend in the posterior wall of the thorax, passing through the diaphragm and reaching the abdominal ganglia. The greater splanchnic nerve ends mostly in celiac and superior mesenteric ganglia. The lesser splanchnic nerve ends primarily in superior mesenteric and renal ganglia. The least splanchnic nerve ends mostly in the renal and inferior mesenteric ganglia. The lumbar splanchnic nerves spread

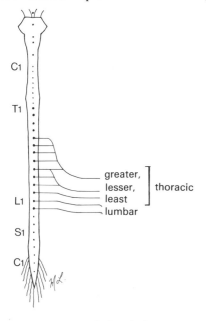

Fig. 10-8. Splanchnic nerves.

through the plexuses of the abdominal and pelvic regions, where there are many minute scattered sympathetic ganglia.

Parasympathetic Nervous System

Cranial Preganglionic Neurons

There are five **parasympathetic nuclei** in the brain stem tegmental region (Fig. 10-9): the **Edinger-Westphal nucleus,** the **lacrimal nucleus,** the **superior salivatory nucleus,** the **inferior salivatory nucleus,** and the **dorsal nucleus of vagus.**

The **Edinger-Westphal nucleus** is located in the midbrain tegmentum. The preganglionic fibers travel with the cranial nerve III (the oculomotor nerve), until they are close to a parasympathetic ganglion, the **ciliary ganglion.** They then leave the cranial nerve III and enter the ciliary ganglion, synapsing in what are known as motor parasympathetic cells.

The **lacrimal nucleus** is situated in the tegmentum of the pons. The preganglionic fibers travel with the cranial nerve VII (the facial nerve). They follow a tortuous route of nerve branches until they end synapsing in the **sphenopalatine ganglion,** also known as the **pterygopalatine ganglion.**

The **superior salivatory nucleus** is located in the tegmentum of the pons. The preganglionic fibers travel with the cranial nerve VII (the facial nerve). They course through a laborious path of nerve branches and finally synapse in the **submandibular** (also known as the **submaxillary) ganglion.**

The **inferior salivatory nucleus** is located in the tegmentum of the pons. The preganglionic fibers travel with cranial nerve IX (the glossopharyngeal nerve) along a twisting roadwork of nerve

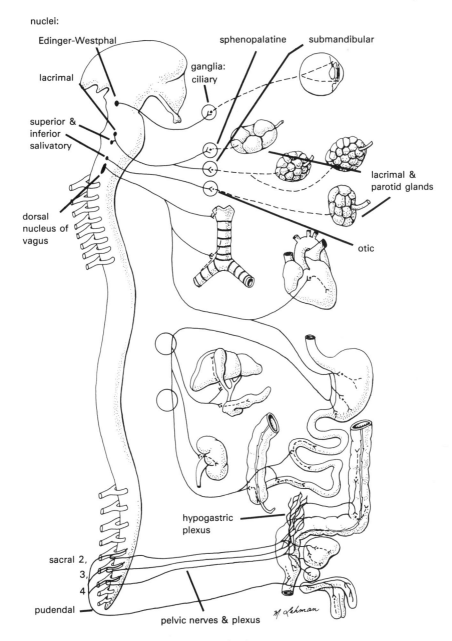

nuclei:

Edinger-Westphal

lacrimal

superior &
inferior
salivatory

dorsal
nucleus of
vagus

sphenopalatine   submandibular

ganglia:
ciliary

lacrimal &
parotid glands

otic

hypogastric
plexus

sacral 2,
3,
4

pudendal

pelvic nerves & plexus

M. Lehman

Fig. 10-9. Parasympathetic nervous system.

branches, ending in the **otic ganglion,**
where they synapse.

The **dorsal nucleus** is situated in the
tegmentum of the medulla oblongata. The
abundant preganglionic fibers contribute
to the formation of the cranial nerve X

(the vagus nerve), which they leave at the
neck, thorax, and abdomen, ending in
parasympathetic ganglia that are attached
to the viscera of these three regions.

There are many small ganglia innervating each organ. These parasympathetic

ganglia are named after the viscera to which they are related and attached, e.g., **cardiac, pulmonary, gastric, parasympathetic ganglia.**

The preganglionic parasympathetic fibers of the vagus spread in the thorax and abdomen, contributing to the formation of many of the plexuses described in previous sections. Hence these plexuses have preganglionic and postganglionic sympathetic fibers and parasympathetic, mainly preganglionic, fibers.

Sacral Preganglionic Neurons

The sacral preganglionic parasympathetic cell bodies are found in clusters forming the intermediate parasympathetic nuclei of segment S2 to S4–5. Their fibers, the preganglionic parasympathetic fibers, travel with the corresponding anterior roots, the spinal nerves and, for a short section, the pudendal nerve as the **pudendal parasympathetic plexus.** They then continue with the pelvic nerves, also known as the pelvic splanchnic nerves or nervi erigentes, subsequently coming into contact with the pelvic plexus and ending in the parasympathetic ganglia attached to the viscera of the pelvic region. Some of the fibers continue ascending uninterrupted through the hypogastric plexus and the inferior mesenteric plexus, reaching the parasympathetic ganglia attached to the descending and sigmoid colon.

Motor Parasympathetic Neurons

The **motor parasympathetic neurons** are within or very close to the organ they innervate. They receive input from the preganglionic cells and form the above-mentioned ganglia, i.e., the **ciliary,** the **sphenopalatine,** the **submandibular,** and the **otic ganglia** in addition to all the specific ganglia for the viscera of the neck, thorax, abdomen, and pelvis.

To complete the study of the autonomic innervation of the visceral body, specifics related to the innervation of each organ follow.

Specific Structures Innervated by the Autonomic Nervous System

Ciliary Muscle

The **ciliary muscle** (Fig. 10-10) has two components: the **radial division,** innervated by the sympathetic postganglionic fibers, and the **circular division,** innervated by the parasympathetic postganglionic fibers.

The ciliary muscle is part of the ciliary body of the eye. The ciliary body is ring-shaped around the lens, which is attached to it by the **suspensory ligament.** When the ciliary body expands, due to contraction of the radial muscle fibers, the suspensory ligament becomes tense and makes the lens less convex, (thinner in its antero-posterior diameter), which is useful in distance vision.

When the ciliary body contracts, due to contraction of the circular muscle fibers,

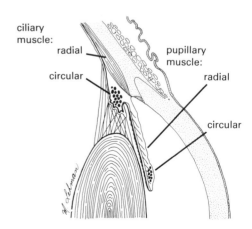

Fig. 10-10. Ciliary and pupillary muscles.

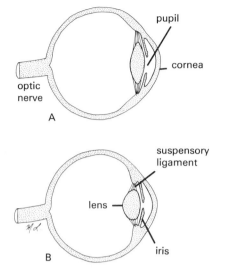

Fig. 10-11. (A) Narrowed lens; (B) thickened lens.

the suspensory ligament relaxes and makes the lens more convex (thicker in its anteroposterior diameter), which is useful in close vision.

Stimulation of the parasympathetic fibers thickens the lens, while stimulation of the sympathetic fibers thins it (Fig. 10-11).

Pupillary Muscle

The **pupillary muscle** is part of the iris, which is ring-shaped in front of the lens.

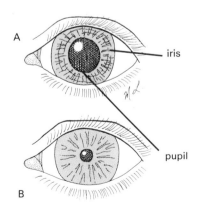

Fig. 10-12. (A) Pupil dilated (mydriasis); and (B) constricted (miosis).

This muscle has two components (Fig. 10-10): (1) the circular **sphincter pupillae,** which is innervated by the parasympathetic fibers and, in action, narrows the pupil **(miosis);** and (2) the radial **dilator pupillae,** which is innervated by the sympathetic fibers and, in action, dilates the pupil **(mydriasis)** (Fig. 10-12).

Parasympathetic Innervation

The parasympathetic pathway for the ciliary and pupillary sphincters consists of

1. preganglionic cells of the Edinger-Westphal nucleus;
2. preganglionic fibers within the cranial nerve III;
3. the ciliary ganglion; and
4. postganglionic fibers forming short ciliary nerves to the sphincters of the ciliary body and the pupillae.

Sympathetic Innervation

The sympathetic pathway for the ciliary and pupillary dilator is composed of

1. preganglionic cells of spinal cord segments T1 and T2;
2. preganglionic fibers through the sympathetic trunk to the superior cervical ganglion; and
3. postganglionic fibers from the superior cervical ganglion traveling with the internal carotid artery and then through short and long ciliary nerves to the dilators of the ciliary body and the pupillae.

Tarsal Muscle

The eyelids have smooth muscle fibers, called **tarsal muscles,** which are innervated by sympathetic fibers. The tarsal muscle of the upper eyelid helps to lift it (Fig. 10-13).

Note: Some schools of thought regard the upper tarsal muscle as a muscle component of the levator palpebrae superioris.

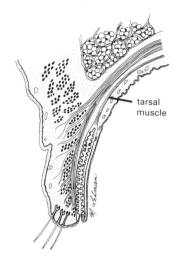

Fig. 10-13. Upper eyelid, tarsal muscle.

Glands of the Head

Parasympathetic Innervation

The **glands of the head** and their parasympathetic innervation are presented in Table 10-1 and Figure 10-14.

Sympathetic Innervation

The sympathetic innervation to the glands is from T1 and T2 spinal segments to the superior cervical ganglion and from there through the internal and external carotid artery plexuses to glands, which vasoconstrict, thus reducing the bulk of secretion.

Heart

Parasympathetic Innervation

The preganglionic cells of the dorsal nucleus of the vagus send their preganglionic fibers with the vagus nerve and then separate from the vagus as the superior and inferior cervical and thoracic cardiac branches of the vagus, reaching the cardiac plexus and heart, where they synapse in postganglionic neurons (Fig. 10-15). In this action, the heart rate is reduced and the coronary vessels vasoconstrict.

Bradycardia (Gr. *bradys* slow) means an abnormally slow and **tachycardia** an abnormally rapid heart rate.

Sympathetic Innervation

The schematic representation of the innervation of the **heart** is shown in Table 10-2.

It is noteworthy that the superior, middle, and inferior cervical ganglia are so far from the heart that their postganglionic fibers form the superior, middle, and inferior cervical sympathetic nerves respectively (Fig. 10-15). The input to the heart from the upper five thoracic ganglia form the thoracic sympathetic cardiac nerves.

Lungs

Parasympathetic Innervation

Preganglionic cells of the dorsal nucleus of the vagus travel with the vagus nerve,

Table 10-1. Parasympathetic Innervation of the Glands of the Head

Nucleus (preganglionic)	Nerve	Ganglion (motor)	Organ	Function
Lacrimal	VII	Sphenopalatine	Lacrimal gland and mucosal glands of nose and palate	Vasodilation and secretion of nasal mucus and tears
Superior salivatory	VII	Submandibular	Submandibular and sublingual salivary glands	Vasodilation and secretion of saliva
Inferior salivatory	IX	Otic	Parotid gland	Vasodilation and secretion of saliva

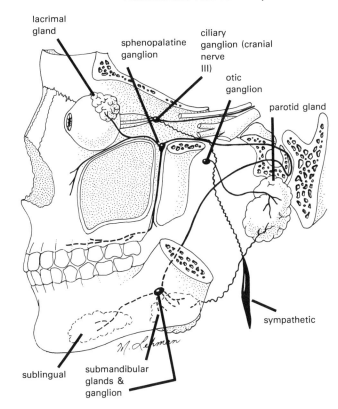

Fig. 10-14. Glands of the head.

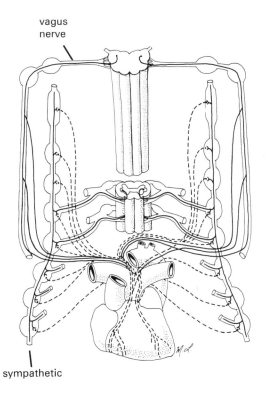

Fig. 10-15. Innervation of the heart.

Table 10-2. Sympathetic Innervation of the Heart

Nucleus (preganglionic)	Ganglion (postganglionic)	Innervation	Function
Spinal segments T1–5	Cervical ganglia and upper five thoracic ganglia	Heart and coronary vessels	Acceleration of rate of heart beat and vasodilation

separate later as pulmonary branches of the vagus, and reach the pulmonary plexus and pulmonary parasympathetic ganglia. Postganglionic fibers reach the trachea and bronchial tree to supply their smooth muscles, glands, and vessels. The parasympathetic innervation produces bronchoconstriction, vasodilation, and secretion.

Sympathetic Innervation

Preganglionic fibers from T2–5 synapse in the inferior cervical ganglion and the upper five thoracic ganglia. Postganglionic fibers reach the trachea and the bronchial tree to supply their respective smooth muscles, glands, and vessels. Their action produces bronchodilation, vasoconstriction, and inhibition of secretion.

Stomach and Intestine As Far As the Splenic Flexure

Parasympathetic Innervation

Vagal preganglionic fibers descend around the **esophagal plexus** and reach the stomach as anterior and posterior gastric cords. From this level on, the fibers spread to the stomach and intestine as far as the **splenic flexure** and the endings, which synapse with the postganglionic neurons located within the wall of the gastrointestinal tract.

The postganglionic neurons form part of two well-developed plexuses, namely, the **myenteric plexus of Auerbach** and the **submucosal plexus of Meissner.** Other neurons of these plexuses contain a variety of neurotransmitter substances. Parasympathetic activity produces vasodilation, glandular secretion, peristalsis, and relaxation of sphincters.

Sympathetic Innervation

Preganglionic fibers travel from spinal segments T6–11 and postganglionic fibers from thoracic trunk ganglia of T6–11, celiac and superior mesenteric ganglia around the vessels of the same name, and reach the stomach and intestine as far as the splenic flexure (flexure of the transverse colon with the descending colon). It produces vasoconstriction, contraction of sphincters, and inhibition of secretion and of peristalsis.

Other Abdominal Viscera

Parasympathetic Innervation

The **pancreas** and the **gall bladder** also receive parasympathetic innervation in a fashion similar to that described for the stomach. It produces secretion and relaxation of sphincters. The parasympathetic innervation of the **spleen, liver,** and **kidneys** is unclear and under debate.

Sympathetic Innervation

The **pancreas, gall bladder, spleen, liver,** and **kidneys** receive sympathetic innervation through their respective plexuses. Its effects are still being explored.

Distal Intestinal Tract (From Splenic Flexure Down) and Pelvic Viscera

Parasympathetic Innervation

Through the corresponding nerves and plexuses, preganglionic fibers from spinal cord segments S1 to S4–5 reach the walls of their target organs and relay in the postganglionic parasympathetic neurons. The functions of this innervation are vasodilation, peristalsis and contraction in the lower bowel, contraction of the detrusor muscle of the bladder, stimulation of glands, and penile erection.

Sympathetic Innervation

Preganglionic fibers from spinal cord segments L1 to L2–3 and their corresponding postganglionic fibers reach through the respective plexuses, the descending colon, the sigmoid colon, the rectum, the urinary bladder, the testes, the seminal vesicles, the prostate, the erectile tissue, the ovaries, the uterus and tubes, and blood vessels, thus supplying these organs. The known functions of this innervation are vasoconstriction, inhibition of peristalsis and of secretion in the lower bowel, contraction of muscle fibers of the vesical trigone, and ejaculation of semen.

Adrenal Gland

The core of the **adrenal gland,** or **adrenal medulla,** does not receive parasympathetic innervation.

The sympathetic innervation is handled directly by preganglionic sympathetic fibers originating in spinal cord segments T10 to L1 and reaching the gland through the adrenal plexus. The reason that there is no postganglionic sympathetic innervation is that the cells of the adrenal medulla, the postganglionic sympathetic fibers, have modified to become a hormonal secretory gland. The adrenal medulla cells release **norepinephrine** into the blood stream, affecting the whole body.

Skin Blood Vessels, Erector Pili Muscles, and Sweat Glands

Skin blood vessels, erector pili muscles, and **sweat glands** have no parasympathetic innervation.

Sympathetic Innervation

Preganglionic fibers from T1 to L2–3 and postganglionic fibers from the sympathetic trunk participate in the innervation of the skin blood vessels. This innervation produces vasoconstriction, stimulates secretion of the sweat glands, and causes contraction of the smooth muscles attached to the hair follicles, namely, the **erector pili muscles,** (causing "goose pimples") (Table 10-3).

Blood Vessels to Skeletal Muscles

Blood vessels irrigating the skeletal muscles do not receive parasympathetic innervation. The sympathetic innervation

Table 10-3. Sympathetic Innervation of Skin Blood Vessels, Erector Pili Muscles, and Sweat Glands

Structure	Preganglionic	Postganglionic
Skin of head and neck	T2–5	Superior and middle cervical ganglia
Upper extremity	T3–6	Inferior cervical ganglion and upper thoracic ganglia of sympathetic trunk
Lower extremity	T10–L2–3	Lower lumbar and upper sacral ganglia of sympathetic trunk

follows a pattern similar to that of the skin, while its effect, however, is opposite—it produces vasodilation.

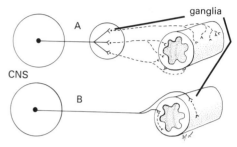

Fig. 10-16. (A) Sympathetic and (B) parasympathetic systems.

Transmitter Substances in Autonomic Nervous System

Synapses

The **neurotransmitter substance** for each type of synapse has been identified, i.e.:

acetylcholine—in synapses between preganglionic and postganglionic neurons, whether sympathetic or parasympathetic;

acetylcholine—in synapses between parasympathetic postganglionic neuron and effector organ; and

norepinephrine (noradrenaline)—in synapses between sympathetic postganglionic neuron and effector organ with two exceptions: the sweat glands (acetylcholine), and the smooth muscles of the vessels to skeletal muscles (acetylcholine).

The preganglionic fibers innervating the adrenal medulla liberate acetylcholine, while the cells of the adrenal medulla release norepinephrine (noradrenaline).

Fibers secreting acetylcholine are called **cholinergic** and those secreting norepinephrine are called **adrenergic fibers.**

Table 10-4. Comparisons Between Sympathetic and Parasympathetic Systems

Basis of Comparison	Sympathetic	Parasympathetic
(1) Position of preganglionic cells	Thoracolumbar	Craniosacral
(2) Types of ganglia	As described	As described
(3) Position of ganglia	Far from organ	In or close to organ
(4) Length of postganglionic fibers	Long	Short
(5) Ratio of preganglionic terminal to postganglionic neurons	1 : 30	1 : 2
(6) Ratio of postganglionic terminal to effector cells	One—many	One—very few
(7) Postganglionic transmitter	Norepinephrine, slowly inactivated	Acetylcholine, rapidly inactivated
(8) Effects	As described	As described

Note: Apart from the differences in specific functions, one can note, based on (5), (6), and (7), that sympathetic functions are spread out and last while parasympathetic functions are localized and of short duration.

Differences Between Sympathetic and Parasympathetic Systems

Important differences between sympathetic and parasympathetic systems (Fig. 10-16) are listed in Table 10-4.

Review of Sympathetic Functions Triggered by Danger from the Outside

1. pale skin—vasoconstriction of skin
2. wet skin—secretion of sweat glands
3. raised hair—constriction of piloerector muscles
4. dilated pupils, mydriasis—dilatation of pupillae muscles
5. raised upper eyelid—constriction of tarsal muscle
6. redistribution of blood from skin and viscera to the brain, the heart muscle, and skeletal muscles—vasodilation of skeletal muscle vessels
7. increased heart rate—activation of heart muscle
8. increased blood pressure—increase in peripheral resistance of arterioles
9. dilated bronchi—dilatation of bronchial smooth muscles
10. diminished intestinal activity and closed sphincters—constriction of intestinal smooth muscles and glands
11. raised blood sugar level—adrenal medulla release of adrenalin, acting on liver; glucogen conversion into glucose
12. dry mouth—constriction of salivary glands.

Suggested Readings

Appenzeller D: The Autonomic Nervous System. An Introduction to Basic and Clinical Concepts. Third Edition. Elsevier BioMedical Press, Amsterdam, 1982.

Brooks CMcC, Koizumi K, Sato A, Eds.: Integrative Actions of the Autonomic Nervous System, Chapter 24, Elsevier/North-Holland, Amsterdam, 1979.

Carpenter MB: Human Neuroanatomy. Seventh Edition. Williams and Wilkins, Baltimore, pp. 191–212, 1976.

Coggeshall RE, Galbraith SL: Categories of axons in mammalian rami communicantes, Part 2, J Comp Neurol 181:349–360, 1978.

Gabella G: Structure of the Autonomic Nervous System, Chapman and Hall, London, 1976.

Gershon MD: The enteric nervous system, Ann Rev Neurosci 4:227–272, 1981.

Johnson RH, Spalding DMK: Disorders of the Autonomic Nervous System, Blackwell, Oxford, 1974.

Pick J: The Autonomic Nervous System: Morphological, Comparative, Clinical and Surgical Aspects, JB Lippincott, Philadelphia, 1970.

Sato A, Ed.: Central organization of the autonomic nervous system, Brain Res 87:137–437, 1975.

11

The Peripheral Nervous System and Related Structures

Clinical Examination of the Body

With a few simple tools and procedures experienced clinicians are able to explore the state of a patient's body and obtain a considerable amount of information.

Two test tubes with warm and cold water, respectively, can help in determining **temperature sensation.** The abnormal sensibility is described as **thermoanesthesia** (absent), **thermohypesthesia** (diminished), and **thermohyperesthesia** (exaggerated) (Fig. 11-1A).

A needle can be employed to explore regional **pain perception.** The abnormal sensibility is described as **analgesia** (absent), **hypalgesia** (diminished), and **hyperalgesia** (exaggerated) (Fig. 11-1B).

Motion and position sense can be tested by flexing and extending one of the patient's fingers and asking her/him to state the initiation and direction of the move-

ment as well as the new position (Fig. 11-1C).

A wisp of cotton or a feather can be used to explore regional **tactile sensibility.** Abnormal sensibility is labeled as **tactile anesthesia** (absent), **tactile hypesthesia** (diminished), and **tactile hyperesthesia** (exaggerated) (Fig. 11-1D).

A compass can be used to explore regional **two-point discrimination** (Fig. 11-1E).

A reflex hammer assists in assessing **stretch reflexes.** The abnormal reaction is described as **arreflexia, hyporeflexia,** and **hyperreflexia** and quantified by gradient numbers (Fig. 11-1F).

A tuning fork can be used to explore **vibratory sense (pallesthesia)** (Fig. 11-1G).

Muscle tone may be investigated by moving the joints with the patient's passive cooperation. Muscle tone is, for clinical purposes, the muscle resistance to passive movement. Abnormal muscle tone is described as **hypotonia** (diminished), **normotonia** (normal), and **hypertonia** (exaggerated) (see Fig. 11-6).

Muscle strength can be tested by evaluating the patient's ability to move a joint while the examiner actively resists (see Fig. 11-9).

By observing surface areas one may detect a great variety of signs regarding the state of the skin, possible muscle waste (atrophy), abnormal locomotion or posture, etc.

These exploratory procedures, which are very revealing to the skillful, experienced clinician, take time and practice to master. This holds especially true for the somatic sensory examination. Practice in developing full support from the patient is

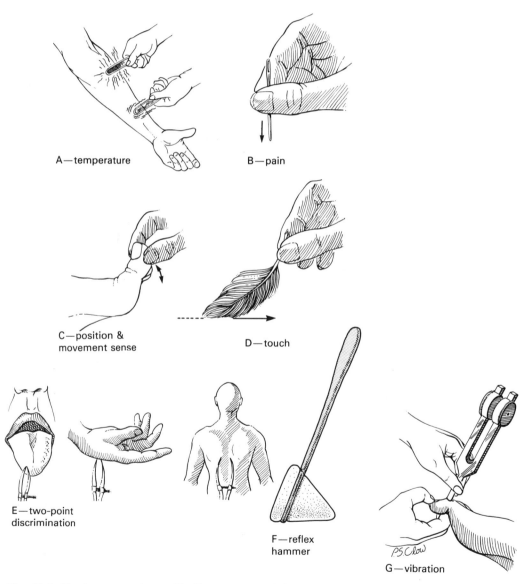

Fig. 11-1. Testing procedures. (A) Temperature; (B) pain; (C) position and movement sense; (D) touch; (E) two-point discrimination; (F) reflex hammer; (G) vibration.

essential for such exploratory procedures to be a reliable part of the clinical investigation.

The basis for establishing a systematic procedure and evaluation of findings require accurate and extensive knowledge of the peripheral nervous system (PNS) and its connections with the central nervous system (CNS).

The student must be aware that a group of neurological signs may be common to a number of diseases that can be differentiated only by a precise record of their history, i.e., their mode of development.

The clinical history is by far the most important element in interpreting dysfunction of the nervous system. It is through a historical perspective, as in any other field of knowledge, that the true value of clinical signs and symptoms can be comprehended. Past and present circumstantial events, as well as patterns and sequence of appearance of signs, are invaluable factors in the making of a correct diagnosis.

Motor Neuron and Motor Unit

An α motor neuron and the muscle fibers it innervates (from one to several hundred) together are defined as a **motor unit.** The motor unit is called small if the α motor neuron innervates only a few muscle fibers and large if it innervates many. Muscles involved in delicate, precise movements, like hand and eye muscles, have small motor units; muscles involved in vigorous movements, like proximal limb muscles, have large motor units. The muscle fibers of a motor unit are most frequently scattered over a given part of the muscle.

Destruction of a spinal motor neuron or its axon produces hypotonia, paralysis, and initiation of degeneration of the muscle fibers innervated. Two weeks after losing their innervation, muscle fibers may contract, twitching spontaneously. They become hypersensitive to direct mechanical, chemical, or electrical stimuli (**denervation hypersensitivity**). Such spontaneous, regular twitching of single muscle fibers is called **fibrillation.**

Irritability

A **fasciculation** is a spontaneous contraction of a motor unit, due to a state of **irritability** of the unit. Irritability in sensory fibers is perceived as **paresthesia,** i.e., spontaneous abnormal sensation, experienced as tingling or crawling when large fibers are involved, and as burning or prickling when the fibers are small.

Neurons or fibers can become irritated by a number of mechanisms, e.g., certain types of mechanical compression.

Spinal Motor Output

When sufficient excitation arrives to the spinal motor neurons, they discharge. Spinal motor neurons handle approximately 100,000 synaptic contacts, some excitatory, some inhibitory, coming from many regions of the CNS, directly or indirectly.

Reflexes

In the very particular case of the excitatory stimulus coming from sensory fibers of a segment to motor neurons of the same segment and making them discharge, a **segmental reflex** response ensues in the corresponding motor organ. This reflex may be **monosynaptic,** if there is no interneuron in the circuit, or **polysynaptic,** if one or more interneurons are involved in the circuit.

Other adjectives can be used to indicate the specific morphological characteristics of a reflex circuit, e.g., **unilateral** (on one side), **bilateral** (on both sides), **ipsilateral** (on one and the same side).

In a **contralateral** (also called **heterolateral** or **crossed**) **reflex** the sensory or input component comes from one side of the body and the motor or output component belongs to the opposite side; the reflex path crosses the midline.

Polysegmental (intersegmental) reflex circuits involve many segmental reflexes.

Stretch Reflex

In general terms, the stretch reflex is the opposing reaction of a muscle to forces that attempt to lengthen it. A muscle positioned with a certain length endeavors to maintain this length and resists any imposed lengthening by increasing its tone.

Four basic elements are involved in the stretch reflex: intrafusal muscle fibers, primary afferent fibers (Ia), α motor neurons, and extrafusal muscle fibers.

The response of extrafusal muscle fibers initiated by afferent discharges due to the stretching of the intrafusal muscle fibers is a stretch reflex (Fig. 11-2). It is, in essence, a feedback mechanism.

When a muscle is stretched, the extrafusal and intrafusal muscle fibers become stretched; the primary afferents (Ia fibers) discharge and stimulate the α motor neuron in such a manner that an increment of tone of the extrafusal muscle fibers **(tonic stretch reflex)** is produced. If the intrafusal muscle fibers are stretched abruptly, on the other hand, the massive afferent discharges, through type IIa, stimulate the α motor neurons so that a strong contraction of the extrafusal muscle fibers results.

The testing of stretch reflexes with a percussion hammer is routine practice in clinical examinations. The hammer strikes a tendon which, in a normal response, abruptly stretches its muscle, triggering

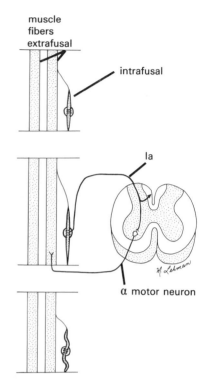

Fig. 11-2. Stretch reflex.

the stretch reflex. Clinicians call this a test for the **deep tendon reflex.** The appropriate term from a physiological point of view is **myotatic stretch reflex.**

The stretch reflex is essentially a monosynaptic, ipsilateral, monosegmental, **myotatic reflex.**

γ Loop

The intrinsic tone of the muscle is indirectly due to the relative tension of the intrafusal muscle fibers which actively maintains the circuit: primary afferents—α motor neurons—extrafusal muscle fiber tone. When for instance in a voluntary muscle contraction the extrafusal muscle fibers contract, the intrafusal muscle fibers would slacken, and the feedback activity contributing to the stimulation of the α fibers would be lost, if it were not for the γ loop phenomenon.

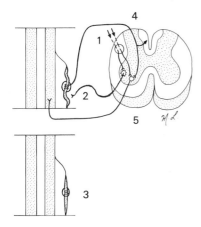

Fig. 11-3. γ loop.

The γ efferents innervate the intrafusal muscle fibers to shorten their length if required to actively maintain the stretch reflex and the tone of the muscle. This regulatory activity of the γ efferents is a necessity for the harmonious sequential contraction of a muscle. The circuit of this loop (Fig. 11-3) is

1. stimulation arrives to the γ neuron;
2. the γ neuron fires;
3. the intrafusal fiber contracts (tension); as a partial consequence of this action, it may be followed by:
4. activation of Ia;
5. activation of α motor neuron; and
6. extrafusal muscle contraction (not represented in the figure).

The γ motor neurons are stimulated and inhibited from many sources in concert with the α motor neurons, and their synchronization is fundamental for the execution of harmonious movement. Movement can be initiated through proper activation of the γ or the α loop.

Golgi Tendon Organs

Golgi tendon organs are tension detectors. Their activity reinforces the activity of the stretch reflex circuit if the muscle is not overly contracted, or reduces it if the muscle is too much contracted. The

change of function is handled by interneurons in the spinal cord segment. In the latter case (Fig. 11-4), the Ib afferents of the Golgi tendon organ send inhibitory impulses to the interneurons, which, effecting a dual function, inhibit its muscle activity and facilitate the action of the antagonist.

The reciprocal innervation operated by these interneurons is very efficient and economical. They switch the activity of α and γ neurons to flexor and extensor muscles as needed.

The myotatic, γ, and Golgi tendon reflexes are fundamental in motor function.

Double Reciprocal Innervation

Groups III and IV afferents operate on interneurons.

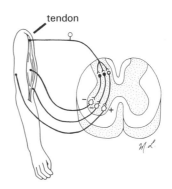

Fig. 11-4. Golgi tendon loop.

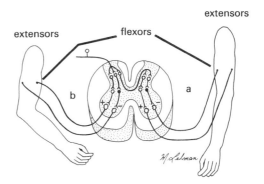

Fig. 11-5. Double reciprocal innervation.

If the interneuronal switch for reciprocal innervation operates ipsilaterally in one direction, e.g., excitation of extensor muscles and inhibition of flexor muscles in one side (a in Fig. 11-5), it operates on the opposite side (b in Fig. 11-5) in the opposite way as inhibition of extensors and excitation of flexors (**double reciprocal innervation**).

Muscle Tone

Muscle tone is directly dependent on the activity of the α motor neurons. In turn, the α motor neuron activity depends on three types of activity:

1. the intrinsic proprioceptive muscle activity, like the loop γ motor neuron, muscle spindle afferents to α motor neuron, or Golgi tendon organ to α motor neuron;
2. sensory (cutaneous, joints, etc.) reflex input to α motor neuron; and
3. CNS influences on α motor neuron.

When describing lower motor neuron lesions, it was emphasized that reduction in muscle tone (hypotonia or flaccidity) ensues because the motor neurons or their reflex loop become disrupted.

Furthermore, cerebellar lesions may also develop hypotonia, due to the fact that proprioceptive cerebellar signals, looping in the cerebellum through the CNS to stimulate α and γ motor neurons, are disrupted.

In lesions of the cerebral motor system, being as varied as they are, one may find resulting hypotonia, normotonia, or hypertonia. As a general rule, it is safe to say that what occurs most frequently is hypertonus of the muscles related to the lesioned region of the cerebral motor system.

Examination of Muscle Tone

Muscle tone is evaluated by the examiner in two different ways which give the same or different "readings": by palpation at rest (which normally reveals a certain tension in the muscle), and by passive movement of joints.

The examiner must keep in mind that the resistance offered by a muscle in response to being pulled may be due either to inherent physical viscoelastic properties of the body tissue or to tension set up by myotatic reflexes in the muscles stretched.

When evaluating normotonic, hypertonic, or hypotonic muscles, it must be done with special consideration to synergic muscles, agonists and antagonists. One may find that a group of agonist muscles (e.g. flexors) displays the same, a higher, or a lower level of tone as compared to its antagonists (in this case, the extensors). In brief terms, the examiner must distinguish between a stable tone, balanced between flexors and extensors; and an unstable tone, not balanced between flexors and extensors.

Three Clinical Signs

Clasp-Knife Phenomenon

When trying to move a patient's joint briskly (with passive participation), the examiner may find an abnormally increased resistance (hypertonus), which suddenly disappears if the examiner sustains his pulling action. This type of muscle reaction is called a **clasp-knife phenomenon** (Fig. 11-6).

Lead Pipe Phenomenon

The **lead pipe phenomenon** constitutes a different response to the examination procedure described above. In this reaction the hypertonus remains when the pulling is sustained.

Cogwheel Phenomenon

A variation of this reaction is the **cogwheel phenomenon** with persistent hyper-

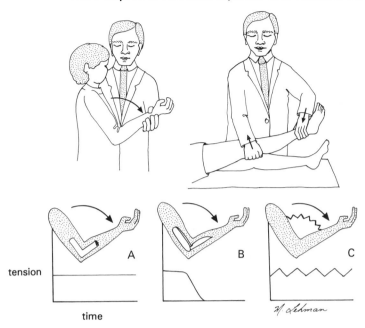

Fig. 11-6. (A) Lead pipe; (B) clasp-knife; (C) cogwheel.

tonus and superimposed rhythmic contractions.

Spasticity and Rigidity

The terms **spasticity** and **rigidity** have been used rather haphazardly and before the underlying mechanisms were understood. To discern the meanings of these two terms in the literature one must be aware of several facts:

1. Essentially, both terms relate to muscle hypertonus, either inherent or triggered.
2. The basic meaning of the term rigidity is stiffness.
3. The stiffness of all the clinical states identified as rigidity may be due either to exaggerated tone of one group of muscles, either flexors or extensors, or to exaggerated tone of both groups at the same time. Unfortunately, no pro-

viso for this difference was made when the term rigidity was coined.

4. Generally, the lead pipe phenomenon and the cogwheel phenomenon may appear when hypertonus (or its substrate) prevails in both muscle groups.
5. Generally, the clasp-knife phenomenon may appear when hypertonus (or its substrate) prevails in one muscle group.
6. The basic meaning of the term spasticity is spasm, a sudden muscle reactive hyperreflexia. This sudden muscle reaction may be one of muscle contraction (clinical spasm) or one of muscle hypertonus (clinical spasticity).
7. The clasp-knife phenomenon is an effect seen as part of spasticity.
8. Based on previous statements (1 to 7), one can understand the apparent terminological paradox of a patient's suffering some types of rigid states and displaying a clasp-knife phenomenon indicative of spasticity. The two terms are not antithetical but different.

Status of the Myotatic Reflexes

Figure 11-7 illustrates methods of testing myotatic reflexes.

Lower motor neuron circuit lesions result in hyporeflexia or arreflexia, which are detected as signs in the response to the percussion of tendons. Also, hyporeflexia and pendular reflexes may result from cerebellar lesions. In cerebral motor system lesions, as a general rule, the reaction most frequently elicited by percussion of tendons is hyperreflexia.

Clonus

In some normal individuals with ongoing raised physiological activity of myotatic reflexes one may find that if a suddenly applied and sustained stretch is imposed to a muscle, it may respond with a few repetitive contractions. This is called a **physiological clonus.**

In hyperreflexive states due to cerebral

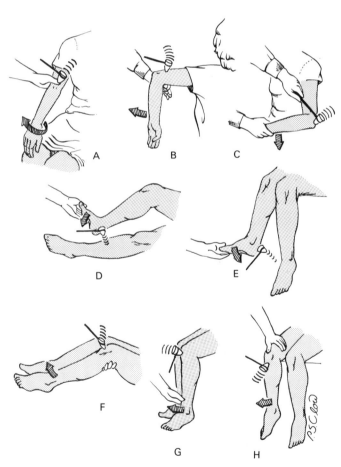

Fig. 11-7. Tests of myotatic reflexes. (A) Biceps; (B) and (C) triceps; (D) and (E) Achilles; (F), (G), and (H) patelar.

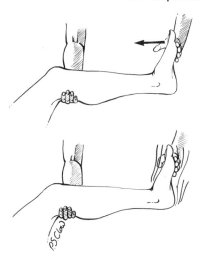

Fig. 11-8. Clonus.

motor system lesions, the clonus may become clearly pronounced, lasting longer (Fig. 11-8).

Tremor

Tremor is a series of involuntary alternating rhythmic contractions of antagonist muscles, producing a trembling or oscillating movement.

The examiner may detect tremor of minimal amplitude with a frequency of 10 cycles per second (c.p.s.) in normal subjects, or higher amplitude in normal subjects affected by routine excesses of normal life, like tension and substantial intake of caffeine, tobacco, alcohol, etc.

The phenomenon of tremor requires the intrinsic neuromuscular loop to be structurally intact. Tremor is due to an exaggerated actvity of the α and γ motor neuron loop.

In cerebellar lesions a tremor of wide oscillations, called **intention tremor,** may appear when the patient tries to perform voluntary movements. This disorder is due to the fact that the proprioceptive information transmitted through the cerebellum and traveling from there toward the CNS is altered, causing the appropriate automatic adjustment (fine-tuning) of muscle movement, regulated by the cerebellum, to become faulty.

In some cases of cerebral motor system lesions, resulting tremor may be due to disordered input signals over the α and γ neurons.

Muscle Strength

The contraction force of a muscle is called **muscle strength.** Terms like "strong muscle," "weak muscle," "normal muscle

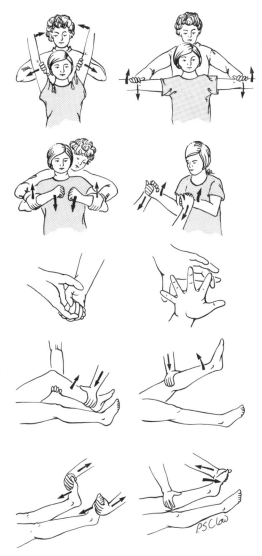

Fig. 11-9. Tests of muscle strength.

strength," refer only to the capability level of muscle contraction. The examiner must be aware that in testing muscle strength (Fig. 11-9), the initial length of the muscle influences the capability of the muscle in displaying its strength. This length-strength relation in muscle contraction follows the rule: The shorter the muscle, the less contraction force can be executed. Nevertheless, when the examiner measures the strength of a muscle, he finds that, due to biomechanical principles like leverage, supporting action of other muscles, blocking of inhibitory proprioceptive feedback mechanisms, etc., the shorter the muscle, the more difficult it becomes for the examiner to stretch it. This fact has practical implications during exploratory procedures, e.g., when it comes to maintaining the same position while comparing strength of left and right muscles.

Muscle Power

The capability of the muscle to execute movements is called **muscle power.** In some texts the term is used synonymously to strength when considering only the contraction phenomenon. It is convenient to distinguish muscle strength (contraction) from muscle power, which specifically refers to the dual capacity of contraction and

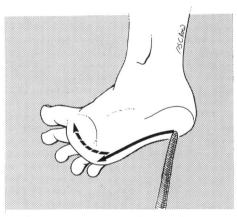

Fig. 11-10. Babinski's sign.

relaxation in the execution of movements.

Palsy is most generally used as meaning loss of power of the muscular system. **Paresis** means reduction of muscle power.

Superficial Reflexes

Muscle responses of a reflex nature elicited by stimulation of surface receptors in skin and mucous membranes are called **superficial reflexes.**

Superficial Plantar Reflex

By stroking a blunt object along the lateral border of the sole of the foot with sufficient pressure to excite nociceptive receptors, muscle contractions are elicited.

The muscles of primary concern to the examiner are the flexor and extensor muscles of the big toe.

In newborn babies this stimulus produces an **extensor plantar response,** i.e., **dorsiflexion of the big toe,** which expresses itself in a defensive withdrawal reaction to the noxious stimulus, executed by the spinal motor segments L4–5 to S1–2.

As the child develops, upper motor neurons modify this reflex circuit to secure stability of the feet during walking, so that minor noxious stimuli, instead of triggering withdrawal, work to improve stability of the feet. In young and adult persons the same stimulus triggers a **flexor plantar response (plantar flexion) of the big toe.** This reflex reaction, imprinted in the upper motor neurons, is lost when they are affected and the original defensive dorsiflexion, the extensor plantar response of the big toe, is released. This abnormality is also known as **Babinski's sign** (Fig. 11-10).

Superficial Abdominal Reflexes

By stroking the quadrants of the abdominal wall in a young or mature person with

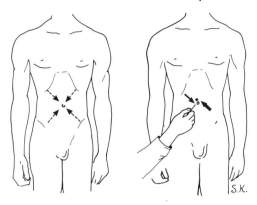

Fig. 11-11. Superficial abdominal reflex.

lower roots are longer than the upper ones.

Spinal Ganglia

Composed by the cell bodies of sensory root fibers, **spinal ganglia** are found in the intervertebral foramina. Within these regions the sensory ganglia and the motor root are cuffed together by the **spinal cord meninges.**

Nerve Trunks and Branches

The sensory and motor fibers, extensions of the roots, exit through the intervertebral foramen. They then become intermingled with and enveloped by the extensions of the spinal meninges, the so-called **perineurium** and **epineurium.** Such mixed bundles of fibers with their coverings are called **spinal nerves** or **spinal nerve trunks** and contain visceral sensory and preganglionic fibers as well as somatic sensory and motor fibers. They are short, only coursing a small distance from the intervertebral foramen and then giving off, in general, **spinal nerve branches.** Each such branch is named after the particular region it innervates, as evident in those described below (Fig. 11-12).

The **meningeal branch** (sensory and vasomotor) courses to the dura mater and blood vessels of the vertebral canal through the intervertebral foramen. It is also known as the **recurrent branch,** as it re-enters the vertebral canal.

The **posterior branch** or **ramus** (motor and sensory) is also known as the **dorsal branch, posterior,** or **dorsal primary division.** It innervates the back of the trunk.

The **anterior branch** or **ramus** (Fig. 11-12) (motor and sensory) is also called the

an object (e.g., a pin), the umbilicus twitches toward the quadrant stimulated (Fig. 11-11). In infants, a massive reaction may be obtained, which affects the whole abdominal wall and leaves the umbilicus centered.

The selective modification of the reaction is due to a more defined segmental organization of the developed nervous system, in which the upper motor neurons exert increasing and selectively segmental influence on the spinal cord reaction. In some cerebral motor system lesions this incremental and selective influence may be lost, and the reaction may fail to be triggered in response to stimulation. This loss, however, is not always permanent but may reverse itself in the course of time.

The cerebral motor system monitors the activity of the lower motor neuron loops through excitation and inhibition.

Spinal Roots

The 31 pairs of **sensory** and **motor spinal roots** situated on each side of the spinal cord and connected to each corresponding segment by **rootlets** are found in most of its length within the vertebral canal. The

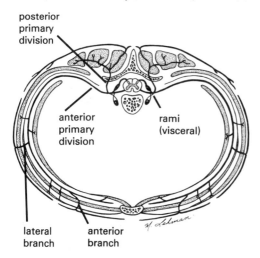

Fig. 11-12. Spinal nerve branches.

ventral branch, anterior, or **ventral primary division** and is the largest of the branches. It innervates the anterior region of the trunk and the extremities.

The **communicating branches** (visceral) are also known as **gray** and **white communicating branches** or **gray** and **white rami** of the visceral nervous system. It must be remembered that there are gray rami in all the spinal nerves but white rami only in spinal nerves at the levels of T1 to L2–3 and S2–4.

Nerve Supply of the Cranial Dura Mater

The rich nerve supply of the cranial dura mater originates principally from cranial nerve V as well as from twigs of the vagus nerve and twigs of the first three cervical spinal nerves entering the posterior cranial fossa through the hypoglossal canal.

Fibers of the ophthalmic nerve innervate mainly the dural lining of the anterior cranial fossa, the vault, falx cerebri, and tentorium cerebelli.

Fibers of the maxillary nerve course with the anterior branch of the middle meningeal artery.

Fibers of the mandibular nerve course through the foramen spinosum with the middle meningeal artery.

Fibers of the vagus nerve do not enter the jugular foramen but innervate the dural lining of the posterior cranial fossa.

Development of Nerve Plexuses

With regard to the development of nerve plexuses from the anterior branch of the spinal nerves, two facts should be stressed: (1) most of the peripheral nerves of the body are branches of the anterior branch of the spinal nerves; and (2) many of them, especially the nerves innervating the extremities, consist of fibers that belong to several segmental roots.

To understand this second fact one must recognize that in the simple segmental organization **(metamerism)** of the embryo, the segmental **mesoderm (somites)** engenders the segmented **myotomes** which receive the corresponding segmental (metameric) spinal innervation.

However, as development progresses, the somites of the extremity, especially the myotomes, re-organize themselves in such a manner that the muscles they originate create a compound, **polymer,** of two or more myotomes. The muscles are then said to be polymerous, i.e., they originate from two or more myotomes. The muscles also carry a polymerous innervation, i.e., each muscle is innervated by nerve fibers coming from two or more spinal cord segments. Such a re-arrangement of the myotomes with their nerve fibers is clearly seen in the formation of nerve plexuses, especially the brachial, lumbar, and sacral plexuses. During development the anterior branches of the "segmental" spinal nerves exchange fibers in their course to

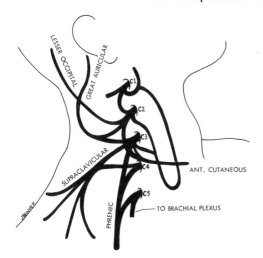

Fig. 11-13. Cervical plexus.

cated in the neck region. This plexus originates a number of peripheral nerve branches to innervate mainly the neck region.

Brachial Plexus

The **brachial plexus** (Fig. 11-14) is made of anterior branches of C5–8 and T1 and may receive contributions from C4 and T2. It is situated in the lower neck region. Attempts have been made to classify all the lesions of the brachial plexus encountered in clinical practice. There is a wide variety of such cases, and in sorting out the situation two practical findings are helpful:

If a lesion of the brachial plexus is present, the deficiencies detected in the periphery are a product of the individual roots and nerves affected.

An upper brachial plexus lesion (C5–6) affects the shoulder muscles and the lateral region of the arm and forearm.

A lower brachial plexus lesion (C8 to T1) affects the hand muscles and the sensation of the medial region of the arm and forearm.

the periphery; the nerve fibers hence maintain their relation to their migrating muscle fibers. Once the plexus is organized, the epineurial connective tissue wraps all the branches of the spinal nerves.

Cervical Plexus

The **cervical plexus** (Fig. 11-13) is made of anterior branches of C1–4 and is lo-

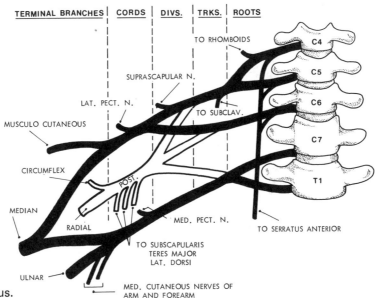

Fig. 11-14. Brachial plexus.

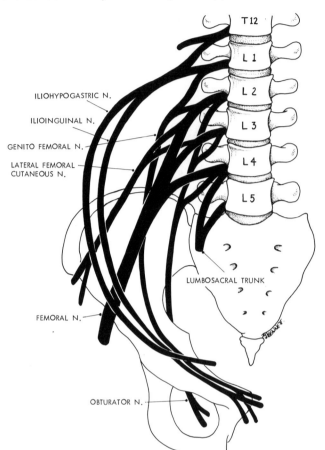

Fig. 11-15. Lumbar plexus.

ILIOHYPOGASTRIC N.

ILIOINGUINAL N.

GENITO FEMORAL N.

LATERAL FEMORAL CUTANEOUS N.

LUMBOSACRAL TRUNK

FEMORAL N.

OBTURATOR N.

T 12
L 1
L 2
L 3
L 4
L 5

Once a lesion of the brachial plexus has been clinically diagnosed, the specialist makes a detailed diagnosis based on the anatomic details of the plexus.

The brachial plexus originates a number of peripheral nerve branches.

Lumbar Plexus

The **lumbar plexus** (Fig. 11-15) is made of anterior branches of L1–4 and sometimes receives fibers from T12. It is located anterior to the transverse processes of the lumbar vertebrae. Due to its deep location, lesions of this plexus occur infrequently. More common are lesions affecting the roots or the nerves related to the plexus.

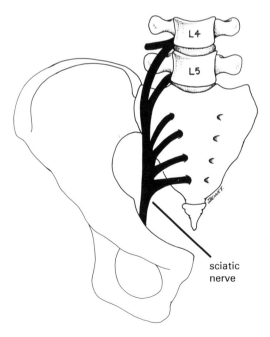

L4
L5

sciatic nerve

Fig. 11-16. Sacral plexus.

The lumbar plexus originates a number of peripheral nerve branches.

Sacral Plexus

With regard to the **sacral plexus** (Fig. 11-16) there are two different views recorded in the literature. One view holds that it consists of anterior branches of L4 to S3, which implies that the pudendal nerve is not included in the sacral plexus. The other view manifests that the sacral plexus is made of anterior branches of L4 to S4 and that the pudendal nerve hence is included.

The sacral plexus is located in the pelvis

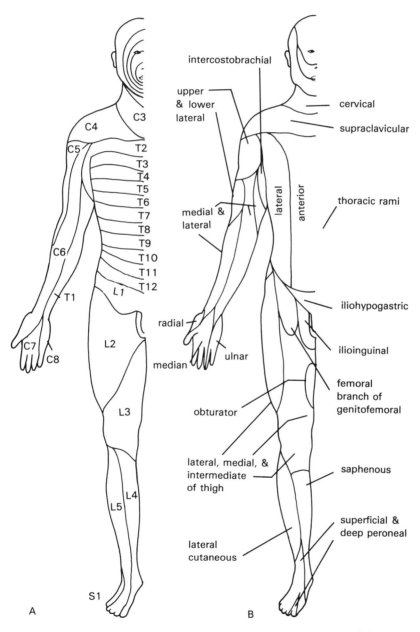

Fig. 11-17. Maps of the body, anterior view. (A) Segmental, radicular map; (B) peripheral nerve map.

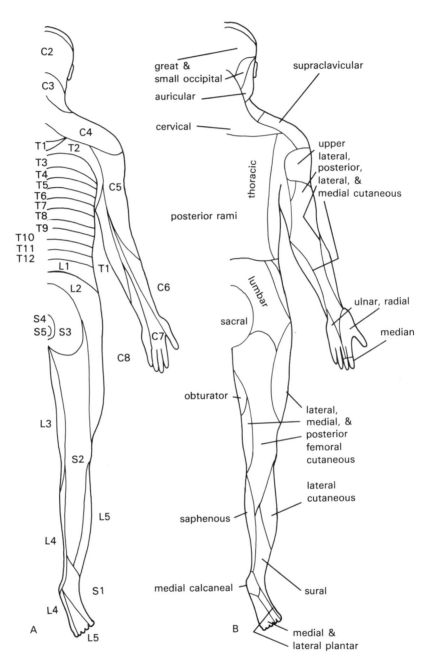

Fig. 11-18. Maps of the body, posterior view. (A) Segmental, radicular map; (B) peripheral nerve map.

minor (the lower region of the pelvis), anterolateral to the edge of the sacrum.

From the sacral plexus originates a number of peripheral nerve branches.

Anatomical Maps in Clinical Diagnosis

The functional loss of peripheral nerve fibers connected to the spinal cord can be mapped in two ways, giving different illustrations of the body and extremities. Thus an analysis can be based on lesions at the spinal root or segment, i.e., **radicular, segmental mapping;** or lesions at the level of the branches of the plexuses, i.e., **peripheral nerve mapping.**

Depending on whether the neurological deficiencies observed in a patient fit the radicular or peripheral nerve map, the lesions will be assumed to be present at the root level or peripheral nerve level, respectively (Figs. 11-17 and 11-18). Needless to say, the precise anatomic localization of a lesion is an important objective of neurologic diagnosis.

Procedure Followed for Localization of a Lesion

In order to localize a lesion the clinician proceeds first to find out where the normal motor and sensory functions are altered or lost. If such deficiencies are found, they are then contrasted with the radicular (segmental) and peripheral nerve maps of the body. Table 11-1 is based on the muscle action to be tested, which in turn is correlated with the muscle, muscle nerve, and spinal cord segments.

Another way of analyzing the segmental innervation of limbs is in terms of joint movement as accounted for in Table 11-2. Figures 11-17 and 11-18 illustrate the maps of cutaneous innervation according to the radicular versus peripheral nerve maps.

The information recorded in these tables and figures is necessary for the localization of peripheral nerve lesions.

Comments Concerning the Evaluation of Results

Sensory

In the literature different authors have reported different dermatomal maps. The discrepancies may be attributed to the procedure followed in determining the dermatomes, e.g., whether an analysis is based on remaining sensibility following root lesions, or on hypalgesia (diminished sensitivity to pain) from compression of single nerve roots. There is overlapping of innervation of contiguous dermatomes, and hence the loss of sensation due to damage to a single dorsal root may be experienced quantitatively by the patient. However, because it is compensated for by the nerve fibers of the contiguous roots, it is not a sensory loss which is qualitatively testable (objective) by ordinary clinical methods.

If two contiguous dermatomes lose their sensory function, the dermatomal sensory loss can be detected by the clinician in the lower half of the upper dermatome lesioned and the upper half of the lower dermatome lesioned (Fig. 11-19).

The region deprived of sensory innervation on account of a peripheral nerve lesion is smaller than the region innervated by the lesioned nerve, since there is some overlapping of neighboring peripheral

(*Text continues on p. 204.*)

Table 11-1. Muscle Innervation and Function

Nerve Muscle	Function	Cervical 5	6	7	8	Thor. 1
Axillary		███	███			
Deltoid	Abducts, flexes, extends, and rotates arm	•	•			
Teres minor	Adducts and rotates humerus laterally	•	•			
Musculocutaneous		███	███	███		
Biceps brachii	Flexes and supinates forearm	•	•			
Brachialis	Flexes forearm	•	•			
Coracobrachialis	Flexes and adducts arm					
Anterior thoracic		███	███	███	███	███
Pectoralis major	Adducts, flexes, and medially rotates arm	•	•	•	•	•
Pectoralis minor	Depresses scapula; pulls shoulder forward	•	•	•	•	•
Long thoracic		███	███	███		
Serratus anterior	Abducts and rotates scapula	•	•	•		
Subscapular		███	███	███	███	
Latissimus dorsi	Adducts, extends, and medially rotates humerus	•	•	•	•	
Teres major	Adducts, extends, and medially rotates humerus	•	•	•		
Subscapularis	Rotates humerus medially	•	•	•		
Supracapular		███	███			
Supraspinatus	Abducts humerus	•	•			
Infraspinatus	Rotates humerus laterally	•	•			
Radial		███	███	███	███	███
Brachioradialis	Flexes forearm	•	•			
Supinator	Supinates hand	•	•	•		
Triceps brachii	Extends forearm		•	•	•	
Extensor carpi radialis	Extends wrist; abducts hand		•	•	•	
Extensor digiti minimi	Extends little finger		•	•	•	
Extensor carpi ulnaris	Extends wrist; adducts hand		•	•	•	
Extensor indicis	Extends proximal phalanx of index finger		•	•	•	
Extensor pollicis L & B	Extend thumb		•	•	•	
Ulnar				███	███	███
Flexor carpi ulnaris	Flexes wrist; adducts hand			•	•	•
Flexor digitorum profundus[d]	Flexes distal phalanges			•	•	•
Flexor digiti minimi	Flexes little finger			•	•	•
Opponens difiti minimi	Adducts, flexes, and rotates fifth metacarpal			•	•	•
Abductor pollicis L & B	Abduct thumb				•	•
Interossei dorsales	Abduct fingers and flex proximal phalanges				•	•
Interossei palmares	Adduct fingers and flex first phalanx				•	•
Flexor pollices brevis—						
Deep head	Flexes and adducts thumb				•	•
3rd & 4th lumbricals	Flex proximal phalanges				•	•
Abductor digiti minimi	Abducts first phalanx of little finger				•	•
Median			███	███	███	███
Pronator teres	Pronates and flexes forearm		•	•	•	•
Flexor carpi radialis	Flexes wrist; abducts hand		•	•	•	•
Abductor pollicis brevis	Abducts thumb		•	•	•	•
Opponens pollicis	Flexes and opposes thumb		•	•	•	•
Flexor pollicis brevis	Flexes first phalanx of thumb		•	•	•	•
Flexor digitorum superficialis	Flexes middle phalanges			•	•	•
*Flexor digitorum profundus	Flexes distal phalanges			•	•	•
Flexor pollicis longus	Flexes thumb			•	•	•
Palmaris longus	Flexes wrist			•	•	•
1st & 2nd lumbricals	Flex first phalanges				•	•

(Continued)

Table 11-1. Muscle Innervation and Function *(Continued)*

Nerve Muscle	Function	Lumbar 1	2	3	4	5	Sacral 1	2	3
Obturator			█	█	█				
Adductor L & B	Adduct, flex, and medially rotate thigh		•	•	•				
Adductor magnus[a]	Adducts, flexes, extends, and laterally rotates thigh		•	•	•				
Gracilis	Adducts thigh; flexes and medially rotates leg		•	•	•				
Femoral			█	█	█				
Iliacus	Flexes thigh and rotates it medially		•	•	•				
Quadriceps	Extends leg		•	•	•				
Sartorius	Flexes thigh and rotates it laterally; flexes leg		•	•	•				
Sciatic					█	█	█	█	
Adductor magnus[a]	Adducts, flexes, extends, and rotates thigh				•	•	•		
Internal hamstrings	Flex and medially rotate knee joint; extend hip joint				•	•	•	•	
Biceps femoris (extensor hamstring)	Flexes leg and extends thigh (rotates leg laterally when knee is flexed)				•	•	•	•	
Common peroneal									
Superficial peroneal					█	█	█	█	
Peroneus longus	Plantar flexes; everts foot					•	•	•	
Peroneus brevis	Plantar flexes; everts foot					•	•	•	
Deep peroneal					█	█	█		
Tibialis anterior	Dorsiflexes and inverts foot				•	•	•		
Extensor digitorum longus	Extends phalanges; dorsiflexes foot				•	•	•		
Extensor digitorum brevis	Extends toes				•	•	•		
Extensor hallucis longus	Extends great toe; aids dorsiflexion of foot				•	•	•		
Tibial					█	█	█	█	
Tibialis posterior	Plantar flexes and inverts foot					•	•		
Soleus	Plantar flexes foot					•	•		
Flexor digitorum longus	Flexes distal phalanges; aids in plantar flexion					•	•	•	
Flexor hallucis longus	Flexes great toe; aids in plantar flexion					•	•	•	
Gastrocnemius	Plantar flexes foot; flexes leg					•	•	•	
Flexor digitorum brevis	Flexes toes						•	•	
Flexor hallucis brevis	Flexes first phalanx of great toe						•	•	
Inferior gluteal						█	█	█	
Gluteus maximus	Extends, adbucts, and laterally rotates thigh; extends lower trunk					•	•	•	•
Superior gluteal					█	█	█		
Gluteus medius & minimus	Abduct and medially rotate thigh					•	•	•	
Tensor fasciae latae	Flexes thigh					•	•	•	

[a] Innervated by more than one nerve.

Table 11-2. Segments Involved in Joint Movements

Upper Body			Lower Body		
Shoulder	Abductors and lateral rotators	C5	Hip	Flexors, adductors, medial rotators	L1,2,3
	Adductors and medial rotators	C6,7,8			
Elbow	Flexors	C5,6		Extensors, abductors, lateral rotators	L5,S1
	Extensors	C7,8			
Foream	Supinators	C6	Knee	Extensors	L3,4
	Pronators	C7,8		Flexors	L5,S1
Wrist	Flexors and extensors	C6,7	Ankle	Dorsiflexors	L4,5
Digits	Long flexors and extensors	C7,8		Plantar flexors	S1,2
Hand	Intrinsic muscles	C8,T1	Foot	Invertors	L4,5
				Evertors	L5,S1

203

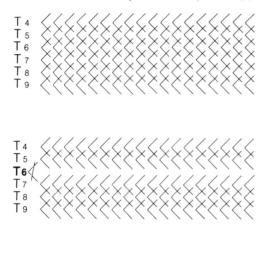

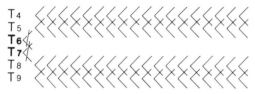

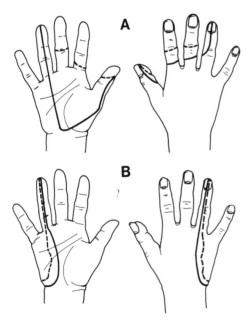

Fig. 11-19. Overlapping of dermatomal innervation.

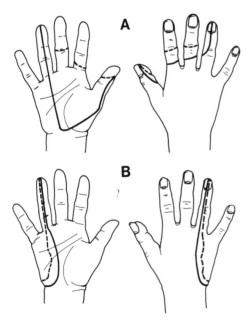

Fig. 11-20. (A) Area of sensory loss in lesion of median nerve; (B) area of sensory loss in lesion of ulnar nerve (touch: continuous line; pin prick: dotted line).

nerves. The region with lost perception of nociceptive signals is even smaller than the region with lost perception of tactile stimuli (Fig. 11-20).

Motor

Suppression of function of the nerve supplying a muscle means paralysis of the muscle. Suppression of function of one of the roots supplying a muscle means a varying degree of weakness of the muscle.

The nutrition (L. *nutrire* to nourish, to feed) of all the body tissues or organs is influenced and supported by their nerve supply. If a tissue or organ loses its nerve supply, i.e., in a case of **denervation,** the **trophic function** of the denervated tissue or organ is handicapped and **atrophy** (reduction in size), as well as other alterations, ensues. The nerves exert a trophic influence in the whole body, directly, physiochemically, by nutritional factors transmitted through the synapses, and indirectly by suppression of function as in muscle contraction, vascular contraction, etc. If a muscle is denervated, it will in time become atrophic.

Long Peripheral Nerves

It is important to keep in mind that an interruption of a nerve may occur at any level along its course and that the corresponding distal portion of the nerve expresses the effects of such a lesion. This fact makes it necessary to know the course of each major nerve and where it branches. The schematic representation in Figures 11-21 and 11-22 is given for this purpose.

There are certain regions in the course of the nerves that make them prone to injury, like the **ulnar nerve** at the posterior elbow region (the medial epicondyle); the **radial nerve** in the radial groove of the humerus; the **median nerve** at the anterior elbow region and carpal region, the **carpal tunnel;** and the **peroneal nerve** close to the head of the fibula.

(Text continues on p. 208.)

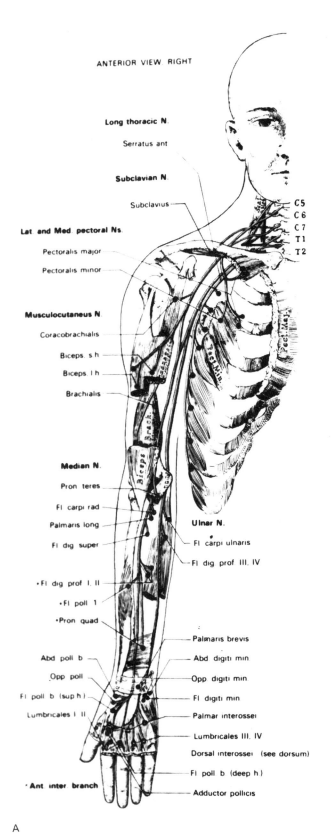

ANTERIOR VIEW RIGHT

Long thoracic N.

Serratus ant

Subclavian N.

Subclavius

C5
C6
C7
T1
T2

Lat. and Med. pectoral Ns.

Pectoralis major

Pectoralis minor

Musculocutaneus N.

Coracobrachialis

Biceps. s h

Biceps. l h

Brachialis

Median N.

Pron. teres

Fl. carpi rad

Palmaris long

Fl. dig. super

·Fl. dig. prof. I. II

·Fl. poll. l

·Pron. quad

Abd. poll. b

Opp. poll

Fl. poll. b (sup h.)

Lumbricales I. II

·Ant. inter. branch

Ulnar N.

Fl. carpi ulnaris

Fl. dig. prof. III. IV

Palmaris brevis

Abd. digiti min

Opp. digiti min

Fl. digiti min

Palmar interossei

Lumbricales III. IV

Dorsal interossei (see dorsum)

Fl. poll. b (deep h.)

Adductor pollicis

A

Fig. 11-21. Peripheral nerves and muscle innervation of upper limb. (A) Anterior view.

(Figure continues)

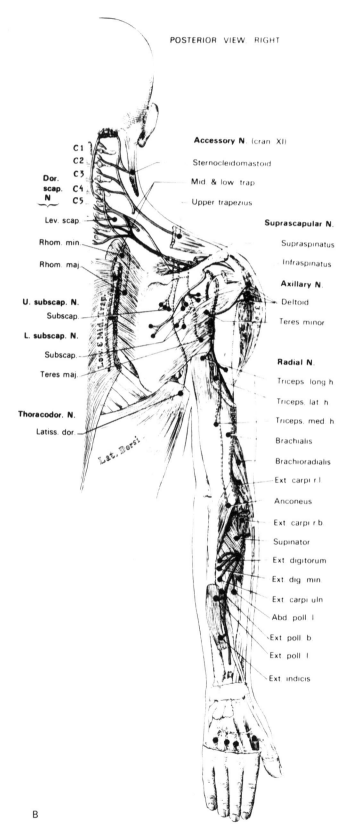

POSTERIOR VIEW, RIGHT

Accessory N. (cran XI)

Sternocleidomastoid

Mid. & low. trap.

Upper trapezius

C1
C2
C3
Dor. scap. N C4
C5

Lev. scap.

Rhom. min.

Rhom. maj.

Suprascapular N.

Supraspinatus

Infraspinatus

Axillary N.

Deltoid

Teres minor

U. subscap. N.

Subscap.

L. subscap. N.

Subscap.

Teres maj.

Low. & Mid. Trap.

Thoracodor. N.

Latiss. dor.

Lat. Dorsi

Radial N.

Triceps long h

Triceps lat h

Triceps med h

Brachialis

Brachioradialis

Ext carpi r l

Anconeus

Ext carpi r b

Supinator

Ext digitorum

Ext dig min

Ext carpi uln

Abd poll l

Ext poll b

Ext poll l

Ext indicis

B

Fig. 11-21 (Continued). (B) Posterior view. (Figs. A & B from Kendall FP, McCreary EK: Muscles—Testing and Function. Third Edition. © 1983 The Williams & Wilkins Co., Baltimore.)

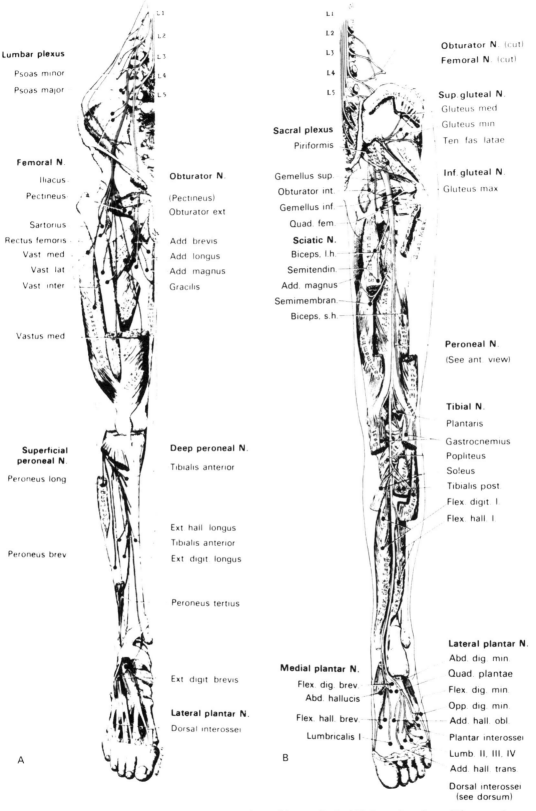

Fig. 11-22. Spinal nerves and motor innervation of lower limb. (A) Anterior view; (B) posterior view. (Figs. A & B from Kendall FP, McCreary EK: Muscles—Testing and Function. Third Edition. © 1983 The Williams & Wilkins Co., Baltimore.)

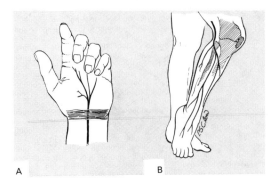

A   B

Fig. 11-23. (A) Compression of median nerve. (B) Lesion of peroneal nerve.

The **transverse carpal ligament (flexor retinaculum)** may compress the median nerve (Fig. 11-23) and produce the **carpal tunnel syndrome,** which starts with pain in the hand followed by muscle weakness of the innervated muscles with thenar atrophy and trophic changes of the last three fingertips. Surgical division of the transverse carpal ligament relieves the nerve compression.

The common peroneal nerve may become lesioned in fractures of the neck of the fibula or in badly applied plaster casts to the leg which compress the nerve (Fig. 11-23). It may induce paralysis of the plantar dorsiflexors with "foot drop" and sensory loss of the dorsum of the foot. To compensate for the foot drop the patient walks with a characteristic high-stepping gait.

Radial Nerve

The area of sensory distribution of the radial nerve is illustrated in Figures 11-17 and 11-18.

The deformity pattern in the hand as an expression of a radial nerve lesion is characterized by the wrist and fingers being flexed in a position described as a "wrist drop" and by adduction of the thumb (Fig. 11-24).

Median Nerve

The area of sensory distribution of the median nerve is illustrated in Figure 11-20.

The deformity pattern in the hand as a result of a total median nerve lesion is the thumb in a fixed position in the plane of the hand and thenar atrophy, resulting in what is termed as "ape hand" (Fig. 11-25). The thumb can adduct and abduct, but it cannot oppose.

Ulnar Nerve

The area of sensory distribution of the ulnar nerve is illustrated in Figure 11-21.

The deformity pattern in the hand as an expression of a total nerve lesion is hy-

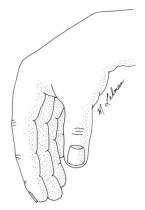

Fig. 11-24. Radial nerve lesion—wrist drop.

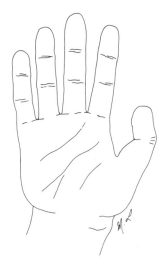

Fig. 11-25. Median nerve lesion—ape hand.

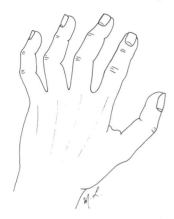

Fig. 11-26. Ulnar nerve lesion—claw hand.

perextension of the metacarpophalangeal joints of the ring and little fingers; semiflexed distal phalanx of the fingers; abduction of the little finger; and atrophy of the interosseus and hypothenar muscles, forcing the hand into the shape of a claw (claw-hand) (Fig. 11-26).

Sciatic Nerve

Injections of chemicals in the buttock may touch and damage the sciatic nerve. Diabetes mellitus, tumors, trauma, and collagen diseases may also affect this nerve.

Disc prolapse in the lower lumbar region is a cause of backache (lumbago) and radic-ular pain in the leg corresponding to the distribution of the sciatic nerve (sciatica). A valuable procedure for testing lumbosacral root lesions or meningeal irritation is the **straight leg raising test (SLR or Lasègue's maneuver).** The examiner lifts the patient's straightened leg slowly, thus flexing the hip. This procedure stretches the roots to the sciatic nerve. Dorsiflexion of the foot increases the tension of the already stretched roots (Fig. 11-27).

Nerve Diseases

To assist in the understanding of the great many different peripheral nerve diseases (neuropathies) encountered in clinical practice, the structural and functional alterations of nerves have been classified in a number of ways. Contributions to the knowledge on neuropathies come from several fields of clinical medicine, e.g., neuropathology, neurology, neurosurgery.

Neuropathies can be classified as **mononeuropathies** (affecting one nerve) or **polyneuropathies** (affecting several or many

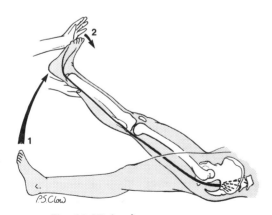

Fig. 11-27. Lasègue maneuver.

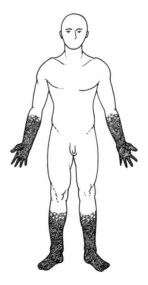

Fig. 11-28. Polyneuropathy.

nerves). In turn, polyneuropathies can be classified according to their etiology into infective, toxic, metabolic, genetic, traumatic, vascular, or others of unknown origin.

A common regional pattern of affliction in polyneuropathies is illustrated in Figure 11-28.

Based on their pathophysiology, the nerve lesions may be classified into diseases of the axons (axolemma, axoplasm) or the myelin sheath.

Some alterations of the nerve function may be due to blockade of the blood supply to the nerve due to compression. The functional alteration may be transitory and is familiarly known as a body part "going to sleep."

Neuromuscular Junctions

The neuromuscular junctions may suffer disorders of their own, like in **myastenia gravis,** a disease which is due to a postsynaptic defect of acetylcholine receptors and is characterized chiefly by weakness and fatigue of skeletal muscles.

Muscles

The muscles may also suffer particular disorders, e.g., muscular dystrophies, which are expressed as weakness of muscles. To distinguish between **neuropathies** and **myopathies** one can make use, although only as a general rule, of the fact that neuropathies in many instances affect the distal muscles initially and remain most severe in those areas. The chances of lesions of a nerve increase with the length of the nerve. A lesion at any level always affects the distal portion. Myopathies, on the other hand, typically affect the proximal muscles (girdle muscles) initially, and are proportional to the muscle power demanded. In neuropathies it is common to find cutaneous sensibility altered, which is rare in myopathies.

Suggested Readings

Barker D: The morphology of muscle receptors. In Hunt CC, Ed.: Handbook of Sensory Physiology, Vol. 3/2: Muscle Receptors, Springer-Verlag, Berlin, 1974.

Basmajian JV: Muscles Alive. Their Functions Revealed by Electromyography. Third Edition. Williams and Wilkins, Baltimore, 1974.

Brooke MH: A Clinician's View of Neuromuscular Diseases, Williams and Wilkins, Baltimore, 1977.

Carpenter MB: Human Neuroanatomy. Seventh Edition. Williams and Wilkins, Baltimore, pp. 159–190, 1976.

Coggeshall RE: Law of separation of function of the spinal roots, Physiol Rev 60:716–755, 1980.

Hagbarth K-E, Wallin G, Löfstedt L: Muscle spindle activity in man during voluntary fast alternating movements, J Neurol Neurosurg Psychiat 38:625–635, 1975.

Hubbard JI, Ed.: The Peripheral Nervous System, Plenum Press, New York, 1974.

Light AR, Perl ER: Reexamination of the dorsal root projection to the spinal dorsal horn including observations on the differential termination of coarse and fine fibers, J Comp Neurol 186:117–132, 1979.

Light AR, Perl ER: Spinal termination of functionally identified primary afferent neurons with slowly conducting myelinated fibers, J Comp Neurol 186:133–150, 1975.

Matthews PBC: Muscle afferents and kinaesthesia, Brit Med Bull 33:137–142, 1977.

Matthews PBC: Where does Sherrington's "muscular sense" originate? Ann Rev Neurosci 5:189–218, 1982.

Perl ER: Sensitization of nociceptors and its relation to sensation. In Bonico JJ, Albe-Fessard D, Eds.: Advances in Pain Research and Therapy, Vol. 1, Raven Press, New York, pp. 17–28, 1973.

Skoglund S: Joint receptors and kinaesthesis. In Iggo A, Ed.: Handbook of Sensory Physiology, Vol. 2: Somatosensory System, Springer-Verlag, Berlin, pp. 111–136, 1973.

Sunderland S: Nerves and Nerve Injuries. Second Edition. Churchill Livingstone, New York, 1978.

van Gijn J: The Babinski sign and the pyramidal syndrome, J Neurol Neurosurg Psychiat 41:865–873, 1978.

12

Spinal Cord

Intersegmental Reflexes of the Spinal Cord

It was mentioned in Chapter 5 that the fasciculus propriospinalis is a massive fasciculus adjacent to the gray matter along the spinal cord, interconnecting the cord segments.

The existence of many intersegmental reflex mechanisms as the basis of patterns of movement intrinsic to the spinal cord has been suspected but not yet defined. Fortunately, research data pertaining to this question are accumulating and a clearer picture is emerging with developmental patterns of locomotion as the primary source of information. Undoubtedly, increased knowledge will eventually translate into improved rehabilitation procedures.

A fact deservedly emphasized in textbooks when dealing with intersegmental cord reflexes is the "priority" of the cervical cord over lower regions in voluntary movement, due to its better developed circuitry and functions as well as to its stronger input from higher centers.

Spinal Cord–Brain Connections

Types of Connections

There are two distinct types of connective paths: **multisynaptic paths,** i.e., paths with multiple synaptic links, and **oligosynaptic paths,** i.e., paths with a few (two to four) synaptic links.

Multisynaptic Paths

Typical of the multisynaptic paths are the **spinoreticulothalamic paths.** Phylogenetically, they are older than oligosynaptic paths and travel bilaterally in the three funiculi, mostly mixed with the fasciculus propriospinalis, but also scattered in the anterior and lateral funiculi and within the gray matter close to the central canal. They are involved in the transmission of "primitive" information, e.g., noxious, alarm signals, from large receptive fields. They reach the brain stem reticular formation, which connects with the intralaminar and midline thalamic nuclei. They are generally called spinoreticulothalamic paths.

Oligosynaptic Paths

Important considerations regarding the oligosynaptic ascending paths from the spinal cord to the brain and vice versa are listed below.

1. Where do the paths originate, or, in other words, where are their cell bodies located?
2. Do the fibers cross to the other side before they ascend in the spinal cord?
3. In which funiculi do they course?
4. Where do they end?
5. What function do they have?

A summary of ascending and descending paths covering these five questions follows below.

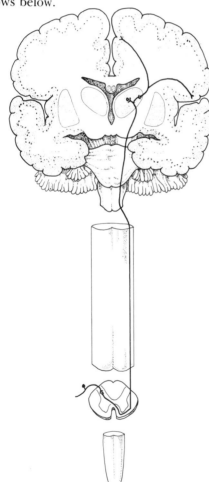

Fig. 12-1. Anterolateral spinothalamic tract.

Ascending Spinal Cord Tracts

Anterolateral Spinothalamic Tract (Fig. 12-1)

Origin—Dorsal horn and intermediate gray matter.
Crossing—Yes, in the anterior spinal commissure. Contralateral.
Spinal cord position—Anterior and lateral funiculi.
Brain stem position—Lateral fibers.
Ending—Thalamus; mainly in the posterior region of the intralaminar nuclei, but also in ventralis posterior.
Types of signals—Nondiscriminative tactile and noxious (pain and temperature).

Spinotectal Tract (Fig. 12-2)

Origin—Dorsal horn and intermediate gray matter.
Crossing—Yes, in the anterior spinal commissure. Contralateral.
Spinal cord position—Anterolateral funiculi.
Brain stem position—Together with the spinothalamic.

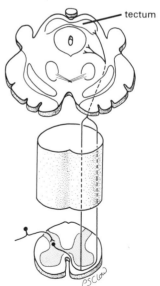

Fig. 12-2. Spinotectal tract.

Ending—Superior colliculus.
Types of signals—Unknown.

Spinoolivary Tract (Fig. 12-3)

Origin—Dorsal horn.
Crossing—Yes, in the anterior spinal commissure. Contralateral.
Spinal cord position—Anterolateral funiculi.
Ending—Inferior olivary nucleus.
Types of signals—Multiple modalities from the body.

Posterior Spinocerebellar Tract (Fig. 12-4)

Origin—Clarke's column.
Crossing—No. It is thus an ipsilateral tract.
Spinal cord position—Lateral funiculus (posterior region).
Medulla oblongata position—Lateral fibers.
Ending—Cerebellum (through the inferior cerebellar peduncle).
Types of signals—Exteroceptive and proprioceptive from ipsilateral lower limb and lower trunk.

Note: The dorsal spinocerebellar tract

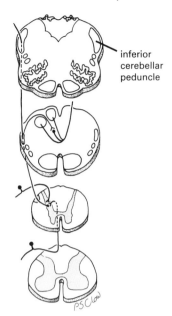

Fig. 12-4. Posterior spinocerebellar tract.

branches off into collaterals to nucleus Z, which is located anterior to the nucleus gracilis. The fibers of this nucleus travel with the medial lemniscus and carry the proprioceptive signals from the inferior limb to the thalamus (conscious path).

Anterior Spinocerebellar Tract (Fig. 12-5)

Origin—Intermediate gray matter from thoracic, lumbar, and sacral regions.
Crossing—Yes, most of the fibers in the anterior spinal commissure.
Spinal cord position—Lateral funiculus.
Brain stem position—See Figure 12-5.
Ending—Cerebellum. The tract reaches the cerebellum through the superior cerebellar peduncle, then crosses the midline within the cerebellum, ending in the opposite cerebellar hemisphere. Because of the double crossing of the fibers (in the spinal cord in one direction and in the cerebellum in the other), the signals coming from one limb end in the cerebellar half of the same side as the source of the signal in the limb.
Types of signals—Exteroceptive and pro-

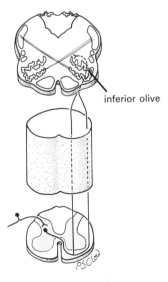

Fig. 12-3. Spinoolivary tract.

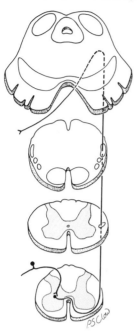

Fig. 12-5. Anterior spinocerebellar tract.

prioceptive from lower limb and lower trunk.

Rostral Spinocerebellar Tract (Fig. 12-6)

Origin—Intermediate gray matter of cervical segments C4–8.

Crossing—No. It is thus an ipsilateral tract.

Spinal cord position—Lateral funiculus.

Brain stem position—Some fibers travel with the posterior spinocerebellar tract and some with the anterior spinocerebellar tract.

Ending—Cerebellum through the inferior and superior cerebellar peduncles.

Types of signals—Exteroceptive and proprioceptive from the upper limb and the neck.

Cuneocerebellar Tract (Fig. 12-7)

Origin—Accessory cuneate nucleus. It receives collateral branches from the fasciculus cuneatus.

Crossing—No. Hence it is an ipsilateral tract.

Brain stem position—Medulla oblongata.

Ending—Cerebellum through the inferior cerebellar peduncle.

Types of signals—Exteroceptive and proprioceptive from the neck and the upper limb.

Spinocervicothalamic Tract (Fig. 12-8)

Origin—Nucleus proprius.

Crossing—No, at the spinal level. Ipsilat-

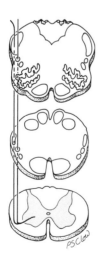

Fig. 12-6. Rostral spinocerebellar tract.

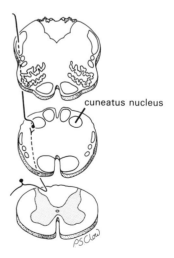

cuneatus nucleus

Fig. 12-7. Cuneocerebellar tract.

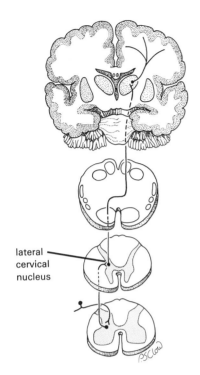

lateral
cervical
nucleus

Fig. 12-8. Spinocervicothalamic tract.

eral. Yes, at the level of the medulla ob-longata. Contralateral.

Spinal cord position—Lateral funiculus. The ascending tract relays in the **lateral cervical nucleus,** which is located in the lower medulla and the cervical segments C1–2, lateral to the tip of the dorsal horn. Cells of this nucleus project their fibers toward the opposite side.

Brain stem position—The tract ascends to-gether with the medial lemniscus fibers toward the thalamus.

Ending—Ventralis posterior nucleus of thalamus.

Types of signals—Discriminative extero-ceptive (tactile, pressure) from the body modulated by ongoing sensory activity of the upper cervical segments.

Fasciculus Gracilis (Fig. 12-9)

Origin—Dorsal root fibers from the coccy-geal segment up to T6 coming from the lower limb and lower trunk and entering the posterior funiculus.

Crossing—No. Hence this is an ipsilateral tract.

Spinal cord position—Ascends in the pos-terior funiculus.

Ending and types of signals—The fibers concerned with signals for discrimina-tive exteroceptive information ascend all the way up the posterior funiculus and relay in the nucleus gracilis.

Note: The fibers concerned with signals for conscious proprioception relay in the nucleus dorsalis (Clarke's column). The signals then travel from Clarke's column through the posterior spinocerebellar tract (in the lateral funiculus) and at the level of the medulla collaterals of this tract reach the nucleus Z in front of the nucleus gracilis.

Fasciculus Cuneatus (Fig. 12-9)

Origin—Dorsal root fibers from T6 up to C2 coming from the neck, upper limb, and upper trunk and entering the poste-rior funiculus.

Crossing—No. It is thus an ipsilateral tract.

Spinal cord position—Ascends in the pos-terior funiculus, lateral to the fasciculus gracilis.

Ending—Nucleus cuneatus.

Types of signals—Discriminative extero-ceptive information and conscious pro-prioception from the neck, upper limb, and upper trunk.

Note Regarding the Medial Lemniscus Components

The signal information collected and modified in the lateral cervical, gracilis, Z, and cuneatus nuclei is transmitted to the thalamus through their fibers, which cross to the opposite side (decussate) and form the medial lemniscus, carrying signals from the contralateral side of the body to-ward the ventralis posterior nucleus of the thalamus.

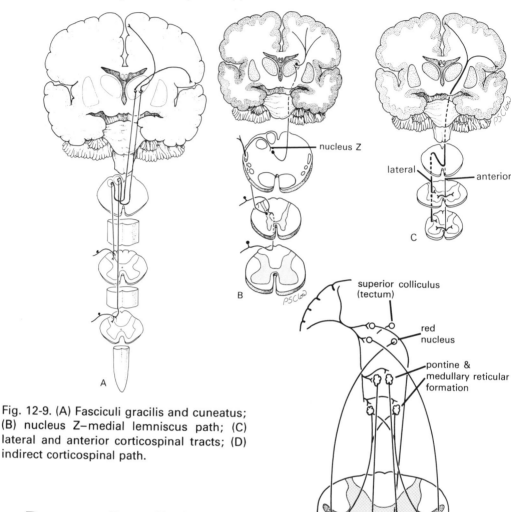

Fig. 12-9. (A) Fasciculi gracilis and cuneatus; (B) nucleus Z–medial lemniscus path; (C) lateral and anterior corticospinal tracts; (D) indirect corticospinal path.

Descending Spinal Cord Tracts

Direct Corticospinal Tracts: Lateral and Anterior Corticospinal Tracts (Fig. 12-9C)

Origin—Mostly from Brodmann's areas 1 to 4 and 6.

Crossing—Yes. Most of the fibers cross at the junction of the medulla–spinal cord, and are known as the pyramidal decussation. Most of the crossing fibers descend in the opposite lateral funiculus, forming the lateral corticospinal tract. A small amount of fibers do not decussate at the level of the pyramidal decussation but continue ipsilaterally downward in the anterior funiculus, forming the anterior corticospinal tract.

Course—Many of the fibers travel through the brain as indicated in Figure 12-9C and form part of different regions.

Ending—Most of the fibers of the corticospinal tracts end along the spinal cord in Rexed's laminae IV to VII, while some end in lamina IX. The lateral corticospinal tract is concerned mostly with the innervation circuitry of the limb muscles.

The anterior corticospinal tract is mostly concerned with the innervation circuitry of the trunk muscles.

Types of signals—Mostly concerned with the control of precision and speed of highly skilled movements.

Indirect Corticospinal Paths: Corticorubrospinal and Corticoreticulospinal Tracts

Although the red nucleus and the reticular nuclei receive a variety of input signals from different brain areas, they are regarded as corticospinal links because of the important role the cortex plays in them in skilled movements.

Corticorubrospinal Path (Fig. 12-9D)

Corticorubral course—Corticorubral fibers descend ipsilaterally together with the direct corticospinal tracts mainly from motor (precentral gyrus) and premotor areas and relay in the red nucleus.

Rubrospinal course—The rubrospinal fibers cross the midline (ventral tegmental decussation of Forel) and descend contralaterally along the brain stem and spinal cord.

Brain stem position—Tegmentum.

Spinal cord position—In the lateral funiculus.

Ending—In laminae V to VII.

Types of signals—Mostly concerned with the innervation circuitry of the flexor muscles of the limbs.

Corticoreticulospinal Tract (Fig. 12-9D)

Corticoreticular course—The corticoreticular fibers originate mostly from areas 1 to 4 and 6, descend with the corticospinal tract, and then reach the reticular nuclei bilaterally. The pontine reticulo-spinal and the medullary reticulospinal tracts are identified as descending from the reticular nuclei to the spinal cord.

Pontine Reticulospinal Tract

The pontine reticulospinal tract originates on the oral and caudal reticular nuclei and descends ipsilaterally, reaching the anterior funiculus where its fibers terminate bilaterally along the spinal cord, synapsing in laminae VII and VIII.

Medullary Reticulospinal Tract

The medullary reticulospinal tract originates on the gigantocellular reticular nuclei of the medulla bilaterally and descends reaching the lateral funiculi where the fibers terminate along the spinal cord, synapsing mostly in lamina VII.

Types of signals—It appears to influence visceral and somatic motor circuitries.

Other Descending Tracts

Lateral Vestibulospinal Tract (Fig. 6-20)

Origin—Lateral vestibular nucleus (of Deiter).

Crossing—No. This is hence an ipsilateral tract.

Spinal cord position—Anterior funiculus.

Ending—In laminae VII and VIII along the spinal cord.

Types of signals—Mainly excitatory of extensor muscles of trunk.

Medial Vestibulospinal Tract (Fig. 6-20)

Origin—Medial vestibular nucleus bilaterally. The descending fibers form the medial vestibulospinal tract. It is also known as the descending portion of the medial longitudinal fasciculus.

Spinal cord position—In the anterior funiculi, ending in laminae VII and VIII of cervical segments.

Types of signals—Influences motor circuitry of neck and shoulder muscles, correlating visual gaze with head, neck, and shoulders in posture and movements.

Tectospinal Tract (Fig. 12-10)

Origin—Superior colliculus.

Crossing—Yes, in the dorsal tegmental decussation of Meynert. Contralateral.

Brain stem position—In the tegmentum anterior to the medial longitudinal fasciculus.

Spinal cord position—In the anterior funiculus, ending in laminae VII and VIII of cervical segments.

Types of signals—Similar to those of the medial vestibulospinal tract.

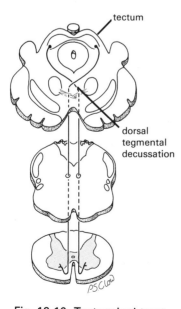

Fig. 12-10. Tectospinal tract.

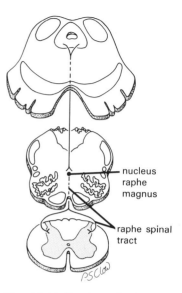

Fig. 12-11. Raphe spinal tract.

Raphe Spinal Tract (Fig. 12-11)

The raphe spinal tract originates in the raphe nuclei, mainly the nucleus raphe magnus and descends in the lateral funiculus, ending along the spinal cord in lamina II. The raphe spinal endings release serotonin and modify the sensory activity of the dorsal horn.

Crossing of Fibers

The crossing of fibers (commissural fibers) from one-half of the nervous system to the other offers an economical and efficient way, in terms of time and wiring, to bring about the harmonious integration in one unit of the two-sided (left-right) input-output processes of the nervous system. Hence, when one-half receives sensory input, it first informs the other half rather than proceeding with the execution of a motor output.

The "normal" activity of monosynaptic reflexes, like the stretch reflex, does not execute movement. Monosynaptic reflexes are followed by movements if the triggering stimulus is noxious or massive (e.g., tendon percussion).

The Study of Paths—Three Main Pathways

Students of a complex subject often lose efficiency in their reasoning, because their efforts are concentrated on memorizing facts. The list of paths presented in the above summary is of use in the elucidation of detailed and complex problems in clinical neurology. For the beginners to medical practice, however, it is better to concentrate first on the most basic and outstanding facts. Once these are familiar, the study of the paths can be approached with added depth of reasoning regarding detail as well as with pertinent comprehensive concepts.

Two individual ascending and all the descending corticospinal paths as a unit are analyzed with regard to their normal characteristics as well as to neurological signs triggered by their interruption.

Anterolateral Spinothalamic Tract

Input to the Tract

The input to the **anterolateral spinothalamic tract** courses through small myelinated and nonmyelinated fibers of the dorsal roots, enters the spinal cord as the **lateral bundle,** and spreads its branches as a fork to one or two contiguous segments through the fasciculus posterolateralis. It then enters the spinal cord gray matter of the same side where it synapses.

Course of the Tract

The cells receiving the stimulus send their axons contralaterally to the anterior and lateral funiculus of the other side of the cord, ascend, pass the brain stem, and reach the posterior region of the intralaminar nuclei and the ventralis posterolateralis nucleus of the thalamus, where their neurons convey information of nondiscriminating touch, pain, and temperature to a variety of cerebral regions, where it becomes conscious.

Of clinical importance is the fact that an interruptive lesion of the anterolateral spinothalamic tract results in loss of pain and temperature sensation originated in the body contralaterally, below the level of the lesion.

The three major consequences of such a lesion are described below.

1. There is no loss of touch, because other pathways convey similar information.
2. The loss of pain sensation is contralateral, because the spinothalamic path carries information from the opposite side of the body.
3. The contralateral information is lost one or two segments below the level of the lesion, because the segmental input to the cord spreads to one or two segments above, where it escapes being interrupted by the lesion.

If one-half (left or right) of the body becomes deprived of pain sensation, the lesion is known to be located in the tract above the spinal cord level.

Posterolateral White Column–Medial Lemniscus Path

Medium and large myelinated fibers of the dorsal roots enter the spinal cord as the **medial bundle** and ascend in the posterolateral white column either without relay or through one or two relays to reach the lower portion of the medulla oblongata. Nuclei of this region, mainly the gracilis and cuneatus, send fibers to the opposite half of the brain stem which ascend as the medial lemniscus and reach the ventralis posterolateralis nucleus of the thalamus where their neurons convey information of discriminative touch, pressure, proprioception (position and movement sense), and vibration to the cortex.

It should be stressed that loss of discriminative touch and pressure (**astereognosis**) and deficiencies in the senses of vibration, position, and movement involve the region of the body ipsilaterally below the level of a posterolateral white column lesion and contralaterally below the level of a medial lemniscus lesion (Fig. 12-12).

Impairment of these sensibilities results in **sensory ataxia**, i.e., disturbance in muscle coordination. A person suffering from this disorder has difficulty maintaining a standing position with the feet together. This imbalance becomes exacerbated when the patient closes his eyes (**Romberg's sign**) (Fig. 12-13).

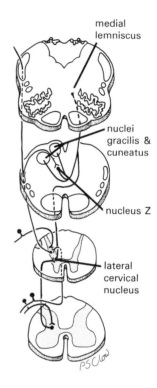

Fig. 12-12. Posterolateral white column–medial lemniscus path. The medial lemniscus is made of fibers from (1) the nuclei gracilis and cuneatus = discriminative touch and pressure from body and proprioception from upper half of body. (2) Nucleus Z = proprioception from lower half of body. (3) Lateral cervical nucleus = modified discriminative touch and pressure.

Direct and Indirect Corticospinal Motor Tracts

For the simultaneous analysis of the direct and indirect corticospinal motor tracts, certain general statements can be useful.

Within these tracts two major functions are carried out, i.e., voluntary movement and modulation of the motor activity of the spinal motor neurons.

Lesions of the corticospinal descending tracts produce an immediate reaction known as **early spinal shock**, which is characterized by paralysis of voluntary movements and lack of modulation of motor activity of spinal motor neurons, which will result in

1. muscle hypertonus, a condition which develops due to the lack of modulatory activity controlling the spinal motor neuron, which hence involves itself in aberrant, biased activity;

2. myotatic hyperreflexia, which develops for the same reason as in (1);

3. abolition of superficial plantar reflex (plantar flexion of the toes) and appearance of Babinski's sign (dorsiflexion of the toes); and

4. abolition of superficial abdominal reflexes.

Only two major regions in the course of these tracts will be analyzed in this context, namely, the cerebrum and the spinal cord regions.

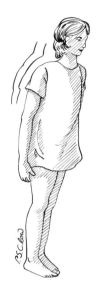

Fig. 12-13. Romberg's sign.

descending tracts at any level within one-half of the cerebrum produces paralysis, hypertonus, and hyperreflexia in the contralateral side of the body (a in Fig. 12-14).

Spinal Cord Level

Most of the descending motor tracts within one-half of the spinal cord convey motor signals toward the motor neurons of that same half of the spinal cord (b in Fig. 12-14). Any unilateral interruptive lesion of the corticospinal (motor) descending tracts at any level within the spinal cord produces (ipsilaterally below the lesion) paralysis, hypertonus, and hyperreflexia.

Level of Cerebrum

The vast majority of the fibers composing the direct and indirect corticospinal motor tracts, which originate in one hemisphere, is concerned with the innervation of contralateral spinal motor neurons.

An interruptive lesion affecting these

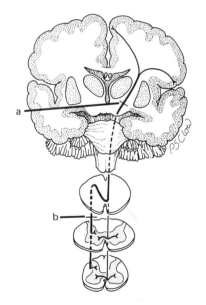

Fig. 12-14. Lesions of the corticospinal tract at brain level (a) and spinal cord level (b).

Spinal Cord Hemisection

By now, the student could use the information collected about the three main paths described above in the following exercise.

Question

What signs would appear in a patient whose spinal cord has been severed on the right side between cord segments T6 and T7? (Figure 12-15.)

Answer

The following signs may appear:

1. hemiparesis or motor paralysis on the right side (below T6); the right leg is paralyzed, hypertonic, hyperflexic; and has elicitable Babinski's sign; corticospinal tracts are interrupted;
2. hemianesthesia, which means that no proprioceptive or stereognostic sensation can be triggered by stimulating the right side of the body (below T6), since the posterior funiculus is interrupted;

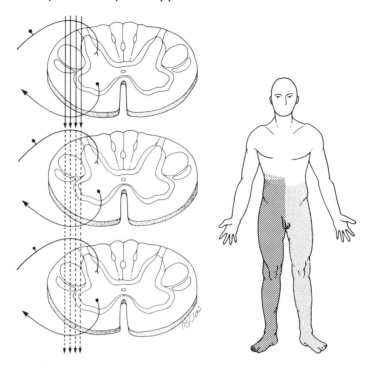

Fig. 12-15. Spinal cord lesion affecting vertical paths.

3. hemianalgesia and hemithermoanalgesia, which means that no painful or temperature sensation can be evoked by stimulating the left side of the body (below T8), since the anterolateral spinothalamic tract is interrupted.

Based on these signs, the clinician makes the diagnosis of a **hemisection** (half section) of the right side of the cord at T6 level.

The term syndrome means a group of symptoms and signs, which, when considered together, characterize a disease or lesion. The signs mentioned above due to hemisection of the spinal cord were described by Brown-Séquard and are together hence known as the **Brown-Séquard syndrome.**

It is unusual for patients to suffer an exact hemisection of the cord. An incomplete syndrome, due to tumor compression, a bullet wound, or other causes, is more frequent.

Combination of Segmental Loop and Vertical Loop Lesions

The effects of interruptive lesions affecting only a number of isolated vertical paths, ascending and descending, were described above. Often patients show signs that indicate a lesion of the descending motor tracts, the corticospinal, and signs that indicate a lesion of the spinal motor neurons (Fig. 12-16).

To distinguish between the signs caused by interruptive lesions, they are presented in Table 12-1 classified into lesions of the corticospinal tract (known in clinical practice as **upper motor neuron (UMN) lesions**) and of the spinal motor neurons and their axons (known as **lower motor neuron (LMN) lesions**).

In the case of Brown-Séquard syndrome produced by a tumor growth damaging

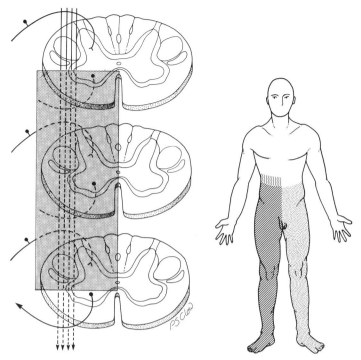

Fig. 12-16. Spinal cord lesion affecting vertical and horizontal paths (segmental loops).

the right side of the cord in segments T6–7, it may involve not only the vertical tracts but also catch the sensory input and motor neuron output of these segments. The patient will present the previously mentioned signs pertaining to hemisection and affecting the ascending and descending tracts, and a zone of total anesthesia and signs of lower motor neuron lesions related to T6 and T7 segments on the right side.

Topographic Organization and Cord Lesions

The examples of spinal cord lesions given until now are only simple problems. The variety of possible clinical signs recorded in clinical practice caused by lesions that a patient can suffer may be diagnosed by the proper use of the knowledge pre-

Table 12-1. Signs of UMN and LMN Lesions

Corticospinal Tracts (UMN)	Spinal Motor Neurons (LMN)
Paralysis	Paralysis
Hypertonia	Hypotonia
No significant muscle atrophy	Significant muscle atrophy
No fasciculation or fibrillations	Fasciculation and fibrillations
Hyperreflexia	Hyporeflexia

sented in the topographical organization of the cord.

One or many tracts may be involved in the pathological process or it may affect one side more than the other, which in turn produces other signs (such as a tumor located outside the cord, compressing it lateromedially).

The three examples below serve well to illustrate the vital importance of keen knowledge of neuroanatomical structures and their functions in a correct analysis of neurological signs.

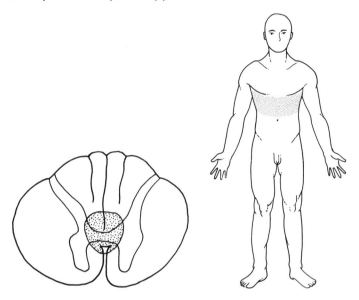

Fig. 12-17. Small internal spinal cord lesion.

Early Spinal Cord Core Lesion

In the case of an **early spinal cord core (internal spinal cord) lesion,** the crossing fibers of the spinothalamic tract are lesioned, producing a region of analgesia (Fig. 12-17), due to a degenerative lesion of the core of the spinal cord **(syringomyelia)** or a tumor within the spinal cord.

Advanced Intramedullary Lesion with Sacral Sparing

In the case of an **advanced intramedullary lesion with sacral sparing,** the lesion has spread and affects most of the ascending spinothalamic fibers, sparing the most peripheral ones. It produces the result illustrated in Figure 12-18.

Remembering that the topographical ar-

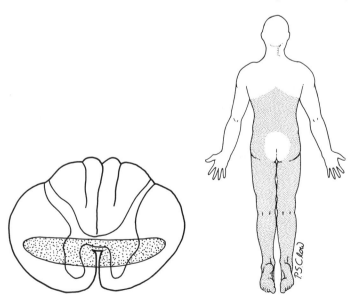

Fig. 12-18. Large internal spinal cord lesion.

rangement of the ascending lateral spino-thalamic tracts is as depicted in Figure 5-32, one may conclude that a lesion within the core of the cord at T4 has affected the central portions of the spinothalamic tracts and has spared the peripheral portions involved in the transmission of noxious signals from the sacral region.

Cauda Equina Lesion

Another example is presented in Figure 12-19 and indicates a lesion of the **cauda equina** or the lower sacral segments.

Syndrome of a Sudden Complete Transverse Section of the Spinal Cord

In the **initial stage** of a sudden complete transverse section of the spinal cord, the

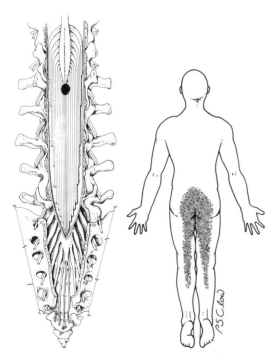

Fig. 12-19. Cauda equina lesion.

following will appear immediately below the lesion:

complete flaccid paralysis of all muscles;
complete anesthesia;
abolition of cutaneous and tendon reflexes;
retention of urine and feces;
abolition of sweat secretion and pili erection; and
temporary drop in blood pressure.

The initial stage is followed by a **recovery stage** where the following changes may be observed:

spontaneous and reflex-induced emptying of bladder and bowel;
reappearance of automatic reflex activity of bladder and rectum and sweat secretion;
regaining of some muscle tone and some muscle reflex activity;
appearance of automatic spinal mass reflexes, e.g., flexion of a leg may empty the bladder;
tendency to retracted position (flexion) of the limbs, e.g., lower limb—hip flexion, knee flexion, plantar dorsiflexion;
hypertonus in flexor muscles;
spastic reaction to passive stretch, especially of flexor muscles;
elicitability of mass myotatic reflexes and clonus (which may even become exaggerated); and
unrelented paralysis of muscles to voluntary movements.

The stage of recovery, better known as the **stage of reorganization,** usually develops over a period of several months. This process is most likely due to the takeover of dorsal roots, interneurons, and terminal buttons on motor neuron cell surfaces left by the degenerated buttons from the supraspinal regions. Depending on the care received by the patient, definitive deviations from these standard changes may occur. For instance, if an infection sets in, the hypertonic retracted paralyzed position returns to the initial flaccid paralysis. If the transection occurs in the upper

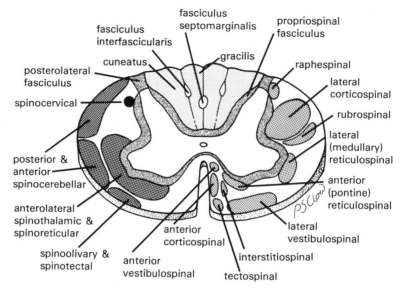

Fig. 12-20. Vertical spinal cord paths.

cervical region, death due to paralysis of respiratory muscles ensues. If it occurs in the sacral region, most of the signs pertain to the lower viscera.

Paraplegia is the term used to indicate paralysis of two symmetrical limbs, i.e., the lower or the upper limbs. The most common occurrence of paraplegia is of the lower limbs.

Quadriplegia (tetraplegia) refers to paralysis of the four limbs.

Hemiplegia is paralysis of one side of the body.

Monoplegia refers to paralysis of one limb.

Progressive, Gradual, Complete Transection of the Spinal Cord

In the case of progressive, gradual, complete transection of the spinal cord, the picture is quite different and shifting. The appearance, sequence, and intensity of the signs depend on which structures are af-

fected first and on the speed at which the transection comes about (Fig. 12-20).

Potentials of Rehabilitation Therapy

Due to the loss of all the supraspinal influences, the spinal sensory motor loops and centers with their intersegmental circuits are left to operate on their own and at the mercy of whatever circumstantial sensory input the body receives.

In the initial stage, the loss of supraspinal influences is expressed by hypoactivity of the spindle loop on α motor neurons. Later on, α and γ loops of some muscle regions of the body become hyperactivated in a vicious circle. As mentioned above, this hyperactivity principally depends on two factors: the stimuli imposed on the body—sensory modalities, intensity, duration, regional body patterns, etc.; and the intrinsic reaction of the spinal cord in handling such stimuli.

The above described pattern of reaction to lesions of the motor system is based on what has been observed in clinical practice. It could be changed in response to proper physiotherapy.

The main objective of such therapy is to counteract the strong tendency toward hypersensitivity due to increased α activity and increased phasic and tonic α activity with a dominating hyperactivity of muscles of certain groups (e.g., the retracting limb muscles) and a recessive activity of their antagonists. The sooner the treatment starts, the smaller the chances are for biased patterns to become established. Extensive knowledge about spinal cord reflexology is indispensable in the design of the therapy, which should take into account monosynaptic reflexes, the contralateral reflexes, polysynaptic reflexes, reciprocal innervation reflexes, mass reflexes, etc.

Suggested Readings

Asanuma H, Zarzecki P, Jankowska E, Hongo T, Marcus S: Projection of individual pyramidal tract neurons to lumbar motor nuclei of the monkey, Exp Brain Res 34:73–89, 1979.

Berkley KJ, Hand PJ: Efferent projections of the gracile nucleus in the cat, Brain Res 153:263–283, 1978.

Boivie J: Anatomical observations on the dorsal column nuclei, their thalamic projection and the cytoarchitecture of some somatosensory thalamic nuclei in the monkey, J Comp Neurol 178:17–48, 1978.

Boivie J: An anatomical reinvestigation of the termination of the spinothalamic tract in the monkey, J Comp Neurol 186:343–370, 1979.

Brown AG: Ascending and long spinal pathways: dorsal columns, spinocervical tract and spinothalamic tract. In Iggo A, Ed.: Handbook of Sensory Physiology, Vol. 2: Somatosensory System, Springer-Verlag, Berlin, pp. 315–338, 1973.

Brown AG: Organization in the Spinal Cord. The Anatomy and Physiology of Identified Neurons, Springer-Verlag, Berlin, 1981.

Carpenter MB: Human Neuroanatomy. Seventh Edition. Williams and Wilkins, Baltimore, pp. 238–284, 1976.

Coulter JD, Ewing L, Carter C: Origin of primary sensorimotor cortical projections to lumbar spinal cord of cat and monkey, Brain Res 103:366–372, 1976.

Denny-Brown D, Kirke EJ, Yanagisawa N: The tract of Lissauer in relation to sensory transmission in the dorsal horn of spinal cord in the Macaque monkey, J Comp Neurol 151:175–200, 1973.

Eklund G: General features of vibration-induced effects on balance, Uppsala J Med Sci 77:112–124, 1972.

Grant G, Boivie J, Silfvenius H: Course and termination of fibres from the nucleus z of the medulla oblongata. An experimental light microscopical study in the cat, Brain Res 55:55–70, 1973.

Henneman E: Principles governing distribution of sensory input to motor neurons. In Schmidt FO, Worden FG, Eds.: The Neurosciences, Third Study Program, The MIT Press, Cambridge, 1974.

Henneman E: Organization of the spinal cord and its reflexes. In Mountcastle VB, Ed.: Medical Physiology, Fourteenth Edition, Vol. 1, CV Mosby, St. Louis, pp. 762–786, 1980.

Hentall I: A novel class of unit in the substantia gelatinosa of the spinal cat, Exp Neurol 57:792–806, 1977.

Kerr FWL: The ventral spinothalamic tract and other ascending systems of the ventral funiculus of the spinal cord, J Comp Neurol 159:335–356, 1975.

Rexed B: The cytoarchitectonic organization of the spinal cord in the cat, J Comp Neurol 96:415–495, 1952.

Snell RS: Clinical Neuroanatomy for Medical Students, Little, Brown and Co., Boston, pp. 305–341, 1980.

Wall PD: The substantia gelatinosa, a gate control mechanism set across a sensory pathway, Trends in Neurosciences 3:221–224, 1980.

Wall PD, Noordenbos W: Sensory functions which remain in man after complete transaction of dorsal columns, Brain 100:641–653, 1977.

Willis WD, Coggeshall RE: Sensory Mechanism of the Spinal Cord, Plenum Press, New York, 1978.

13

Cranial Nerves III to VI

Cranial Nerves III, IV, and VI

Cranial nerves III (oculomotor), IV (trochlear), and VI (abducens) are concerned with the innervation of the intrinsic and extrinsic muscles of the eye and the levator palpebrae superior.

The Eye

The **eye** is a highly specialized end-organ for vision. Operating like a spherical photographic camera, the eyeball has two intrinsic and two extrinsic adjustable sets of components.

Intrinsic Eye Components

1. An aperture, the pupil, regulated in its size by a diaphragm, i.e., the **iris,** to adjust to light intensity. This regulation is carried out by circular muscle fibers **(sphincter pupillae)** and radial muscle fibers **(dilator pupillae).**
2. A lens, adjustable to near and far vision by changes in its refractive power. Such lens changes are executed by the ciliary muscle with circular muscle fibers to thicken the lens for near vision and radial muscle fibers to thin the lens for far vision.

Extrinsic Eye Components

1. A set of six extrinsic muscles attached to the eyeball, to move the eyeball.
2. Two muscles on the superior eyelid, the tarsal muscle and the levator palpebrae, to lift the upper eyelid to uncover the eyeball.

Eye Function

When light reaches the eye, it enters the eyeball through the pupil and lens, stimulates the neuronal cells of the retina or light receptor layer, and is transported through the optic nerve to two distinct regions of the brain:

1. the visual cortex of the cerebral hemispheres via the thalamus; the signals,

which travel along the sensory conscious visual path, will become conscious;

2. the brain stem, to trigger all the appropriate reflex mechanisms; this is the reflex visual path, which has these components:

A. the sensory, from the retina to the brain stem;

B. the sensorimotor center (interneuronal);

C. the motor neurons from the brain stem to the extrinsic muscles of the eye; these are the motor neurons which make up the motor nuclei of the ocular nerves;

D. efferent visceral neurons making up the Edinger-Westphal nucleus;

E. the ciliary ganglion; and

F. intrinsic muscles of the eye.

Connections of Reflex and Conscious Visual Path

A number of links are established between the cortical and brain stem visual regions, enabling a continuous and harmonious interaction between the conscious and reflex visual neural paths.

Structural Components and Functions of Cranial Nerves III, IV, and VI

In the context of reflex and conscious visual paths, related structural components and functions of the cranial nerves III, IV, and VI can be presented schematically as shown in Table 13-1.

Eyeball Movements

The eyeballs are always **conjugating,** i.e., synchronizing, their movement. There are two distinct types of eyeball movement, namely, **parallel eye movement** and **convergent eye movement.**

Parallel Eye Movement

In parallel eye movement the two eyeballs move while maintaining their axis parallel.

Parallel Horizontal Gaze

The two eyes may look to the left or to the right. This is expressed as a **conjugate**

Table 13-1. Structural Components and Functions of Cranial Nerves III, IV, and VI

Cranial Nerve	Nucleus	Ganglion	Muscle Innervated	Function*
III Oculomotor	Edinger-Westphal (parasympathetic)	Ciliary	Ciliary (circular fibers)	Thickens lens
		Ciliary	Sphincter pupillae	Constricts pupil
	Oculomotor		Levator palpebrae superior	Lifts upper eyelid
			Superior rectus	Moves eyeball upward
			Medial rectus	Moves eyeball medially
			Inferior rectus	Moves eyeball inferiorly
			Inferior oblique	Moves eyeball upward
IV Trochlear	Trochlear		Superior oblique	Moves eyeball downward
VI Abducens	Abducens		Lateral rectus	Moves eyeball laterally

* Movements are referred to in the "straight ahead" position.

parallel horizontal gaze (look) **to the left or right.**

Parallel Vertical Movement

The two eyes can also look upward or downward in what is called a **conjugate parallel vertical gaze upward** or **downward.**

Intermediate stages of parallel gaze movement are cases of **parallel gaze upward and to the left; downward and to the left; upward and to the right,** and **downward and to the right.**

Convergent Eye Movement

In conjugate **convergent eye movement,** the two eyes gaze toward the midline. Two variations of such movement are both eyes gazing toward the midline and up, and both eyes gazing toward the midline and down.

Examination of Function of the Muscles of the Upper Eyelid

Two of the muscles of the eyelid, namely, the **superior tarsal smooth muscle** innervated by the **sympathetic** and the **levator palpebrae superioris,** have as their function to elevate the upper eyelid and expose the eye. Drooping eyelids, **ptosis,** may be due to paralysis of one of the two muscles. The distinction between levator

Table 13-2. Primary Action of Extrinsic Eye Muscles

Muscle	Primary Action
Medial rectus	Medial
Lateral rectus	Lateral
Superior rectus	Up
Inferior rectus	Down
Superior oblique	Down
Inferior oblique	Up

Table 13-3. Function of Extrinsic Eye Muscles

Muscle	Primary Action	Oriented Position
Superior rectus	Up	Lateral
Inferior rectus	Down	Lateral
Superior oblique	Down	Medial
Inferior oblique	Up	Medial

and tarsal muscle weakness addresses mainly the degree of droop and associated signs. If the ptosis is non-existent or reduced when the patient looks upward, the causal lesion is known to be in the smooth muscle.

Examination of Function of Extrinsic Eye Muscles

Each extrinsic muscle of the eye exerts a **primary action** (primary movement) of the eyeball (Table 13-2).

One can observe that the superior rectus and inferior oblique muscles have similar functions, as do the inferior rectus and the superior oblique muscles. To differentiate the functions of these pairs, i.e., to best observe each primary action, the eye has to be oriented first to one side (laterally or medially) as shown in Table 13-3.

Note: One can, in this manner, distinguish between the "up" pair (superior rectus → lateral; inferior oblique → medial) and the "down" pair (inferior rectus → lateral; superior oblique → medial).

Muscles Involved in Eyeball Oriented Position in Parallel Gaze

With reference to the respective muscles involved, the diagram of Table 13-4 depicts the orientation of the eyes in six directions.

Table 13-4. Orientation of the Eyes

Right	Eye	Left	Eye
Up-right			Up-left (2)
Right	Sup. rec. (5) ⟶ (2) Inf. obl. / Lat. rec. (4) ⟶ (1) Med. rec. / Inf. rec. (6) ⟶ (3) Sup. obl.	Inf. obl. (5) ⟶ (2) Sup. rec. / Med. rec. (4) ⟶ (1) Lat. rec. / Sup. obl. (6) ⟶ (3) Inf. rec.	Left (1)
Down-right			Down-left (3)

In the testing of the individual eye muscles the patient's eyes must follow the examiner's finger as it is moved into each of the six positions shown in Table 13-5 and Figure 13-1. The muscles tested are indicated in each of the given positions.

Testing Convergence of Eyes

In testing the convergence of the eyes the patient's eye follows the examiner's finger as it approaches the eyes in a midline (position A of drawing) (Fig. 13-2). The finger is then moved upward (position B) and downward (position C). In each of these positions the following muscles are tested: A—medial recti; B—inferior oblique muscles; C—superior oblique muscles.

Strabismus

A lack of parallelism of the ocular axes, commonly referred to as "cross eyed" or "lazy eye," is called **strabismus** (Gr. strabis-

mos squinting), **heterotropia,** or **heterophoria** by the neuroscientist. It may be due to paralysis or weakness (paresis) of the ocular muscles and is qualified as **convergent** or **divergent** according to the angle it

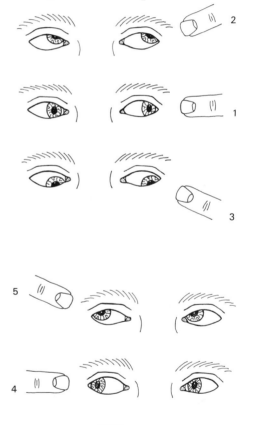

Fig. 13-1. Testing eye movement.

Table 13-5. Testing Individual Eye Muscles

(1) Left	-left lateral rectus and right medial rectus
(2) Upper left	-left superior rectus and right inferior oblique
(3) Lower left	-left inferior rectus and right superior oblique
(4) Right	-right lateral rectus and left medial rectus
(5) Upper right	-right superior rectus and left inferior oblique
(6) Lower right	-right inferior rectus and left superior oblique

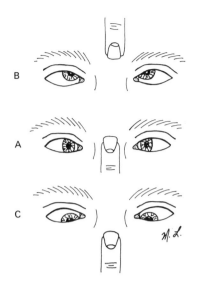

Fig. 13-2. Testing convergence of eyes.

forms with the ocular axes. A common consequence of strabismus is **diplopia** or **double vision.** If the diplopia is due to strabismus, both the diplopia and the strabismus are most pronounced when the patient looks toward the field of action of the weak muscle.

Diplopia is a sign of recent muscle imbalance. Patients with chronic strabismus do not complain of diplopia, since they learn to suppress one image.

Nystagmus

Nystagmus is a disturbance of the ocular posture characterized by a more or less rhythmical oscillation of the eyes. This word may be used in association with a few dozen different terms, some of which are descriptive of the rhythm of the oscillation, e.g., **pendular nystagmus** (movements of equal velocity to and fro) and **jerking nystagmus** (slow movement in one direction and fast return movement). Some are descriptive of the direction of the oscillation, e.g., **vertical, horizonal,** and **rotatory nystagmus,** some of its etiology, e.g., **caloric nystagmus** (induced by applying heat or cold to the ear), **optokinetic nystagmus** (induced by looking at a moving object), or

etiopathologic like **labyrinthine vestibular nystagmus** (due to vestibular disturbance).

Note: In jerking nystagmus the direction of the nystagmus is by conventional rule expressed by the direction in which the fast movement is executed.

Examination of Function of Intrinsic Eye Muscles

Light Reflexes

By shining a bright light to one eye, both pupils should become smaller. Two terms are used to describe this reaction, namely, **direct light reflex,** for the pupil illuminated, and **consensual light reflex,** for the pupil not illuminated.

Loss of direct light reflex may be due to a lesion of the sensory (optic) or motor (oculomotor) nerve component of the reflex path on the same side.

Loss of the consensual light reflex may be due to a lesion of either the optic nerve on the side illuminated or of the oculomotor nerve on the side where the consensual reflex is absent.

The normal substrate of the light reflexes is the adjustment of the pupil to avoid too much light. The reflex path is the optic nerve, the Edinger-Westphal nucleus, and its efferent fibers traveling with the oculomotor nerve relaying in the ciliary ganglion and ending up by constricting the sphincter pupillae.

Note: Fibers of the optic nerve toward the Edinger-Westphal nucleus course through the pretectal area.

In darkness, this activity is inhibited and natural dilation of the pupil occurs. If a person in darkness is in a state of fear, the sympathetic system may stimulate the dilator pupillae and further dilation **(mydriasis)** occurs. The stimulus is mediated through the cervical sympathetic pathway.

Ciliospinal Reflex

One way of testing the integrity of the cervical sympathetic pathway is to pinch the skin of the neck vigorously, which in a normal response triggers ipsilateral pupillary dilation. The reactive mechanism is called a **ciliospinal reflex.**

Accommodation Reflex for Near Vision

When a person looks quickly at a near object, i.e., 15 to 20 cm from the face, three mechanisms are in operation to ensure proper vision of the object: convergence of the eyes to achieve visual alignment, **miosis** or narrowing of the pupils to narrow the field of vision, and thickening of the lens to adjust the focal distance.

These integrated events form the **accommodation reflex.** The three together establish visual acuity. Just how they are integrated is still a matter of controversy.

Horner's Syndrome

A lesion at any level of the sympathetic path toward the head may present the four signs that characterize **Horner's syndrome** (Fig. 13-3): ptosis, miosis, decrease in sweating on the same side of the face as the lesion **(anhydrosis),** and enophthalmus.

Argyll-Robertson Pupil

The **Argyll-Robertson pupil** describes a pupillary abnormality characterized by the following.

The pupil is small and unaltered by light or darkness. It contracts even more in convergence of the eyes and returns to its previous size when the eyes recover the paral-lel position. Four facts are of applied practical importance: the pupil is small, it does not react to light, the pupil constricts normally in the accommodation reflex, and this abnormality is nearly always associated with neurosyphilis.

Different explanations have been suggested as to where the syphilitic lesion resides for these signs to develop: (1) in some interneurons of the upper brain stem, i.e., the pretectal region; (2) in the parasympathetic fibers for light reflex but not in the fibers for accommodation reflex; or (3) in the sympathetic fibers.

The third explanation is supported by a number of facts. The abnormal pupillary reaction is commonly associated with ptosis and with atrophy of the radial fibers of the iris, and the topical application of chemical mydriatics has poor reactive effect.

Note: Although the Argyll-Robertson pupil is described in most textbooks, it is a rare clinical finding.

Another pupillary abnormality is **Adie's pupil,** which usually affects one eye. It is due to an affection of the postganglionic parasympathetic fibers constricting the pupil. The syndrome consists of enlargement of the pupil, very slow pupillary reaction to light and to accommodation. These signs may appear in association with absence of myotatic stretch reflexes. The patient may complain of slight blurring of vision due to the uneven accommodation. The disorder usually begins abruptly, but from all available data it represents a mild polyneuropathy.

Malfunction of the Eye Motor System

A malfunction of the eye motor system may be due to a lesion of

1. the visual path (sensory);
2. the descending motor path from the cortex;
3. the interneurons in the brain stem re-

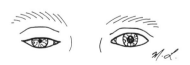

Fig. 13-3. Horner's syndrome.

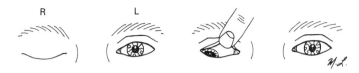

Fig. 13-4. Lesion of right cranial nerve III.

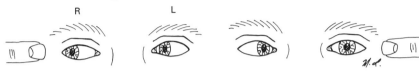

Fig. 13-5. Lesion of left cranial nerve VI.

lated to eye motor neurons;

4. the motor neurons of the eye, either their cell bodies (nuclei and ganglia) or their fibers (nerves) (**Note:** It must be remembered that besides the parasympathetic neurons cited in relation with cranial nerve III there are sympathetic fibers traveling with the internal carotid artery);
5. the extrinsic and intrinsic muscles of the eye;
6. the upper eyelid.

To find the level where the lesion is producing paralysis of ocular muscles, or **ophthalmoplegia,** a systematic procedure must be followed as described in the previous chapter.

If upon testing the muscle function deficiencies typical of myopathies are found that cannot be explained in terms of neurological lesion, one must search for a muscle disease.

Lesion of Cranial Nerve III

Complete paralysis of cranial nerve III causes widely dilated pupil and no accommodation or reaction to light; complete ptosis of the upper eyelid; paralysis of superior, medial, inferior recti, and inferior oblique muscles; outward and downward deviation of the eye (**exotropia),** strabismus, diplopia, and loss of visual acuity (Fig. 13-4).

Lesion of Cranial Nerve IV

Paralysis of the superior oblique muscle creates weakness or inability to orient the

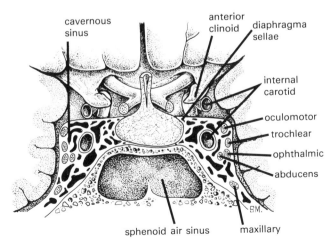

Fig. 13-6. Coronal section through cavernous sinus with outlines of more anterior structures. Dural attachment to anterior clinoids is not shown.

eye inward-downward. Diplopia is manifested when looking inward-downward.

Lesion of Cranial Nerve VI

Paralysis of the lateral rectus muscle causes inward deviation of the eye (**esotropia**), strabismus, and diplopia (Fig. 13-5). This nerve is very long and may be affected by many causes.

Combination of Lesions of the Three Ocular Nerves

Within the region of the cavernous sinus (Fig. 13-6) the three ocular nerves huddle close together. Pathology in this area (internal carotid artery, pituitary) may affect any or all of these nerves as well as branches of the trigeminal.

Ophthalmoplegias

Ophthalmoplegia means ocular muscle paralysis. In ophthalmoplegias due to lesions of the motor nuclei or their fibers

within the brain stem, the paralytic effects are similar to those of cases involving lesions at the peripheral nerve level (outside the brain stem), which were described under lesions of cranial nerves III, IV, and VI. In addition, however, the patient may display other signs related to other damaged near-by structures. In this context sound knowledge of the regional topography of the brain stem is indispensable.

Internuclear Ophthalmoplegia

To understand so-called **internuclear ophthalmoplegia** one must recall certain information.

Three types of conjugate movement, i.e., convergent, parallel vertical, and parallel horizontal, were described previously.

The conjugate convergent as well as the vertical movements involve two pairs of nuclei that are situated close together, i.e., the oculomotor nuclei and the trochlear nuclei. The conjugate horizontal or lateral gaze movement involves a pair of nuclei which are far apart from each other, i.e., the abducens (right or left) and the oculomotor (left or right) (Fig. 13-7). It appears

1. that the cortical descending motor fibers stimulate the superior colliculus and that the superior colliculus sends fibers to a nucleus of the opposite side, i.e., the **parabducens nucleus,** which is

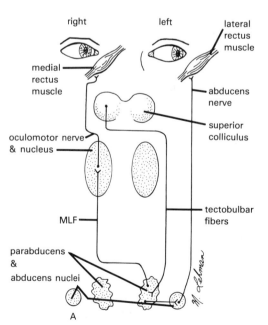

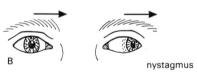

Fig. 13-7. (A) Pathway for lateral conjugate gaze; (B) right internuclear ophthalmoplegia.

located in the **paramedian pontine reticular formation (PPRF),** close to the abducens nucleus; and

2. that the parabducens nucleus stimulates the near-by abducens nucleus (concerned with the lateral rectus muscle) and also, through a path with other different fibers, the medial longitudinal fasciculus (MLF), the portion of the opposite oculomotor nucleus concerned with the medial rectus muscle.

A lesion of the MLF (affecting the path between the parabducens and oculomotor nuclei) produces internuclear ophthalmoplegia. The most common cause is multiple sclerosis.

If a lesion occurs in one MLF, e.g., the right MLF as in Figure 13-7, it is manifest when the patient tries to look laterally to the side opposite of the lesion. The medial rectus on the side of the lesion does not adduct; the abducting left eye moves laterally and displays **horizontal nystagmus** in **lateral gaze.** These signs of internuclear ophthalmoplegia are also known as **medial longitudinal fasciculus syndrome,** which usually is bilateral, affecting both MLF. This is an important syndrome as its verification pinpoints the causal lesion very precisely in a specific region of the brain stem, i.e., the region of the MLF in the upper

pons between the abducens and oculomotor nuclei.

A test to substantiate the diagnosis of internuclear ophthalmoplegia, when the described signs have appeared, consists in verifying that the patient is able to converge the eyes and make vertical movements of the eyes. A case of internuclear ophthalmoplegia affecting both MLF is illustrated in Figure 13-8.

Supranuclear Ophthalmoplegias

There are two types of **supranuclear ophthalmoplegias,** which are described below.

Upper Midbrain Lesion

An **upper midbrain lesion** involves the pretectal region. It may cause the **Parinaud's syndrome,** which is characterized by an inability to look up and down (conjugate vertical movement), and sometimes by dilatation of the pupils.

The pretectal region lies immediately rostral to the superior colliculus and below the posterior commissure. There are a number of nuclei in this region and ventrocaudally to it, intermediary in the execution of eye reflex coordination and movement, like pupillary light reflex in vertical gaze, raising the eyeball, and dropping the upper eyelid during sleep.

These interneuronal nuclei receive stimuli from the various brain stem regions and the brain cortex and send patterned stimuli to the oculomotor nuclei.

Cerebral Cortex Lesion

Different regions of the cortex are involved in ocular movement.

Neurons from the visual cortex (area 17) and the motor cortex (area 4) send fibers to interneuronal nuclei connected with the ocular motor nuclei to adjust visual acuity.

The **frontal eye field cortex** is a region

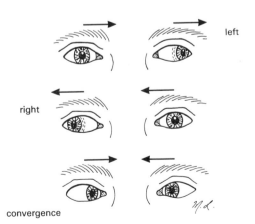

left

right

convergence

Fig. 13-8. Bilateral internuclear ophthalmoplegia.

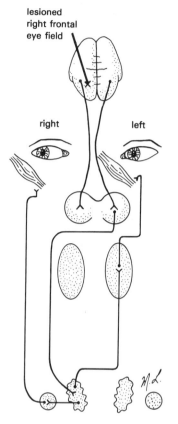

lesioned
right frontal
eye field

right   left

Fig. 13-9. Right supranuclear ophthalmo-plegia.

expected to show up, do not, as they are compensated for by reflex mechanisms.

Irritation of area 8 may produce the opposite sign, i.e., irritation of the left area 8 deviates the eyes to the right and vice versa. Lesions of the descending fibers from the visuomotor cortex present different signs in accordance with the level at which they are damaged.

Trigeminal Nerve (V)

The **trigeminal nerve** is the sensory nerve for most of the head and the motor nerve for the muscles of mastication. As the name denotes, it has three branches.

Ophthalmic Nerve

The **ophthalmic nerve** (Fig. 13-10) has several branches for the sensory innervation of the forehead; the frontal, ethmoidal, and sphenoidal sinuses; the eye, nose,

of area 8 involved in the control of eye movement. Some of its connections are with the visual cortex, the motor cortex, and the superior colliculus. The action of the visuomotor cortex is a subject of debate. Some scientists claim that it sends signals to the interneurons connected with the ocular nuclei. Others maintain that it receives information of muscle eye movements to program eye movements through the motor cortex.

A lesion of the frontal eye field results in an inability to gaze laterally toward the opposite side, i.e., a lesion in the left hemisphere causes an inability to look to the right and vice versa. Such a lesion frequently causes deviation of the patient's eye toward the side of the lesion (see Fig. 13-9). Many other defects that would be

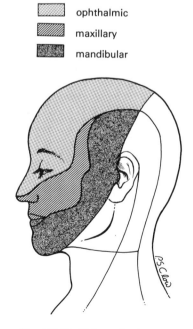

▨ ophthalmic
▧ maxillary
▩ mandibular

Fig. 13-10. Trigeminal nerve.

and nasal mucosa; and the dural region where the nerve passes through.

The **corneal reflex** is triggered by touching the cornea. Touch stimulates endings of the ophthalmic nerve, through which the stimulus travels to the brain and activates motor neurons of cranial nerve VII (facial) on the left and the right, bringing about closure of the eyelids of both eyes.

Maxillary Nerve

The **maxillary nerve** has several branches to make sensory innervation of the maxilla, upper teeth, vestibule of the nose, upper lip, cheeks and palate, maxillary sinus, and the dural region where the nerve passes through.

Mandibular Nerve—Sensory Fibers

The **mandibular nerve** has several branches to make sensory innervation of the anterior two-thirds of the tongue; mandible and lower teeth; lower lip; part of the cheek; anterior portion of the tympanic membrane and anterior portion of the external auditory meatus; temporomandibular joint; and the dural region where the nerve passes through. There are also proprioceptive (sensory) fibers from the muscles of mastication.

Mandibular Nerve—Motor Fibers

The motor fibers of the mandibular nerve form several branches to innervate the four main muscles of mastication, i.e., the **temporal,** the **masseter,** the **lateral (external) pterygoid,** and the **medial (internal) pterygoid.**

They also innervate the **tensor tympani, tensor veli palatini, mylohyoid** and the **anterior belly of digastric muscle.**

The main functions of the lateral pterygoid muscle are lateral movements and opening of the jaw. The main role of the other muscles of mastication is to close the jaw.

Central Connections of the Trigeminal Nerve

The three sensory branches of the trigeminal nerve, i.e., the ophthalmic, maxillary, and mandibular, have their cell bodies in the trigeminal ganglion attached to the pons by the root of the nerve. The fibers inside the pons travel to the target nuclei as follows:

To the mesencephalic nucleus—Fibers carrying proprioceptive signals from muscles travel through fibers of the mandibular nerve. The cell bodies of these fibers are an exception to the rule and, instead of being located in the ganglion, they form the mesencephalic nucleus.

To the main sensory nucleus—Fibers carrying discriminative touch and pressure signals from the head through the three branches.

To the trigeminospinal nucleus—Fibers carrying light touch, pain, and temperature signals from the head through the three branches. The topographical distribution of the fibers in the nucleus, important in diagnostic and surgical procedures, has been mapped. Three portions are distinguished in the nucleus from rostral to caudal, i.e., the **oral, interpolar,** and **caudal** portions.

The nociceptive fibers from the ophthalmic, maxillary, and mandibular nerves end ventrally, intermediately, and dorsally, respectively, through the length of the nucleus (Fig. 13-11).

A lesion restricted to the caudal portion

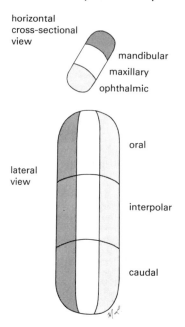

horizontal
cross-sectional
view

mandibular

maxillary

ophthalmic

lateral
view

oral

interpolar

caudal

Fig. 13-11. Trigeminospinal nucleus.

of the nucleus produces facial analgesia, as observed in clinical cases.

Motor Nucleus of Cranial Nerve V (Masticatory Nucleus)

The motor neurons of the masticatory nucleus innervate the above-mentioned muscles of mastication.

Jaw Jerk Reflex

To test the **jaw jerk reflex,** the examiner places his left thumb on the midline of the patient's mandible and taps it lightly with the reflex hammer. A slight outward and upward movement of the jaw is normally elicited, sometimes with difficulty and sometimes not at all. The stimulus signals travel from the muscle stretch receptors to the mesencephalic nucleus and continue to the motor nucleus, which signals to the muscles to contract through the α motor fibers.

Malfunction of Muscles of Mastication

In a case involving malfunction of the muscles of mastication, the causal lesion may be at the level of the muscles, the motor neurons or the "upper motor neurons." If one finds other myopathic deficiencies, one must search for a muscle disease or neuromuscular junction disease such as, for instance, myasthenia gravis or tetanus.

In the case of a unilateral masticatory motor neuron lesion the ipsilateral masticatory muscles display paralysis and, eventually, atrophy. Upon opening the mouth, the mandible deviates ipsilaterally and the patient is unable to move the jaw contralaterally.

In the case of a unilateral "upper motor neuron" lesion, the jaw reflex is not usually affected and no major deficiency in the mastication is manifest, because the motor neurons receive innervation from both hemispheres.

Lesions of the Trigeminal Sensory Paths

A lesion of the trigeminal sensory paths may affect the peripheral nerves or the central components.

Peripheral Nerves

To check for a lesion affecting the **peripheral nerves,** one proceeds by testing the different modalities of sensibility (touch, pain, and temperature) in each branch region.

A lesion of the ophthalmic branch abolishes the corneal reflex and is verified by stimulating the cornea of the affected side, which will not make either eye blink. Stimulation of the other cornea (not affected)

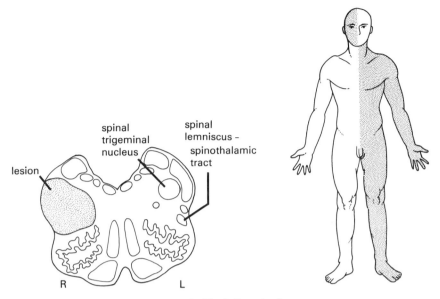

Fig. 13-12. Medullary lesion.

closes both eyes if the facial nerve is normal.

Sound knowledge of the path followed by the three branches of the trigeminal nerve through the skull is essential when localizing lesions within their regional path.

Pain in the region of distribution of the maxillary and mandibular branches is most commonly due to tooth infections. The term **trigeminal neuralgia (tic douloureux)** means a pattern of repetitive painful sensations characterized as brief but excruciating. The etiology is still debated.

Central Components of the Trigeminal Sensory Path

A number of facts related to the topography of the trigeminal components within the central nervous system are very useful

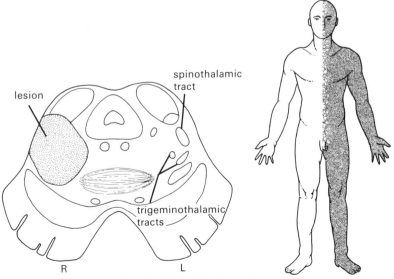

Fig. 13-13. Midbrain lesion.

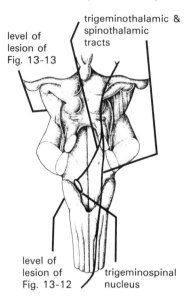

level of
lesion of
Fig. 13-13

trigeminothalamic &
spinothalamic
tracts

level of
lesion of
Fig. 13-12

trigeminospinal
nucleus

Fig. 13-14. Levels of lesions of Figures 13-12 and 13-13.

in the localization of lesions. Some of these facts are listed below.

1. As the trigeminal nerve enters the brain stem, the different sensibilities become separated and distributed to the corresponding nuclei. Loss of one type of sensibility, e.g., noxious, while the sense of another, e.g., touch, is preserved, indicates a nuclear lesion of the spinal trigeminal.

2. If the lesion is situated in the region of the medulla and lower pons on one side involving the trigeminal nuclei and the spinothalamic tract, loss of noxious sensation affects the face ipsilaterally and the body contralaterally (Fig. 13-12).

3. When loss of sensation on one and the same side of the body and the face is manifest, the lesion is known to be lo-

cated contralateral to the affected side and anywhere from the upper pons up, along the lemniscus paths (trigeminal, medial, and spinal) (Figs. 13-13 and 13-14).

Suggested Readings

Bannister R: Brain's Clinical Neurology. Sixth Edition. Oxford University Press, Oxford, 1984.

Bickerstaff ER: Neurological Examination in Clinical Practice. Third Edition. Blackwell Scientific Publications, Oxford, 1974.

DeJong R: The Neurologic Examination. Fourth Edition. Harper and Row, Hagerstown, pp. 40–80, 1979.

DeMyer W: Technique of the Neurologic Examination. Third Edition. McGraw-Hill Book Co., New York, 1980.

Macleod J, Ed.: Clinical Examination. Fifth Edition. Churchill Livingstone, Edinburgh, pp. 243–257, 1979.

Mayo Clinic and Mayo Foundation: Clinical Examinations in Neurology. Fourth Edition. WB Saunders, Philadelphia, 1976.

Samii M, Jannetta PJ, Eds.: The Cranial Nerves: Anatomy, Pathology, Pathophysiology, Diagnosis, Treatment, Springer-Verlag, New York, 1981.

Sears ES, Franklin GM: Diseases of the cranial nerves. In Rosenberg RN, Ed.: Neurology, Vol. 5 of The Science and Practice of Clinical Medicine, Grune and Stratton, New York, pp. 471–494, 1980.

Simpson JF, Magee KR: Clinical Evaluation of the Nervous System, Little, Brown and Co., Boston, pp. 29–45, 1973.

Van Allen MW: Pictorial Manual of Neurologic Tests, Year Book Medical Publishers, Inc., Chicago, 1969.

14

Cranial Nerves VII to XII

Facial Nerve (VII)

The structural arrangement and function of the facial nerve fibers is presented in Table 14-1.

Muscles of Facial Expression

To mention a few, some of the **muscles of facial expression** are

the **frontalis muscle,** to frown and elevate the eyebrows;

the **orbicularis oculi muscle,** to close the eye and wink;

the **perioral muscles,** to close the lips, smile, show the teeth, whistle, etc.;

the **buccinator muscle;** and

the **platysma muscle,** to stretch the skin of the neck.

Testing Muscle Function

Two distinct regions must be explored separately to test muscle function: the **upper face region** (frontalis and orbicularis

Table 14-1. Facial Nerve Fibers

Nucleus	Function and Region	Root	Sensory Ganglion Cells
Sensory solitary	Taste from the anterior ⅔ of the tongue	Intermediate	Yes
Sensory V	Small area of skin behind the ear	Intermediate of Wrisberg	Yes
Motor parasympathetic Lacrimal	Mucosa of nasal cavity and palate (secretion)	Intermediate of Wrisberg	No
	Lacrimal gland (tears)	Intermediate of Wrisberg	No
Superior salivatory	Submandibular and sublingual glands (saliva)	Intermediate of Wrisberg	No
Motor facial	Muscles of facial expression and a few other muscles	Motor	No

Note: The intermediate nerve, or the **nerve of Wrisberg,** is the visceral subdivision of cranial nerve VII.

243

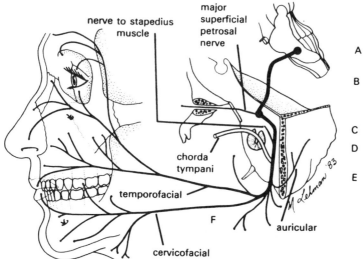

Fig. 14-1. Facial nerve.

oculi) like the motor component of the corneal reflex (both orbicularis oculi contract); and the **lower face region** (the perioral muscles and the platysma muscle). A weakness of one corner of the mouth is an important clue.

Topography of Facial Nerve

Since the topography of these components of the facial nerve is important in clinical diagnosis, a topographical representation of the nerve from the center to the terminals is shown in Figure 14-1. Key regions in facial nerve lesions are lettered.

A—Within the Pons

The motor fibers are hooked around the VI motor nucleus producing a small elevation on the floor of the fourth ventricle called **facial colliculus.** This bending of the fibers of cranial nerve VII is called **internal genu of the facial nerve.**

To know the position and relation of each component to neighboring structures is indispensable in pinpointing and demarcating a pontine lesion.

B—The Root Region, from the Inferior Border of Pons to the Geniculate Ganglion

The fibers are packed in two bundles, the motor root (large) and the intermediate of Wrisberg (small) with sensory and parasympathetic fibers. They enter the internal auditory meatus in company of cranial nerve VIII. The facial nerve then bends **(external genu of the facial nerve)** and the cell bodies of the sensory fibers form the geniculate ganglion. A lesion in region B may damage all the components of the nerve.

Between B and C regions, a bundle of mostly parasympathetic fibers separates, forming the **major superficial petrosal nerve.** These fibers relay in the pterygopalatine ganglion, which innervates the lacrimal, nasal, and palatine glands. The paralysis of this region results in a reduction of glandular secretion.

C—The Upper Facial Canal Region

The facial nerve continues within the temporal bone, backward, and downward in the **facial canal.**

Between C and D regions, the facial

nerve gives off a branch to the **stapedius muscle,** which dampens excessive movement of the auditory ossicles during loud sounds. When it is paralyzed, the patient may report that ordinary sounds are uncomfortably loud **(hyperacusis** or **auditory hyperesthesia).**

D—The Lower Facial Canal Region

The facial nerve continues downward in the lower facial canal region.

Between D and E, the facial nerve gives off another bundle of fibers, forming the **chorda tympani.** It consists mainly of parasympathetic and sensory fibers carrying taste signals. The fibers sensing taste reach the anterior ipsilateral two-thirds of the tongue. The parasympathetic fibers relay in the submandibular ganglion, which reaches the submandibular and sublingual glands.

Lesions of the chorda tympani nerve suppress taste from the ipsilateral anterior two-thirds of the tongue and reduce secretion of the submandibular and sublingual glands.

E—The Lowermost Facial Canal Region

The facial nerve continues descending in the lowermost facial canal region and exits the bone through the stylomastoid foramen.

Between E and F, the facial nerve gives off branches to a small area of the skin behind the ear, to the stylohyoid muscle, to the posterior belly of the digastric muscle, and to the occipital belly of the occipitofrontalis muscle.

F—Face Region

The motor nerve passes through the parotid gland. Its two main branches, the temporofacial and cervicofacial branches, innervate the muscles of facial expression ipsilaterally.

Lesions at this level produce paralysis of the innervated muscles.

Localization of Level of Lesion Along the Course of the Nerve

The localization of a lesion is guided by the verification of malfunction of the nerve branches (Fig. 14-2).

1. A lesion in F produces malfunction only of muscles of the face.

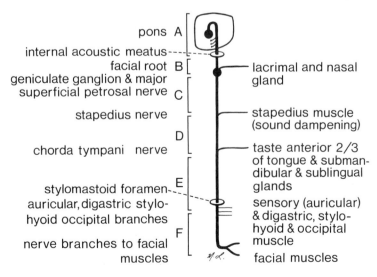

pons A
internal acoustic meatus
facial root B
geniculate ganglion & major
superficial petrosal nerve C

— lacrimal and nasal gland

stapedius nerve
D
— stapedius muscle (sound dampening)

chorda tympani nerve
— taste anterior 2/3 of tongue & submandibular & sublingual glands

stylomastoid foramen
E
auricular, digastric stylo-
hyoid occipital branches
— sensory (auricular) & digastric, stylo-hyoid & occipital muscle

F
nerve branches to facial muscles
— facial muscles

Fig. 14-2. Regions of the facial nerve.

2. A lesion in E produces, in addition to the signs of (1), malfunction of the branches given off after their exit through the stylomastoid foramen.
3. A lesion in D provokes, in addition to the signs of (1) and (2), such signs as those described for lesions of the chorda tympani.
4. A lesion in C causes, apart from the signs of (1) to (3), hypersensitivity to normal sounds.
5. A lesion in B produces the signs of (1) to (4) and a deficit of the superficial petrosal nerve, which results in all the activities of the nerve being damaged.
6. A lesion in A within the brain stem causes all the signs of (1) to (5) in addition to other signs whose nature depends on which facial nuclei are affected and which other surrounding structures are involved.

Middle ear infections may spread to the facial canal and affect the nerve at that level. Infections of the parotid gland may also affect the nerve in its course.

Idiopathic Facial Paralysis—Bell's Palsy

Idiopathic facial paralysis, also called **Bell's palsy,** is of acute onset, almost always affecting one side of the face. It results from a facial nerve lesion within the facial canal or close to the stylomastoid foramen. Its etiology is debated. In some cases, when the affection subsides, a phenomenon called "crocodile tears" may appear, characterized by secretion of tears when eating. It is thought that some parasympathetic fibers have regenerated and established contact with the lacrimal gland instead of the salivary glands which were originally innervated.

Facial Motor Neuron Lesions

A **motor neuron lesion** damaging the motor nucleus or the whole nerve is principally characterized by the fact that it affects one whole side of the face ipsilaterally (Fig. 14-3).

"Upper Motor Neuron" Lesions

In the case of an **"upper motor neuron" lesion** in one cerebral hemisphere there is a loss of voluntary movement of the muscles of the lower half of the face (perioral muscles) contralaterally. A patient with a right "upper motor neuron" lesion is able to close the eyes and frown, but is unable

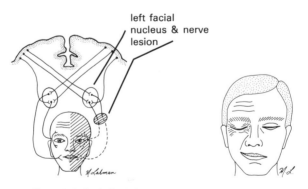

left facial nucleus & nerve lesion

Fig. 14-3. Left facial nerve lesion with paralysis of left side of face.

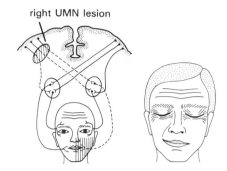

right UMN lesion

Fig. 14-4. Right upper motor neuron lesion with paralysis of left lower quadrant of the face.

to move the left oral commissure. Figure 14-4 intends to help explain why it is restricted to the contralateral lower half of the face muscles.

The restriction of this loss of function to the lower half of the face stems from the fact that the nuclear region concerned with the upper half of the face receives bilateral innervation from the two cerebral hemispheres.

Note: If a patient with an "upper motor neuron" lesion affecting the input to the facial nucleus becomes emotionally overwrought, he or she may be able to mobilize the paralytic muscles due to the activity of the reticular formation involving the opposite corticoreticular path which has bilateral connections with the nuclei.

Vestibulocochlear Nerve (VIII)

As its name indicates, the vestibulocochlear nerve has two components, which are sufficiently distinct to warrant that they be studied independently.

Vestibular Nerve

The **vestibular nerve** is a sensory nerve involved in equilibrium. Information re-

lated to the position and movements of the head is recorded in the vestibular apparatus and conducted through the vestibular nerve to the brain, which reacts to achieve equilibrium by influencing balance, through position and movement of the body and orientation in space. It entails that the spinal cord (position and movements), the cerebellum (automatic balance), the ocular system (orientation in space), and the cerebral cortex receive information from the vestibular nerve and react to it. The first three are unconscious functional levels, the state of which the cortex is informed. They operate as reflex mechanisms. The cortex integrates all the information and discharge signals through the motor cortex. When the stimulus from the vestibular nerve is normal the cortex integrates and controls the information. If, however, the stimulus is persistent (sea sickness) or pathological (nerve irritation), the spinal cord, cerebellum, and ocular reflex mechanisms become overloaded and react out of control of the cortex.

Primary Sensory Neurons

Primary sensory neurons are bipolar cells, whose cell bodies form the vestibular ganglion in the auditory bony canal. One cell process is connected to the vestibular organ. The other process forms the vestibular nerve, which exits from the auditory canal through the internal auditory meatus at the side of cranial nerve VII and reaches laterally the upper medulla spreading upward and downward to end in four vestibular nuclei. Some fibers continue to the cerebellum.

Vestibular Nuclei

The **vestibular nuclei** also receive inputs from the cerebellum, the reticular formation and, through the **medial longitudinal fasciculus (MLF),** the interstitial nucleus of Cajal, located in the periaqueductal gray of the midbrain.

The vestibular nuclei send fibers to the cerebellum, to the spinal cord (through the vestibulospinal tracts), to the motor nuclei of the cranial nerve III, IV, and VI (through the MLF), to the reticular formation, and to the parietal cortex (area 40 of Brodmann) through the ventral posterior nucleus of the thalamus.

Lateral Vestibulospinal Tract

Stimuli travel via the **lateral vestibulospinal tract** from the lateral vestibular nucleus through the anterior funiculus to all segments of the spinal cord to stimulate proximal extensor (antigravity) muscles (Fig. 14-5).

Medial Vestibulospinal Tract

Stimuli travel via the **medial vestibulospinal tract** from the medial and inferior vestibular nuclei through the anterior funiculus to upper spinal cord segments C1 to T6 to influence neck muscles.

These two vestibulospinal tracts are involved in many reflexes like the **labyrinthine righting reflex,** which brings the head into the upright position, and the **tonic labyrinthine reflex,** a postural reflex that increases the extensor muscle activity by stimulating their motor neurons.

Medial Longitudinal Fasciculus

The vestibular nuclei send fibers through the MLF to the nearby reticular formation to conjugate the motor nuclei of cranial nerves III, IV, and VI. The centers of conjugation are thus activated in keeping with the pattern of the stimulus coming from the vestibular organ. In consequence, the eyes move in the same direction of displacement of the head to maintain their straight position. The reticular formation contributes fibers to the MLF to reach other somatic and visceral regions of the brain stem.

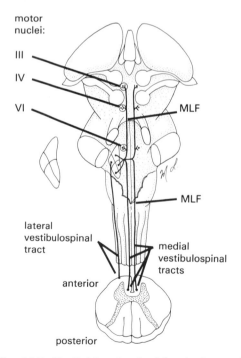

motor nuclei:

III

IV

VI

MLF

MLF

lateral vestibulospinal tract

medial vestibulospinal tracts

anterior

posterior

Fig. 14-5. Medial longitudinal fasciculus and vestibulospinal tracts.

Hyperexcitation or Malfunction of the Vestibular System

Due to the connections of the vestibular nuclei, hyperexcitation, like in motion sickness, or malfunction of the vestibular system may produce postural deviations, nystagmus, vertigo, visceral dysfunctions (nausea, vomiting, sweating, pallor, hypotension), and anxiety.

Cochlear Nerve

The **cochlear nerve** is the sensory nerve for hearing.

Primary sensory neurons are bipolar cells. One cell process picks up sound stimuli from the organ of hearing and the other forms the cochlear nerve which follows the same route as that of the vestibular nerve, ending in the ventral and dorsal cochlear nuclei.

Hearing Paths from Cochlear Nuclei

A simple descriptive illustration of the hearing paths from cochlear nuclei is presented in Figure 14-6.

As explanatory comments to this figure some functional aspects ought to be clarified.

Bilaterality

The fibers from the cochlear nuclei ascend bilaterally. This means that a lesion within the central nervous system (CNS) beyond the cochlear nuclei does not produce deafness. The patient may even be unaware of a reduction in his hearing sensibility.

Parallel Fiber Connections in Series

The parallel fiber arrangement in series of these paths makes it possible to analyze the information of the signals with regard to pitch, intensity, tone, noise discrimination, and, together with bilaterality, stereophonic sensation.

Topography

There are two regions which are of consequence in hearing deficiency:

the **lateral lemniscus,** whose considerable length and dense population of hearing fibers makes it particularly vulnerable (hearing impairment but not deafness is the result of such a lesion); and

the **nerve** and **nuclei region,** a total lesion of which produces deafness.

Reflex Auditory Path

The reflex auditory path is made up of

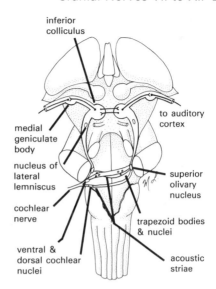

Fig. 14-6. Auditory paths.

fibers reaching the inferior colliculus from where reflex motor reactions are initiated through the appropriate paths, i.e., the tectobulbar, tectospinal, and tectoolivary tracts).

Conscious Auditory Path

Through the brachium of the inferior colliculus and the medial geniculate body, the conscious auditory path reaches the temporal lobe, the cortical auditory areas 41 and 42, and neighboring regions. Irritation of the auditory cortex may produce auditory hallucination. A temporal lobe lesion does not produce deafness unless it is bilateral.

Glossopharyngeal (IX) and Vagus (X) Nerves

Because of the close regional and functional relations of the glossopharyngeal (IX) and vagus (X) nerves, the introduc-

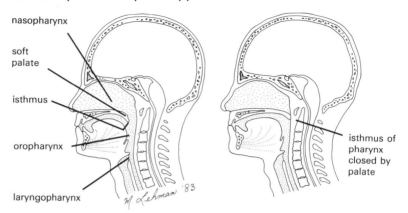

nasopharynx

soft
palate

isthmus

oropharynx

laryngopharynx

isthmus of
pharynx
closed by
palate

H. Lehman '83

Fig. 14-7. Regions innervated by cranial nerves IX and X.

tory analysis of these two nerves is presented in conjunction.

Regions of the body related to these nerves are represented in Figure 14-7 and are subdivided as follows:

Posterior Region of the Oral Cavity

Two distinct structures form the posterior region of the oral cavity.

Soft Palate

The sensory innervation of the soft palate is brought about by cranial nerves VII and IX. Its motor innervation is carried out mainly by the vagus (X), except for one muscle, i.e., the tensor veli palatini. When relaxed, the soft palate hangs down.

Posterior One-third of the Tongue

The sensory and taste innervation of the posterior one-third of the tongue is carried out by the glossopharyngeal nerve.

Pharyngeal Region

Three levels of the pharyngeal region are distinguished, namely, the **nasal pharynx,** the **oral pharynx,** and the **laryngeal pharynx.**

The partition between the nasal and oral pharynges is called the **isthmus of the pharynx,** which closes when the soft palate swings upward and backward. The sensory innervation of the pharynx is carried out by cranial nerve IX and the motor innervation by cranial nerve X. The muscles of the pharynx are called **pharyngeal constrictors** and their repeated contractions propel ingested food downward.

Laryngeal Region

This region is situated above the trachea and its sensory and motor innervation is carried out by cranial nerve X. Two principal activities are carried out by the larynx. One consists of discerning air from liquids and solids, thus making respiration possible while avoiding passage of food into the trachea by closing up. The other is to phonate, i.e., to produce sounds.

Deglutition

The following mechanisms are involved in **deglutition,** the act of swallowing, with reference to the respective participatory nerves:

the jaws close (V);
the lips close (VII);

Table 14-2. Functional Modalities of the Glossopharyngeal Nerve

Nucleus	Ganglion	Function	Region of Supply
Solitary	Inferior	Touch and pressure	Posterior oral cavity and pharynx (posterior ⅓ of tongue)
Trigeminospinal (V)	Superior	Nociceptive	Posterior oral cavity and pharynx (posterior ⅓ of tongue)
Solitary	Inferior	Taste	Posterior ⅓ of tongue
Solitary and reticular formation	Inferior	Blood pressure	Baroceptor organ and chemoceptor organ
Ambiguus		Motor	Stylopharyngeus
Inferior salivatory	Otic (motor)	Parasympathetic	Parotid (salivary) gland through otic ganglion and mucous glands of the pharynx through scattered (parasymp.) ganglia in the pharyngeal plexus

the tongue moves backward (XII);

the isthmus of the pharynx closes by the tensor veli palatini (V), stylopharyngeus (IX), and the X for the remaining muscles;

the constrictors of pharynx propel (X); and

the larynx closes (X).

Simultaneously, the sensory information of the anterior oral cavity (V) and the palate (VII and IX), the posterior one-third of the tongue, the pharynx (IX), and larynx (X) conveys whether the coast is clear for the act of swallowing. Warning signals reverse the process and produce vomiting. A noxious stimulus in the oropharynx or posterior oral cavity produces **archades,** whereas a tactile stimulus of the oropharynx produces the **gag reflex.**

The sensory component is part of cranial nerve IX and the motor component mostly of cranial nerve X. These components consist in the elevations of the soft palate and the contraction of the oropharynx, respectively.

Faulty closure of the isthmus of the pharynx by the palate (mostly X) permits the passage of food to the nasopharynx. Faulty closure of the larynx (X) permits the passage of food to the trachea and results in asphyxia.

Needless to say, the proper function of cranial nerves IX and X is essential in the vital functions of respiration and deglutition.

Phonation

The sound produced in the larynx (X) is articulated (Gr. *arthria* articulation) by a certain positioning of the palate (V, but mostly X), tongue (XII), jaws (V), and lips (VII). Malfunction in the articulation of sounds in speech expresses itself in **dysarthria** (Gr. stuttering), the nature and severity of which depends on which of the nerves (V, VII, IX, X, XII) and/or muscles are affected. With so many components employed in the normal function, it is logical that there are many types of dysarthrias. One is **nasal vocalization,** produced by the escape of air to the nasopharynx during vocalization due to improper closure of the isthmus of the pharynx by the soft palate.

Once the most important facts about cranial nerves IX and X have been introduced, these nerves can be studied independently in more detail.

Glossopharyngeal Nerve (IX)

The functional modalities of the glossopharyngeal nerve (IX) are presented in Table 14-2 with their nuclear, ganglionic, functional, and regional relations.

The regional topography and functional connections of the nuclei are important for the understanding of the structures involved in lesions of the **medulla oblongata.**

The nerve is attached to the lateral surface of the medulla oblongata, dorsal to the inferior olivary nucleus, and exits the cranial cavity through the jugular foramen, where, slightly below it, the nerve has two ganglia, i.e., the superior (nociceptive) and the inferior (sensory and taste). Below it the nerve branches out to reach the appropriate regions.

Sensory information (touch and pressure, etc.) from the regions innervated by cranial nerve IX reaches the solitary nucleus. The signals proceed in reflex and conscious paths: in reflex circuitry involving the appropriate motor nuclei, and in conscious circuitry, ascending through the reticular formation to the thalamus, from where they spread to other regions.

Nociceptive signals picked up by the glossopharyngeal nerve reach the trigeminospinal nucleus and proceed from there through reflex and conscious paths.

Taste sensation signals from the posterior one-third of the tongue reach the solitary nucleus and reticular formation, from where they proceed through reflex and conscious paths. The course of the conscious path for taste within the tegmentum is still debated.

The **carotid sinus** is a pressure receptor organ (baroreceptor) located on the wall of the internal carotid. A rise in blood pressure activates the sensor. The signal travels through the glossopharyngeal nerve to the medulla oblongata, where it stimulates the vagus nerve to decelerate the heart rate, inhibit the sympathetic innervation, and relax the blood vessel walls. These actions reduce blood pressure, which in turn reduces the activity of the sensor. This carotid sinus reflex becomes a blood pressure monitoring feedback mechanism.

The **carotid body,** or **glomus caroticum,** is a chemoreceptor organ located in the bifurcation of the common carotid, which monitors oxygen tension in the circulating blood. Fibers of the glossopharyngeal nerve conduct the signals to the solitary nucleus and to a region of the reticular formation of the medulla, namely, the respiratory center.

Vagus Nerve (X)

The functional modalities of the vagus nerve (X) are presented in Table 14-3 with their nuclear, ganglionic, functional, and regional relations.

The vagus nerve is attached to the lateral surface of the medulla oblongata, dorsal to the inferior olivary nucleus, and exits the cranium (piercing the dura and giving off branches) through the jugular foramen, where, just below it, the nerve has two ganglia, namely, the superior ganglion (sensory cell bodies from skin and meatus) and the inferior ganglion (sensory cell bodies from larynx and viscera). Further below, the nerve branches off to reach the appropriate regions. The vagal sensory fibers from skin and meatus reach the trigeminospinal nucleus from where neurons send fibers to establish the reflex and conscious paths.

Table 14-3. Functional Modalities of the Vagus Nerve

Nucleus	Ganglion	Function	Region of Supply
Trigeminospinal	Superior	Sensory somatic	Retroauricular and posterior wall of external auditory meatus
Solitary	Inferior	Sensory visceral	Larynx, trachea, esophagus, and thoracic and abdominal viscera
Dorsal nucleus of X	Parasymp. ganglia in viscera	Visceral motor	Trachea, esophagus, and thoracic and abdominal viscera
Ambiguus	None	Motor	Soft palate, pharynx, and larynx

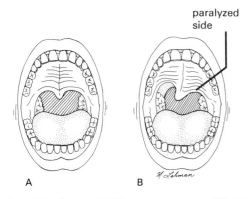

Fig. 14-8. Normal (A) and paralyzed (B) left half of soft palate.

Note: The sensory innervation of the external ear region, the soft palate, and the uvula is carried out by cranial nerves VII (visceral from glands and mucosa), IX (touch and pressure), and X (proprioception). Reflex reactions of the soft palate and uvula may be initiated by the stimulation of their respective receptors.

The afferents from the larynx, the trachea, the esophagus, and the thoracic and abdominal viscera reach the solitary nucleus. From there several reflex paths are established with the nucleus ambiguus, the dorsal nucleus, and the reticular formation. Information of these afferents travels to the thalamus through the reticular formation.

Given the fact that the cranial nerves IX and X are involved in phonation and articulation of speech sounds, signs like **aphonia** (absence of any phonation), **dysphonia** (ill voice, e.g., hoarseness), **anarthria** (lack of speech or articulation, due to motor neuronal or muscle lesions), **dysarthria** (faulty speech articulation due to motor neuronal or muscular lesions), etc., should be suspected to be associated with pathologies of these nerves, as should signs related to deglutition, e.g., **aphagia** (inability to swallow) and **dysphagia** (faulty swallowing).

The gag reflex or the reaction of the palate to the vocalization of the sound "Ah" is very informative and can reveal tell-tale signs of lesions in the participatory muscles, the reflex circuit, sensory neuron, motor neuron, or the "upper motor neuron."

If one side of the palate elevates poorly (Fig. 14-8) when the patient says "Ah" but elevates normally when it is touched, this indicates an "upper motor neuron" lesion. If both reflex and volitional activities are abolished, it is indicative of a motor neuron or muscle lesion. The motor nuclei of these nerves receive bilateral innervation from "upper motor neurons." It is the reason why a unilateral "upper motor neuron" lesion produces weakness only of a transitory nature.

The **cardioaortic body,** or **glomus aorticum,** is a chemoreceptor similar to the carotid body located at the base of the subclavian artery. The afferent fibers travel with the vagus.

Bilateral lesions of the cranial nerve X may be fatal. Alternate means of feeding and handling secretions must be applied.

Exploration of the larynx (with a laryngoscope) is very informative. Paralysis of the right vocal cord is illustrated in Figure 14-9.

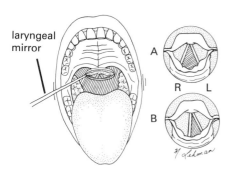

Fig. 14-9. Laryngoscopy: (A) normal and (B) paralyzed right vocal cord.

Spinal Accessory Nerve (XI)

Cranial nerve XI has two components, namely, the accessory (to the vagus) and the spinal. The accessory component arises

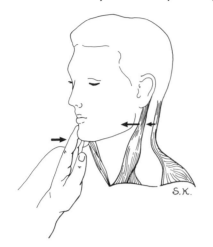

Fig. 14-10. Testing sternomastoid muscle.

Action of the Sternocleidomastoid Muscle

The sternocleidomastoid muscle is capable of executing three types of movements: ipsilateral tilting of the head, contralateral rotation of the head, and forward thrust of the head.

To test these functions, the examiner must offer resistance to each independent movement.

Trapezius Muscle

The **trapezius muscle** (Fig. 14-11) originates from the occiput and spinous processes of cervical and thoracic vertebrae and inserts into the clavicle and scapula.

Action of the Trapezius Muscle

The action of the upper portion of the trapezius muscle consists of elevating the shoulders. In paralysis of this muscle there is sagging of the shoulder on the affected side (Fig. 14-11). The muscle can be tested by observing the ability of the patient to elevate the shoulder (Fig. 14-12).

Path of the Spinal Portion

The path of the spinal portion of cranial nerve XI originates from motor cells in the anterior horn of the upper five cervical segments. Exiting on the lateral aspect of the spinal cord between the anterior and

from the caudalmost part of the nucleus ambiguus, travels for a short distance with the spinal component and then continues with the vagus to innervate the larynx.

The spinal component is the "true" element of the spinal accessory nerve. This component innervates the sternocleidomastoid muscle and the upper part of the trapezius muscle.

Sternocleidomastoid Muscle

The **sternocleidomastoid (sternomastoid) muscle** (Fig. 14-10) originates from the sternum and clavicle and inserts in the mastoid process.

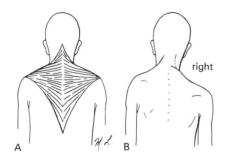

Fig. 14-11. (A) Trapezius muscles; (B) right trapezius paralyzed.

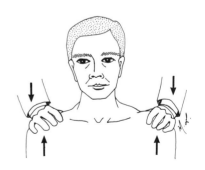

Fig. 14-12. Testing trapezius muscles.

posterior roots, it ascends entering the skull through the foramen magnum and exits the cranium through the jugular foramen in company of the cranial nerves IX and X.

A lesion of the spinal portion of this nerve is not evident unless the strength of the muscles innervated by the nerve is tested, because other muscles compensate for head positioning.

The motor neurons of this nerve receive bilateral innervation, which explains why a unilateral "upper motor neuron" lesion is manifest only in moderate and transient weakness of the muscle.

Hypoglossal Nerve (XII)

Cranial nerve XII, the **hypoglossal nerve** (Gr. *hypo* below; *glossa* tongue), innervates the intrinsic and extrinsic muscles of the tongue.

The motor nucleus of this nerve is situated in the tegmentum of the medulla (Fig. 14-13). The fibers proceed ventrally, lateral to the MLF, and exit on the anterior surface of the medulla, between the pyramid and the inferior olive, leave the cranium through the hypoglossal foramen, and reach the tongue from below.

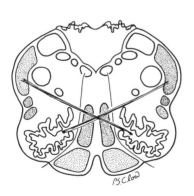

Fig. 14-13. Hypoglossal nerve.

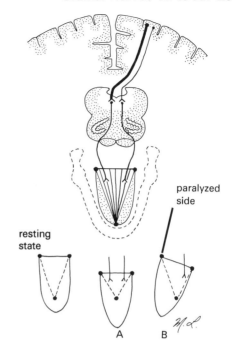

Fig. 14-14. Innervation of tongue muscles; (A) normal and (B) paralyzed side of tongue.

Genioglossus Muscle

The largest extrinsic muscle of the tongue, the **genioglossus muscle,** originates from the apex of the mandible and inserts into the base of the tongue through its base fibers.

When the tongue protrudes, the base fibers of this muscle contract, bringing the tongue forward.

When the basal portion of the left and right genioglossus muscles contract evenly, the tip of the tongue is in a midline protrusion (Fig. 14-14).

In a case of a deficiency in one of the genioglossus muscles, the tip of the tongue is deviated to the side of the deficient genioglossus. In other words, in the presence of a unilateral motor neuron or muscle lesion the tip of the tongue points to the deficient genioglossus that is situated on the same side as the lesion.

A lesion of the intrinsic muscles of the tongue or its motor neurons causes the

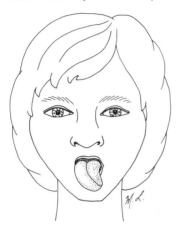

Fig. 14-15. Paralysis and atrophy of left half of tongue.

tongue to atropy, while a lesion of the extrinsic muscles or its motor neurons both shrinks and alters the position of the tongue (Fig. 14-15).

An intramedullary lesion may affect not only the hypoglossal fibers but also neighboring structures like the pyramids. Such a lesion produces a clinical syndrome called **inferior alternating hemiplegia,** which is characterized by contralateral hemiplegia (corticospinal path), and ipsilateral paralysis of the tongue (lower motor neuron).

The hypoglossal nuclei receive bilateral "upper motor neuron" innervation, which explains why a unilateral "upper motor neuron" lesion produces moderate and transient weakness of the tongue, detectable in speech.

The sensory innervation of the tongue is illustrated in Figure 14-16.

Brain Stem Circuitry—Centers

Once again it is convenient to insist that accurate knowledge of nervous system topographical circuitry is essential for the understanding of its functions and for the localization of lesions. This circuitry is still not fully known, but continuous progress is being made in its study.

In earlier analysis of functions like sleep, swallowing, and respiration, a very simplistic view was proposed in which one specific region of the brain stem was thought to exclusively monitor sleep and wakefulness, another swallowing, and another respiration; it was conceived that the proper reaction was triggered by a simple reflex mechanism. These hypothetical regions were called **centers of sleep-wakefulness, of swallowing, of respiration,** etc.

Later on, it was discovered that stimulation of a certain specific area of the brain stem produced sleep, while stimulation of another distinct specific area produced awakening. These areas were then conceived of as a sleep and the other as a wakefulness center. Complicating the picture, however, continued research revealed several "centers" producing sleep and several others producing wakefulness. Some such centers were even found to be unpredictably ambivalent, producing either sleep or wakefulness.

This development of knowledge as described with regard to sleep-wakefulness has evolved in a similar manner also concerning other "centers" of function, e.g.,

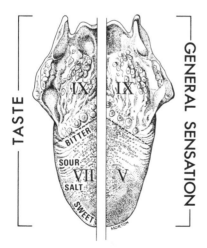

Fig. 14-16. Sensory innervation of tongue.

respiratory, swallowing, vasomotor, cardiovascular, vomiting, mastication, etc. These centers are generally known as **vital centers** because of their role in vital functions.

Today the concept of any specific function is viewed as a more or less complex set of subfunctions requiring the involvement and intimate collaboration of a number of regions of the CNS to coordinate their responses.

These new findings have been interpreted in the literature in three ways. One view maintains that the very concept of centers is invalid. Another view affirms that there are many centers for each function, and yet another affirms that there is one center for each function, the center being a network unit spread through the nervous system, connecting specific areas to permit their interactive coordinated operations, which results in the modulation of a particular function.

It has also been verified that specific areas are linked, not to one network unit only, but to a few or many. This means that each area of the nervous system may be involved in several or many behavioral functions. This finding reinforces the concept of the integrative functions of the nervous system based on anatomical substrates.

Schematic Diagrams of Some Centers

In recent scientific literature there has been an abundance of reports on models of the centers of the nervous system. Some models, using modern computer methods, are impressively elaborate. They are not yet of practical use, but they are edifying the foundations for a new exciting mode of studying the nervous system.

A schematic diagram of a center is shown in Figure 14-17. In the diagram only a few of the components are represented for the sake of simplification. An important fact is that the reticular forma-

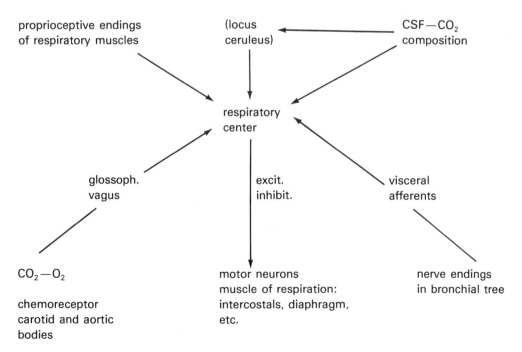

Fig. 14-17. Centers in brain stem tegmentum.

tion is involved in all of these centers. It is currently being studied with great interest and related findings are reported continuously. As the structure and function of the reticular formation are complex, however, it is still far from being clearly understood.

Suggested Readings

Bannister R: Brain's Clinical Neurology. Sixth Edition. Oxford University Press, Oxford, 1984.

Bickerstaff ER: Neurological Examination in Clinical Practice. Third Edition. Blackwell Scientific Publications, Oxford, 1974.

DeJong R: The Neurologic Examination. Fourth Edition. Harper and Row, Hagerstown, pp. 40–80, 1979.

DeMyer W: Technique of the Neurologic Examination. Third Edition. McGraw-Hill Book Co., New York, 1980.

Macleod J, Ed.: Clinical Examination. Fifth Edition. Churchill Livingstone, Edinburgh, pp. 243–257, 1979.

Mayo Clinic and Mayo Foundation: Clinical Examinations in Neurology. Fourth Edition. WB Saunders, Philadelphia, 1976.

Samii M, Jannetta PJ, Eds.: The Cranial Nerves: Anatomy, Pathology, Pathophysiology, Diagnosis, Treatment, Springer-Verlag, New York, 1981.

Sears ES, Franklin GM: Diseases of the cranial nerves. In Rosenberg RN, Ed.: Neurology, Vol. 5 of The Science and Practice of Clinical Medicine, Grune and Stratton, New York, pp. 471–494, 1980.

Simpson JF, Magee KR: Clinical Evaluation of the Nervous System, Little, Brown and Co., Boston, pp. 29–45, 1973.

Van Allen MW: Pictorial Manual of Neurologic Tests, Year Book Medical Publishers, Inc., Chicago, 1969.

IV

Sensory and Motor Systems

15

Cerebellum and Motor Systems

To properly understand the role of the cerebellum in posture and movement it is convenient to clarify a few basic concepts.

Synergy (Gr. *syn* together; *ergon* work) is the cooperation of several structures to perform an action. In the context of the motor system, synergy means the cooperation of muscles to achieve a posture or movement.

The **synergic muscles** involved in any specific posture or movement are grouped in their work into **agonists** (or movers) and **antagonists** (or opponents to the agonists).

During a rhythmic alternating movement, like supinating and pronating a hand, the two groups of muscles in action alternate their role as agonists (excited) and antagonists (inhibited).

Role of Proprioceptors in Synergy

The sensory fibers carrying information from the extrafusal and intrafusal muscle fibers to the central nervous system (CNS) are essential for the execution of synergic motor actions. The information needs to be linked in a very precise manner to the motor neurons so that these can activate (excite or inhibit) the two groups of synergic muscles.

Equilibrium

Equilibrium (L. *aequus* equal; *libra* balance) is a state of balance, a condition in which opposing forces exactly counteract each other.

In reference to the equilibrium of the body, the counteracting forces are the gravitational force and the muscle activity that is opposed to gravitation to gain or retain a specific position or develop a movement in space.

In a state of equilibrium, e.g., in a standing position, the agonist (excited) muscles are (in simple terms) the extensor muscles of the lower limbs and trunk, which (also in simple terms) can be called antigravity

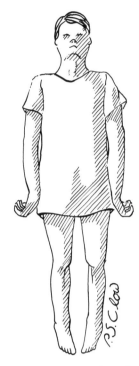

Fig. 15-1. Hyperactivity of antigravitational muscles in trunk and legs.

the awareness of the position of the body in its surroundings.

Intelligent Movements

The cerebrum is able to develop the capacity to perform skilled, voluntary movements to achieve very difficult tasks like, for instance, repairing the machinery of minute wrist watches. Most of these refined, skilled movements are concentrated in (but not restricted to) the hands, the mouth and larynx (speech), and the eyes. For the success of such sophisticated actions the cerebral hemispheres need to receive very specific information from proprioceptors, the vestibular organ, and any other sensory information source pertinent to the execution of intelligent motor acts.

Cerebellum

The cerebellum is an organ which

muscles. The antagonists are thus the flexor (inhibited) muscles (Fig. 15-1).

Excessive extension activity shifts the center of gravity of the body, causing some flexors to contract and some extensors to inhibit their activity to regain balance between gravitational forces and desired body position.

1. receives information from the vestibular apparatus;
2. receives information from the muscle proprioceptors;
3. receives information from other sensory modalities;
4. contributes automatically to the required synergic muscle tone;
5. informs the cerebrum of the status quo of its activity; and
6. receives command from the cerebral cortex to automatically change, prepare, and adjust the required muscle synergies to perform a voluntary or necessary movement.

Organ of Equilibrium

The **vestibular organ,** or **vestibular apparatus,** is the primary area to inform the nervous system of the position of the head in space. The vestibular nerve carries such information to the spinal cord, cerebellum, brain stem, and cerebrum.

The information regarding orientation of the head in space becomes associated with other sensory information (e.g., visual space orientation, sound, tactile, proprioceptive within the cerebrum to refine

Main Functions of the Cerebellum

Before indulging in any detailed analysis of the cerebellum, one must recognize that

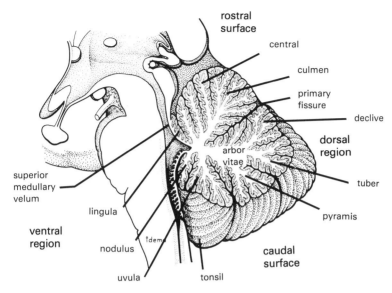

Fig. 15-2. Midsagittal section of the cerebellum.

the six above-mentioned abilities of this organ have a common objective, i.e., to monitor the required synergic tone of the muscles in any circumstances. In some conditions, for instance, a patient resting in bed, the efficiency of the cerebellum in monitoring muscle synergy is not very visible to the observer, whereas in other conditions like, for example, walking, the proficiency of the cerebellum in regulating the same task regarding equilibrium, posture, and movement can be readily appreciated by the observer. The cerebellum is the main automatic center of synergic muscle tone of the whole body.

Structure of the Cerebellum

It has already been mentioned that the cerebellum is a mass of neural tissue attached to the dorsum of the brain stem by three (cerebellar) peduncles, namely, the superior, also called the brachium conjunctivum, oriented with the mesencephalon and the upper pons; the middle, or brachium pontis, oriented with the bulk of the pons; and the inferior, or restiform body, oriented with the lower pons, the medulla, and the spinal cord. These peduncles contain the fibers entering and exiting the cerebellum.

The interval between the two superior cerebellar peduncles is bridged by a sheath of pia and ependyma called **superior medullary velum.** The **inferior medullary velum** is the sheath between the cerebellum and medulla.

The cerebellar mass can be divided in different ways. A midsagittal section of the cerebellum (Fig. 15-2) permits the observer to distinguish an upper, rostral, and lower caudal surface. If one were to flatten the cerebellum and display its entire surface (Fig. 15-3), the following details would be visible: a **vermis** (L. a wormlike structure) in the midline, a **nodule,** two **flocculi** (L. tufts of flakes), and two large **cerebellar hemispheres.**

Two flocculi and the nodulus form the **flocculonodular lobe.**

Across the upper surface of the cerebellum there is a cleft called **primary fissure** (Figs. 15-3 and 15-4), which is used as a

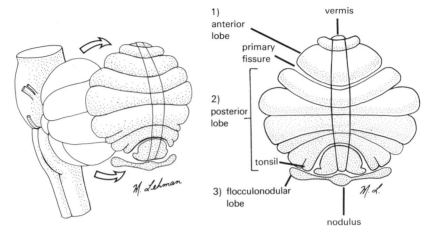

Fig. 15-3. Sketch of flattened cerebellar surface.

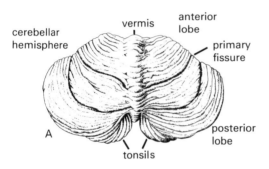

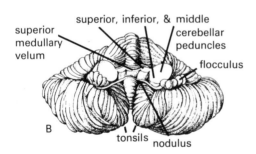

Fig. 15-4. Cerebellum. (A) Superodorsal view; (B) ventral view.

landmark to divide the cerebellar hemispheres into the **anterior** and **posterior lobes.** There are two bulging masses in the inferior portion of the posterior lobe called **cerebellar tonsils.**

A midsagittal section of the cerebellum (Fig. 15-2), i.e., cutting in halves the vermis and the nodulus lengthwise in the midline, displays a number of arborizations, together called **arbor vitae** (L. tree of life). The only ones of concern in this text are the **nodule,** the **uvula,** and the **pyramis** (on the inferior surface). The **lingula** is attached to the superior medullary velum, which is the caudal continuation of the tectum of the mesencephalon between the superior cerebellar peduncles.

A section across the whole cerebellum in the plane of the superior cerebellar peduncle (Fig. 15-5) reveals **gray** and **white matter.**

The gray matter forms the surface or the cortex with three types of cell layers and four pairs of nuclei in the core of the cerebellum, namely, the **fastigial,** the **globose,** the **emboliform,** and the **dentate nuclei.** The globose and emboliform nuclei are together also known as the **nucleus interpositus.**

The cerebellar white matter is located under the cerebellar cortex, around the nuclei, and in the cerebellar peduncles connecting the cerebellar cortex and the cerebellar nuclei with other CNS structures.

If straightened out, the numerous infoldings of the cerebellar cortex forming the **folia (laminae)** are calculated to measure frontocaudally approximately 1 m.

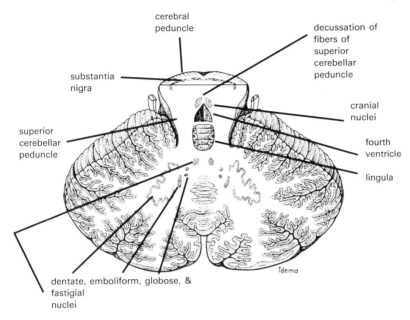

cerebral peduncle

decussation of fibers of superior cerebellar peduncle

substantia nigra

cranial nuclei

superior cerebellar peduncle

fourth ventricle

lingula

dentate, emboliform, globose, & fastigial nuclei

ĭdema

Fig. 15-5. Cross-section of cerebellum.

Divisions of the Cerebellum

With these internal and external views of the cerebellum in mind, one can now classify the structures into three divisions.

The **vestibulocerebellum,** also known as the **archicerebellum,** consists of the flocculonodular region.

The **spinocerebellum,** also known as the **paleocerebellum,** is made of the anterior lobe region, including the lingula plus the pyramis, and the uvula.

The **pontocerebellum,** also known as the **neocerebellum,** consists of the posterior lobe (exclusive of the pyramis and the uvula).

General Rule of Cerebellar Circuitry

As a rule, signals from different regions of the CNS reach the cortex of the cerebellum, where they relay onto cortical cells, which transmit signals through complex processing to the appropriate nucleus or nuclei. The nuclei then send signals to regions outside the cerebellum to the CNS.

Vestibulocerebellar Loops

Fibers from the vestibular nuclei reach the flocculonodular cortex, which connects with the fastigial nucleus. This nucleus then returns signals to the vestibular nuclei. As an exception to this rule, some fibers of the vestibular nerve and nuclei connect directly with the fastigial nucleus.

As was mentioned in the previous chapter, the activity of the vestibulocerebellum, through the vestibular nuclei, bears indirectly on the spinal cord, through the vestibulospinal tracts, and on the reticular formation and cranial nerve nuclei through the medial longitudinal fasciculus (MLF). The vestibulocerebellum is concerned with signals informing of the position of the head in space. The fastigial nucleus also makes connections with the superior colliculus.

The main function of the vestibulocerebellum is to respond in a reflex manner to gravitational stimuli of the vestibular apparatus.

Spinocerebellar Loops

The four tracts that ascend from each side of the spinal cord to the cerebellum are described below.

1. The **posterior spinocerebellar tract (ipsilateral lateral funiculus),** along which fibers travel from the column of Clarke (T1 to L2) and reach the paleocerebellum through the inferior cerebellar peduncle. These fibers convey proprioceptive information of the lower half of the body.
2. The **anterior spinocerebellar tract (contralateral lateral funiculus),** along which fibers travel from the intermediate and anterior spinal gray of the spinal cord and reach the spinocerebellum

through the superior cerebellar peduncle. These fibers transmit proprioceptive information of the lower half of the body. Due to the double decussation (Fig. 15-6), the input to the cerebellum is ipsilateral.

3. The **cuneocerebellar tract,** along which fibers are sent from the accessory cuneate nucleus (also known as the external or lateral cuneate nucleus) to reach the paleocerebellum ipsilaterally through the superior and inferior peduncles. These fibers transport proprioceptive information of the upper half of the body.
4. The **rostral spinocerebellar tract (ipsilateral),** along which fibers travel from the gray matter of the upper spinal cord and reach the spinocerebellum through the upper and lower peduncles. These fibers carry proprioceptive information of the upper part of the body.

The essential task of these paths is to transmit to the spinocerebellum pro-

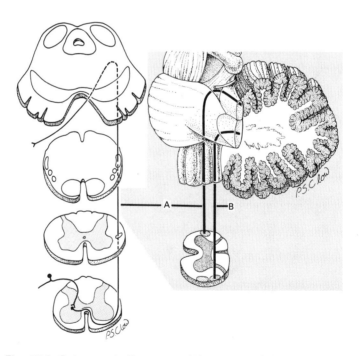

Fig. 15-6. Spinocerebellar tracts. (A) Anterior; (B) posterior.

prioceptive information of the muscles of the body.

The spinocerebellum finds its output through the nucleus interpositus (globose and emboliform) mainly to the red nucleus and the reticular formation, but also to the nucleus ventralis lateralis of the thalamus to inform the cerebrum through the superior cerebellar peduncle.

The main function of the spinocerebellum is synergic monitoring of "basic" postures and movement.

Pontocerebellar Loops

Important input to each side of the pontocerebellum comes from the contralateral cerebral cortex through the massive corticopontine as well as some tectal fibers, which synapse in the pontine nuclei ipsilaterally. These nuclei send fibers across the pons to reach through the middle cerebellar peduncle the opposite pontocerebellar hemisphere (Fig. 15-7).

Some important facts about the pontocerebellum ought to be emphasized:

1. The input from the pontine nuclei to the pontocerebellum is concerned with complex patterns of synergic coding affecting groups of muscles. It operates mainly under the control of the cerebral cortex.
2. The output of the pontocerebellum through the dentate nucleus is mainly to the ventralis lateralis nucleus of the thalamus to inform the cerebral cortex and to the brain stem to enhance and refine the activity of the nuclei (red nucleus, cranial nerve nuclei, reticular nuclei), thus ensuring optimally coordinated synergy of the muscles employed in skilled movement.
3. Pontocerebellar fibers connect mainly with the pontocerebellum, but also with the spinocerebellum and the vestibulocerebellum.
4. The main function of the pontocerebellum is the adjustment of synergy in voluntary skilled movement.

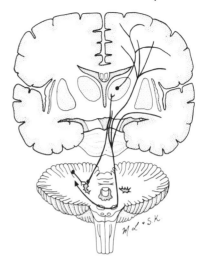

Fig. 15-7. Corticopontocerebellothalamocortical loop.

Other Connections of the Cerebellum

The cerebellum (Fig. 15-8) is also connected with the following structures.

Inferior Olive

Strong feed-back connections are established between each inferior olive and its contralateral (principally) and ipsilateral cerebellar half, through the olivocerebellar and cerebelloolivary tracts.

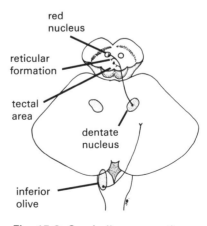

Fig. 15-8. Cerebellar connections.

Red Nucleus

Connections are established with the red nucleus through the rubrocerebellar and cerebellorubral tracts.

Tectum of the Midbrain

Connections are established with the tectum of the midbrain through the tectocerebellar tracts.

The tectum has connections with the reticular formation, cranial nerve motor nuclei, pontine nuclei, inferior olives, and spinal cord.

Reticular Nuclei

Connections are established with the reticular nuclei through the reticulocerebellar and cerebelloreticular paths.

Faced with these profuse connections, the student may fail to identify the main organizational circuitry of the cerebellum as a component of the nervous system unit. In order to gain the required perspective, it is convenient to focus the attention on the corticocerebellocortical loop.

Corticocerebellocortical Loop

The cerebellum is indirectly but strongly linked with the cerebral cortex. This link is the corticopontocerebellothalamocortical loop, comprehensively called the **corticocerebellocortical loop,** in which the cerebellum plays a key role.

Components of the Corticocerebellocortical Loop

As illustrated in Figure 15-7, the cerebral cortex sends bundles of fibers from the different lobes to the pontine nuclei ipsilaterally. The pontine nuclei process the signals and send fibers to the opposite cerebellar hemisphere, which integrates them with those coming in from other sources, and subsequently send the appropriate coded information mostly to the ventralis lateralis but also to the ventralis anterior nuclei of the thalamus. These "proprioceptive" association nuclei finally inform the motor areas 4 and 6 of the actual state of the motor system.

This loop not only has the role of informing the motor cortex but also makes it possible for the cerebellum to adjust the activity of the red nucleus, tectum, reticular nuclei, and vestibular nuclei, so that these structures may cooperate in harmony with the direct and indirect outputs of the cerebral cortex to the spinal cord and cranial nerve nuclei.

In essence, this loop could be known as the corticocerebellocortical motor setting loop, as it sets up proper dynamic conditions in four main structures and informs the cortex of what is happening in their neural links. It has been ascertained that practically any kind of sensory stimuli influences the electrical activity of the cerebellum. How this information is used by the cerebellum is still a matter of conjecture. Its role may be to improve the processing of information related to any sensorimotor activity in the whole body.

Five Signs of Cerebellar Lesions

Asynergia—lack of muscle coordination; incoordination.

Ataxia—(Gr. *taxis* order) lack of organized movement. In essence it means the same as asynergia, i.e., lack of muscle coordination. **Cerebral ataxia** is due to cerebral damage. Incoordination of movements may exhibit a number of peculiarities that can indicate which part of the nervous system is the source of it.

Hypotonia—reduced tonus of the muscles. This condition is present in most cases of cerebellar lesions.

Asthenia—reduced strength of the muscle.

Fatigability—increased tendency of the muscle to easily become tired.

Expression of the Four Cerebellar Signs in Posture

In a standing position, the patient may express the cerebellar deficiency in that he/she shows "weakness" in posture and sways as an expression of imbalance. (There is an attempt to compensate for this unsteadiness, i.e., insecurity of retaining the erect position, by broadening the base of support, which the patient does by assuming a broad-based stance.

Expression of the Four Cerebellar Signs in Movement

In movement, the signs observed regarding posture may be exaggerated, and additional signs may appear, namely,

1. tremor (shaking), when the patient attempts voluntary movements, for which reason it is called **intention tremor.** The oscillations of the tremor are usually coarse (ample and slow);
2. poor gait (i.e., manner or style of walking); in a patient with a cerebellar lesion the gait is clumsy, staggering, lopsided, and broad-based;
3. speech disturbances; and
4. nystagmus.

Signs (1) and (2) become exaggerated when the patient closes his/her eyes.

The particular type of these four signs varies with the type of lesion.

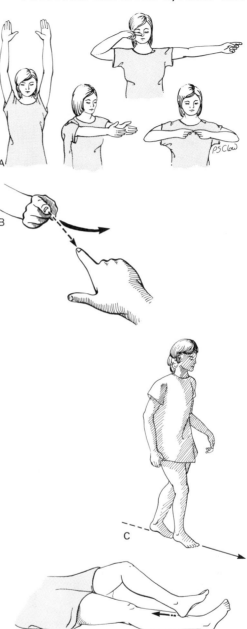

Fig. 15-9. Testing motor functions. (A) Position and movement test; (B) finger-finger test; (C) tandem walk test; (D) heel-shin test.

Tests for Cerebellar Function

By asking the patient to perform a precise task like touching the tip of the examiner's finger or his/her own nose with the index finger with his/her eyes closed (Fig. 15-9), one may witness in cases of impaired cerebellar function the following signs, apart from clumsiness and tremor:

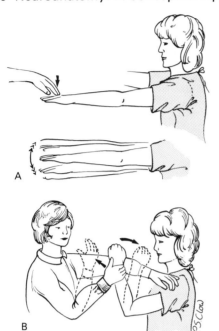

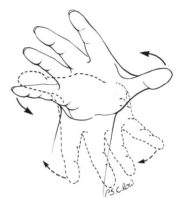

Fig. 15-11. Diadochokinesis.

Fig. 15-10. Testing motor functions. (A) Rebound effect; (B) overshooting.

1. decomposition of movements; the movement is carried out in steps in an attempt to correct errors observed by visual clues;
2. **dysmetria;** this disorder expresses itself in faulty measure of distance and position; and
3. **past point sign;** the finger misses the tip of the nose and touches the face.

To test the so-called **rebound effect** (Fig. 15-10), indicative of malfunction, the patient is asked to keep his/her arms elevated straight forward and the examiner applies a quick push to lower the arms. In the case of a rebound effect, the ensuing response is an up and down oscillation of one or both arms.

To test for **overshooting** (Fig. 15-10), the patient is asked to keep the forearm semiflexed in a fixed position. The examiner applies pressure to extend the fore-

arm and then quickly lets go of the arm. In response one may observe an overflexion of the forearm, which is called overshooting.

Diadochokinesis (Gr. *diadochos* succeeding; *kinesis* movement) is a term describing the function of alternating organized movements like those in quick pronation and supination of the hands (Fig. 15-11). In **dysdiachokinesis (adiadochokinesis)** the patient performs such movements poorly.

In cerebellar malfunctions the myotatic reflexes are most frequently reduced, while they may exhibit a pendular reaction (Fig. 15-12).

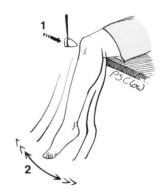

Fig. 15-12. Pendular reaction.

Three Cerebellar Syndromes

Flocculonodular Syndrome—Axial Ataxia

In the **flocculonodular syndrome,** or **axial ataxia,** there is obvious disturbance of equilibrium, affecting the body (head axis synergy). The patient sways when standing and walks unsteadily because of imperfect coordination of the axis of the body. Nystagmus may develop. If the fastigial nucleus is involved, hypotonia appears. Irritation of the flocculonodular region produces vertigo.

Spinocerebellar Syndrome—Limbs Ataxia

In the **paleocerebellar syndrome,** or **limbs ataxia,** hypotonia and asynergia of posture and movement appear, affecting the lower limbs and trunk. If the lesion extends to the most posterior regions of the anterior lobe, it also affects the upper limbs.

Pontocerebellar Syndrome

In the **pontocerebellar syndrome** the four cerebellar signs described above, i.e., ataxia, hypotonia, asthenia, and fatigability, with their expressions in posture as well as movement, appear positive, especially if the onset of the lesion is quick.

One-Sided Cerebellar Lesions

The cerebellar signs appear ipsilaterally in cases of one-sided cerebellar lesions.

Note: Ataxia of the limbs, ataxia of gait and posture, and intention tremor are the hallmarks of cerebellar disease.

Cerebellar Cortex

Among the billions of neurons composing the cerebellar cortex, the five main types are: granule, Golgi, Purkinje, basket, and stellate cells. These neurons are arranged systematically, contributing to a pattern of three cortical layers (Fig. 15-13). From the innermost to the outermost, the names of these layers and their cell body contents are

granular layer—granule and Golgi neural cell bodies;
Purkinje layer—Purkinje neural cell bodies; and
molecular layer—stellate and basket neural cell bodies.

The arrangement of these neurons is schematically represented in Figure 15-14.

Axonal Features

Some of the axonal features of the cortical cellular arrangement are listed below.

1. The axons of granule cells reach the molecular layer where they typically bifurcate in a T-shape and arrange themselves along the longitudinal axis of the cerebellar folia in a manner similar to the wires of telephone lines and synapse with dendrites of Purkinje cells. Their arrangement gives them the name **parallel fibers.**
2. The axons of Golgi cells synapse with the dendrites of granule cells, which are surrounding afferent fiber terminals. This complex, i.e., the afferent fiber terminal, the dendrites of granule cells, and the axon terminals of Golgi cells, is called **glomerulus** (Figs. 15-14A and 15-14B).
3. The axons of Purkinje cells make an inhibitory synapse with neurons of cerebellar nuclei.
4. The axons of basket cells make an inhibitory synapse with Purkinje cell

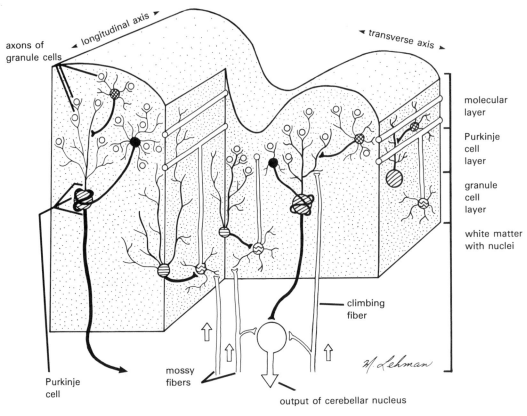

Fig. 15-13. Cytoarchitecture of cerebellum.

bodies, forming around each one of them a basket-like nest.

5. The axons of stellate cells make an inhibitory synapse with the apical dendrites of Purkinje cells.

Afferent Types of Fibers to the Cerebellum

There are two well-known types of fibers coursing to the cerebellum, i.e., **mossy fibers** and **climbing fibers.**

The mossy fibers come from many areas, e.g., the spinal cord, vestibular ganglion and nuclei, reticular formation, trigeminal nuclei, and pontine nuclei. These are excitatory fibers giving off collaterals to the cerebellar nuclei and terminal branches to the granule cells.

The climbing fibers make a typical input to the cerebellum from the inferior olive. They climb along the dendritic arborization of the Purkinje cells.

A less documented and more recently discovered input to the cerebellum is made by the aminergic fibers, originating from raphe nuclei and locus ceruleus.

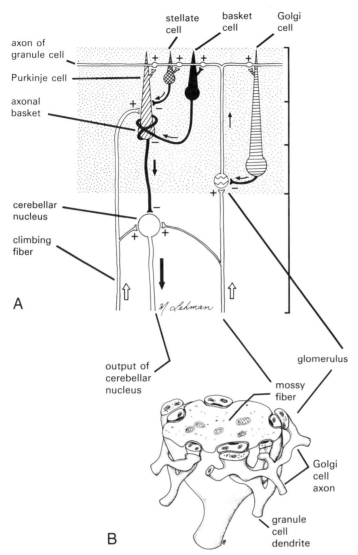

Fig. 15-14. (A) Circuitry of cerebellum; (B) glomerulus.

Cerebellar Cortex Laminar Arrangement

The connectivity between the cerebellar cortex and cerebellar nuclei follows a laminar arrangement as depicted in Figure 15-15.

Perpendicular Arrangement Between Olivocerebellar and Other Inputs

The distribution of fibers from the inferior olive to the cerebellum (climbing fi-

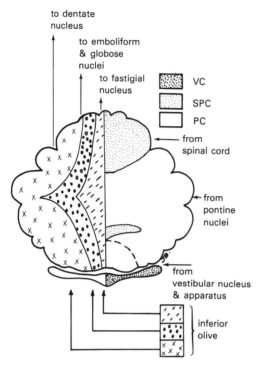

Fig. 15-15. Corticonuclear laminar arrangement.

Cerebellar Circuitry

The excitatory impulses reaching the cerebellum stimulate through collaterals the neurons of cerebellar nuclei and through terminals the Purkinje and granule cells.

The granule cells are excitatory to the other four types of neurons (Fig. 15-14), while the other four types of neurons are inhibitory. The outcome of this circuitry is projected by the Purkinje cells through their axons toward the neurons of the cerebellar nuclei. By the inhibitory action of the circuitry, it modulates the key output of the cerebellum to the CNS through the cerebellar nuclei.

bers) closely follows the laminar organization.

The distribution of fibers from the pontine nuclei, vestibular system, and spinal cord to the cerebellum (mossy fibers), in relation with the climbing fibers, is currently being debated. It is suggested that their arrangement follows a perpendicular pattern.

Somatotopic Mapping of the Cerebellar Cortex

Figure 15-16 illustrates how the different regions of the body and head are represented following a somatotopic organization in both regions, i.e., the anterior lobe and the posterior lobe. This correlation is still being investigated.

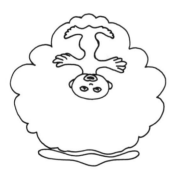

Fig. 15-16. Cerebellar cortex body mapping.

Suggested Readings

Armstrong DM, Schild RF: An investigation of the cerebellar corticonuclear projections in the rat using an autoradiographic tracing method. 2. Projections from the hemisphere, Brain Res 141:235–249, 1978.

Barr ML, Kiernan JA: The Human Nervous System. Fourth Edition. Harper and Row, Philadelphia, pp. 157–175, 1983.

Batini C, Corvisier J, Destombes J, Gioanni H, Everett J: The climbing fibers of the cerebellar cortex, their origin and pathways in the cat, Exp Brain Res 26:407–422, 1976.

Carpenter MB: Human Neuroanatomy. Seventh Edition. Williams and Wilkins, Baltimore, pp. 399–434, 1976.

Chan-Palay V: Cerebellar Dentate Nucleus: Organization, Cytology and Transmitters, Springer-Verlag, Berlin, 1977.

Colin F, Manil J, Desclin JC: The olivocerebellar system. 1. Delayed and slow inhibitory effects: An overlooked salient feature of cerebellar climbing fibers, Brain Res 187:3–27, 1980.

Cooper IS, Riklan M, Snider RS, Eds.: Cerebellum, Epilepsy, and Behavior, Plenum Press, New York, 1974.

Cooper IS, Ed.: Cerebellar Stimulation in Man, Raven Press, New York, p. 222–232, 1978.

Gilman S, Bloedel JR, Lechtenberg R: Disorders of the Cerebellum, FA Davis, Philadelphia, 1981.

Heimer L: The Human Brain and Spinal Cord, Springer-Verlag, New York, pp. 211–224, 1983.

House EL, Pansky B, Siegel A: A Systematic Approach to Neuroscience. Third Edition. McGraw-Hill, New York, pp. 320–349, 1979.

King JS, Andrezik JA, Falls WM, Martin GF: The synaptic organization of the cerebello-olivary circuit, Exp Brain Res 26:159–170, 1976.

Larsell O, Jansen J: The Comparative Anatomy and Histology of the Cerebellum, The Human Cerebellum, Cerebellar Connections, and Cerebellar Cortex, University of Minnesota Press, Minneapolis, 1972.

Nyberg-Hansen R, Horn J: Functional aspects of cerebellar signs in clinical neurology, Acta Neurol Scand, Suppl 51:219–245, 1972.

Palay SL, Chan-Palay V: Cerebellar Cortex: Cytology and Organization, Springer-Verlag, Heidelberg, 1974.

Walberg F, Brodal A: The longitudinal zonal pattern in the paramedian lobule of the cat's cerebellum: an analysis based on a correlation of recent HRP data with results of studies with other methods, J Comp Neurol 187:581–588, 1979.

16

Motor System

As the brain works as a unit, it follows from this fact that faulty motor components and also faulty sensory information may compromise the efficiency of motor coordination.

Given the vast number of neural motor and sensory components, the number of lesions, combinations of lesions, and consequent clinical signs is immense, stretching far beyond the comprehensive scope of textbooks. Therefore, it is essential that the student become aware of the meaning of certain terminology and the importance of a clear understanding of the characteristics of the signs of motor system malfunctions to find out how and where a motor disorder is rooted.

Terminology

The terms **sensory** and **motor neurons** describe neurons which compose the spinal and cranial nerves.

To varying degrees, the sensory and motor neurons are continuously interacting through their loops. The activity of the sensorimotor loop is constantly under the influence of other neuronal groups, classified as components of the sensorimotor system, within the central nervous system (CNS).

To distinguish the motor neurons from the other neuronal groups influencing them, these terms were taken into use: **lower motor neurons** = the motor neurons, and **upper motor neurons** = the ones influencing the lower motor neurons (Fig. 16-1).

At a time when the knowledge of the motor system was limited to the motor cortex and the motor neurons, these two terms were clear and useful. As the number of components added to the concept motor system increased, the clarity of the term upper motor neuron began to become doubtful.

Today the term is riddled with question marks and could imply so many different things that its use would be confusing in a rigorous discussion. Some scientists have therefore opted for discontinuing the use of the terms upper and lower motor neurons. Other scientists advocate that the meaning of the term upper motor neuron lesion be restricted to refer to a lesion of the neurons of the cerebral cortex forming

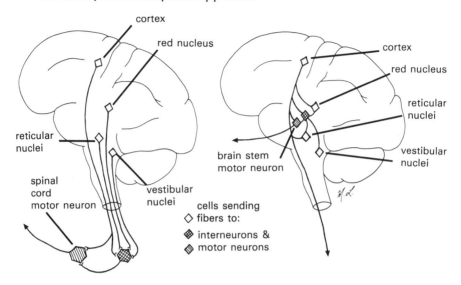

Fig. 16-1. Upper and lower motor neurons.

the direct and indirect paths to the spinal and cranial nerve nuclei. All facts considered, the two terms remain useful in general clinical practice, because they distinguish two major groups of clinical signs, even if the term upper motor neuron lesion is vague when not further specified.

The lower motor neurons are the cell units forming the **final common pathway,** a term which emphasizes its role as final common output of the CNS activity.

The terms direct and indirect corticospinal and corticocranial nerve nuclei paths were introduced and defined in Chapters 12 to 14 as particular components of the motor system.

The term corticocerebellocortical motor setting loop was identified in Chapter 15 as another component of the motor system.

Another important loop, also defined as a component of the motor system, is the corticosubcorticocortical motor setting loop.

Note on Two Terms

The terms **pyramidal tract, path,** and **system** relate to the corticospinal and corticobulbar tracts or their components.

The terms **extrapyramidal tracts, paths, and system** have referred to different components at different historical times. The term extrapyramidal disease is conventionally used in clinical practice in reference to a group of diseases with common clinical signs, some of which are related to the basal ganglia. In this perspective, the term remains useful among clinicians. Largely speaking, however, these terms encompass all nonpyramidal tracts that influence motor activity. Within this general concept the corticosubcoticocortical and the corticocerebellocortical loops are components of the extrapyramidal system.

Leading scientists advocate that the usage of the terms pyramidal and extrapyramidal be avoided altogether because of their vagueness.

Malfunction of the Motor System

Signs of motor malfunctions appearing in lesions affecting muscles, peripheral nerves, the spinal cord, cranial nerves, and the cerebellum have been described in previous chapters. At this point it is convenient to introduce a few clinical concepts of motor dysfunction in order to illustrate the consequences of lesions of cerebral structures, even before analyzing the structural components of the corticosubcorticocortical loop.

Voluntary Movements in Cerebral Lesions

In any type of cerebral motor system lesions, the amount and/or efficiency of voluntary skilled movements is reduced if not abolished. The motor malfunction becomes aggravated during emotional stress.

Dyskinesias: Hyperkinesias and Hypokinesias

Dyskinesia means impairment of the power of voluntary motion. There are two types: paralytical disorders, also known as **hypokinesias,** which are manifest in abnormal decreased muscular movements; and non-paralytical disorders, also known as **hyperkinesias,** which are evident in the execution of involuntary, inefficient movements. The hyperkinesias (involuntary movements) may occur either superimposed on voluntary movements or independently.

Bradykinesia (Gr. *bradys* slow) means abnormally slow muscle contraction.

Not included in the dyskinesias, by definition, is any exaggerated muscular hyperactivity which is due only to emotional causes, even if the movements become abnormal.

A clear understanding of these defined terms makes it possible to conceive that a dyskinetic patient can show signs of hypokinesia and hyperkinesia simultaneously.

Types of Dyskinesias

Parkinsonism or Paralysis Agitans

Parkinsonism or **paralysis agitans** is a disease characterized by three cardinal signs: balanced hypertonus (flexor and extensor hypertonus), i.e., rigidity, tremor (hyperkinesia), and impoverished voluntary movements (hypokinesia).

The voluntary movements of hypokinetic patients are characterized by a delay in their onset and slowness in their execution.

The balanced hypertonus of flexor and extensor muscles is due to an increased positive input from higher centers over the α and static γ motor neurons. This hyperactive state of the motor neurons may be unstable and in such a case cause a muscular tremor to develop when the patient is at rest, due to a continuous alternating adjustment of the myotatic reflex. The tonic properties of the stretch reflex are exaggerated in flexors and extensors. This activity produces a stiffness, rigidity of the muscles (flexors and extensors).

When the examiner tries to stretch a muscle, he/she may witness the lead pipe phenomenon (if there is no strong resting tremor) or the cogwheel pheomenon (especially if there is obvious tremor at rest).

Peculiarities of this tremor at rest of a frequency of 5 cycles per second (c.p.s.) in this disease are that it is regular and has low amplitude and it disappears during sleep and in the execution of voluntary movements.

In parkinsonism the voluntary movements of the patient are slow, retarded. When walking, the patient takes short steps with no arm movements. There is no facial mimic **(mask face),** and the speech is slow and monotonous. This impoverished state of voluntary movements is due to the systemic hypertonicity.

The muscular strength may well be preserved, but the muscle power to execute ample movements is diminished. The variance in degree of intensity and predominance of any of the three cardinal signs in individual cases is ample.

Chorea

Chorea (Gr. *choreia* dance) is a motor disorder characterized by frequent, random, quick movements of short duration, executed alone or superimposed on voluntary movements. There are different types of chorea, clinically identified on the basis of their differences regarding the etiology, intensity, and other aspects of the motor disorder.

Athetosis

Athetosis (Gr. *athetos* without position; *osis* condition) is a motor disorder characterized by recurrent, slow, and continual writhing movements (contortions) affecting the body and the extremities, particularly the distal muscles of the upper limb.

Dystonia

Dystonia (Gr. *dys* bad; *tonos* tone) is a motor disorder characterized by (1) very slow, alternating contraction-relaxation of agonist and antagonist muscles and (2) long (several minutes or longer) sustained contractions of a group of muscles that maintain the region of the body involved in a bizarre position.

Dystonia affects any part of the body, but most frequently the axial body and basal apendicular regions. The biased intensity and duration of these muscular contractions end up deforming the body skeleton. Usually, during the first stages of the disease the pattern described above in

(1) predominates, while (2) takes over as the disease advances.

Hemiballism

Hemiballism (Gr. *hemi* half; *ballismos* jump, throw) is a motor disorder characterized by sudden, quick, violent, spasmodic, flinging movements of the extremities, affecting one side of the body only (left or right).

Corticosubcortico-cortical Loop and Motor Disorders Due to its Lesions

In primitive animals like reptiles and birds, the corpus striatum, together with other subcortical nuclei, acts as the highest motor center regulating the coordination of their motor activity.

The cerebral cortex in man has taken over this task of coordination among

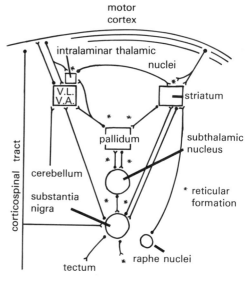

Fig. 16-2. Diagram of corticosubcorticocortical loop.

others while still leaving many other important concerns to the subcortical nuclei, which are looped through the thalamus into the cortex and constitute another intermediate circuit (like the corticocerebellocortical loop) of the whole neural system to perform, among others, motor functions.

In the diagram of Figure 16-2, the following components are represented:

1. cortical areas projecting to subcortical nuclei;
2. striatum;
3. pallidum;
4. ventral lateral and ventral anterior thalamic nuclei;
5. intralaminar nuclei;
6. reticular formation;
7. subthalamic nucleus;
8. substantia nigra; and
9. sensorimotor cortex (projecting toward spinal and cranial nerve nuclei).

For the sake of conceptualization we can consider that the main loop is cortex → striatum → pallidum → thalamus → cortex, the other structures being modifiers of this main circuit.

The structures listed above from (2) to (8) have usually been included as components of the basal ganglia, and their malfunction is classified as disorders of the basal ganglia. Given the current definition of ganglion and the inconsistency regarding which structures are included in the term basal ganglia, many scholars have recommended that this term be abandoned.

Corticostriatal Projections

Connections between cortical areas and the subcortical nuclei have been debated in the literature. A list of the most widely accepted connections is presented in Table 16-1.

The most massive and best known connection is the corticostriatal path. Fibers of this tract come from all the hemispheric lobes. These fibers arrive at the striatum in

Table 16-1. Connections of the Cerebral Cortex Related to the Corticosubcorticocortical Loop

Caudate nucleus
Putamen
Substantia nigra
Reticular formation
Thalamus

a topographically organized manner, e.g., frontal lobe to head of caudate and parietal lobe to body. It has been suggested that the coded information arriving at the striatum contains sensory as well as motor information of programmed learned patterns.

Striatum

The striatum, i.e., caudate and putamen nuclei, acts as a processor of the sensorimotor input and channels it to the pallidum. Most of the input from the caudate to the pallidum courses through the putamen. The putamen is assisted in its processing task by additional information, which it receives from other centers (Table 16-2). The inputs that the caudate and putamen receive equip them for their undertaking of fine processing of information toward the sensorimotor cortex (mainly area 4) through the pallidum and thalamus. The input from the substantia nigra is dopaminergic and the input from the raphe nuclei is serotoninergic.

Table 16-2. Connections of the Striatum Related to the Corticosubcorticocortical Loop

Afferents		Efferents
Cerebral cortex		
Substantia nigra (dopaminergic)		
Raphe nuclei (serotoninergic)	→ Striatum →	Substantia nigra Pallidum
Reticular formation		
Intralaminar thalamic nuclei		

The striatum is the brain structure with the highest concentration of serotonin. The efferent connections of the striatum to the pallidum and the substantia nigra transmit **gamma-aminobutyric acid** (GABA).

In experiments where the striatum of mammals has been stimulated electrically, a variety of reactions have been obtained. Low-frequency stimulation produces arrest of any ongoing behavioral movement. High-frequency stimulation produces head turning and circling movements toward the side opposite of the striatum stimulated. If, through conditioning, the stimulus becomes associated with reward, it can serve as a signal to initiate the learned behavioral response without display of dyskinesia.

Stimulation of the striatum in man has produced psychic responses (e.g., smiling, confusion, anxiety, and slurred speech), indicating the importance of this structure not only in motor functions but also in many aspects of sensorimotor integration.

The hyperkinetic syndrome of choreas has been found to be associated first and foremost with alterations of the striatum. It is logical to assume that the various choreas are related to various degrees and particular types of disturbances of the striatum, from inflammatory to degenerative conditions. In Huntington's chorea, for example, a decrease in the level of GABA which is attributed to a reduction of cholineacetyltransferase has been verified.

In postmortem examinations of patients with hyperkinetic dystonia, lesions have been found located in the striatum but also affecting many sites of the brain other than the striatum itself.

To sum up, chorea, athetosis, and dystonia have been associated with malfunctions of the striatum. However, neither of these disorders exclusively involve the striatum, nor is it conclusive that the original cause of the malfunctions is rooted in the striatum.

Globus Pallidus

The **pallidum,** another link in the corticosubcorticocortical circuit, has a number of connections, which are presented in Table 16-3.

The main input comes from the striatum with GABA as the neurotransmitter.

The main output travels to the thalamus via two bundles of fibers, the **ansa lenticularis** and the **lenticular fasciculus,** which together form the **thalamic fasciculus.** (The thalamic fasciculus becomes reinforced by the cerebellothalamic fibers.) Most of the fibers of the thalamic fasciculus end in the ventralis lateralis and ventralis anterior nuclei of the thalamus, while a few fibers terminate in the intralaminar thalamic nuclei (centromedian).

The ansa lenticularis courses around the internal capsule. The lenticular fasciculus courses across the internal capsule through **Forel's field H_2.** The ansa lenticularis and the lenticular fasciculus converge in **Forel's field H (prerubal field)** and continue as the thalamic fasciculus through **Forel's field H_1** (Fig. 16-3).

The pallidum modulates the signals arriving from the striatum. In order to manage this, the pallidum establishes reciprocal connections with two structures, namely, the subthalamic nucleus and the reticular formation. The subthalamic nucleus feed-back connection to the pallidum appears to be strongly inhibitory. Experimental bilateral lesions of the pallidum in animals result in markedly poor movement.

Table 16-3. Connections of the Pallidum Related to the Corticosubcortico-cortical Loop

Afferents		Efferents
Striatum		Thalamus (VA
Subthalamic		and VL)
nucleus	→ Pallidum →	Intralaminar nuclei
Reticular		Subthalamic nucleus
formation		Reticular formation

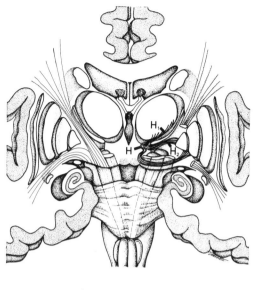

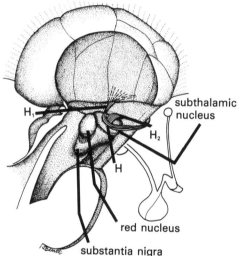

Fig. 16-3. Forel's fields.

Table 16-4. Connections of the VL and VA Nuclei of Thalamus Related to the Cortico-subcorticocortical Loop

Afferents		Efferents
Pallidum		Reticular
Reticular formation		formations
Intralaminar nuclei	→ VL and	Intralaminar
Cerebral cortex	VA nuclei →	nuclei
VP of thalamus		Cerebral cortex
Cerebellum		VP of thalamus
(ccc loop)		

the motor cortex. All the input from the pallidum and cerebellum, as well as proprioceptive information from the ventralis posterior, is integrated within these two nuclei. They also receive feed-back information from the motor cortex.

Electrical stimulation of the ventralis lateralis and ventralis anterior thalamic nuclei increases tonic stretch reflexes via the motor cortex.

Intralaminar Nuclei

It is noteworthy that the intralaminar nuclei send fibers crossing the internal capsule to reach the striatum, especially the nucleus centrum medianum, since it is believed that these nuclei process interoceptive and nociceptive as well as other signals (Table 16-5). By their input, the nuclei are able to influence the processing of signals in the striatum.

Ventralis Lateralis and Ventralis Anterior Thalamic Nuclei

The various connections reported in the literature are listed in Table 16-4. It can be noticed that the ventralis lateralis and ventralis anterior thalamic nuclei constitute the final link between the corticosubcortical and the corticocerebellar loop toward

Table 16-5. Connections of Intralaminar Nuclei of Thalamus Related to the Cortico-subcorticocortical Loop

Afferents		Efferents
Cerebral cortex		
Reticular formation		
Pallidum		
VL and VA	→ Intralaminar	Striatum
Spinothalamic	nuclei →	VL and VA
tract		
Trigeminothalamic		
tract		

Reticular Formation

Three important facts about the reticular formation in relation to the corticosubcorticocortical loop are listed below.

1. It establishes connections with all the components of the loop.
2. The reticular formation plays an important regulatory excitatory and inhibitory role, influencing the lower motor neuron centers.
3. Given the many excitatory and inhibitory roles of this structure in the whole nervous system, scientists have supported the view that it is involved in practically all functions and states of the nervous system, e.g., sleep-wakefulness, emotional stress, distress, depression, REM (rapid eye movement during sleep), and sleep-walking. How these structures become involved in such a variety of behavioral aspects is currently being researched.

Subthalamic Nucleus

The **subthalamic nucleus** is apposed to the substantia nigra (of which it is considered to be a continuation by some scientists) and has connections with the reticular formation (Table 16-6).

The fiber connections from the subthalamic nucleus to the substantia nigra are well-documented, whereas in the reverse they are not.

This nucleus regulates by inhibitory action the activity of the pallidum through the pallidosubthalamopallidal loop. Destruction of this nucleus produces the hyperkinetic syndrome of hemiballism, caused by the ensuing lack of regulatory inhibitory influence on the corticosubcorticocortical loop through the pallidum, permitting the arrival of massive signals to the motor cortex.

In interrupting its connection with the reticular formation, the destruction of the subthalamic nucleus may also disrupt the balance of the reticulospinal tracts. In ex-

Table 16-6. Connections of Subthalamic Nucleus Related to the Corticosubcorticocortical Loop

Afferent		Efferent
Pallidum Reticular formation	→ Subthalamic nucleus →	Pallidum Reticular formation Substantia nigra

perimental animals with hemiballism, a transection of the lateral funiculus in the upper cord segments causes the signs to disappear, which thus indicates that the disorder is attributable to a malfunction of the descending tract(s).

Substantia Nigra

The **substantia nigra** has achieved its highest development in man. In the last decade, it has been the subject of intense studies using a wide range of histochemical and physiological techniques. It has been found to have a very large number of connections (Table 16-7).

Given these numerous connections, it appears to play a far more complex role than that of simply contributing to the regulation of the corticosubcorticocortical loop activity.

It is recognized that the substantia nigra is concerned with the adjustment of muscle tone of all muscles, extensors and flexors alike, enhancing or reducing it in both groups in the same direction.

The substantia nigra not only links up with the corticosubcorticocortical loop, as

Table 16-7. Connections of Substantia Nigra Related to the Corticosubcorticocortical Loop

Afferents		Efferents
Striatum		Striatum
Reticular formation		Reticular formation
Cortex	→ Substantia nigra →	Cortex
Subthalamic nucleus		Thalamus
		Amygdala
Amygdala		Tectum

already mentioned above, but it also has strong connections with the mesencephalic reticular, the tectal, and pretectal regions.

The syndrome of paralysis agitans (parkinsonism) has been found in post-mortem studies to be related to degenerative lesions of the substantia nigra bilaterally, when the signs affect the whole body, or contralaterally, when only one side of the body is affected.

Patients with parkinsonism have abnormally low levels of dopamine. Treating such patients with L-dihydroxyphenylalanine (L-DOPA, a precursor in the synthesis of dopamine) is most effective against akinesia, less against rigidity, and least against tremor. Apomorphine (a specific dopamine receptor agonist) is most effective against tremor, less effective against rigidity, and least against akinesia.

The dysfunction of the substantia nigra and clinically associated signs must not be looked upon simply as a nigrostriatal malfunction. The presence of other dopaminergic pathways and the connections of the substantia nigra must be taken into consideration.

The different connections established via the reticulospinal tracts and the tectal region impose different effects on the nervous system.

Surgical Lesions in Hyperkinetic States

The interruption of the corticospinal paths eliminates any hyperkinesia but produces paralysis of voluntary movements. A surgical lesion in the pallidum in a patient suffering from parkinsonism is effective in relieving the patient from rigidity; it reduces the exaggerated tonic component of the stretch reflexes but does not change the state of the phasic component of the stretch reflexes. A surgical lesion in the ventralis anterior or Forel's field H_1 has a relieving effect on tremor and rigidity but none on akinesia.

A large experimental bilateral lesion in the substantia nigra brings about pronounced hypokinesia with immobility in postures.

Irritation of the Sensory Motor Cortex Projecting to Spinal and Cranial Nerve Nuclei

A pathologic irritative process in or near the primary sensory motor cortex may produce what is known as **jacksonian fits.** It may start by clonic contractions locally in one part of the body and propagate segmentally to other parts, e.g., it may propagate from foot to calf to thigh to trunk, and even continue farther. If the propagation ends up affecting the whole body, loss of consciousness will result. The starting point of the convulsion may give an indication of the site of the cortex focally irritated. This type of focal seizures forms part of a wide variety of convulsive disorders called **epilepsies.**

Lesions of the Sensory Motor Cortex—Decorticate Rigidity

A lesion of the sensorimotor cortex may be more or less extensive and pronounced. For instance, it may be circumscribed to one small region or it may affect larger areas or even the whole sensory motor cortex of both hemispheres (Table 16-8).

Complicating matters even further, destruction and irritation of nearby regions may occur in combination. The smaller the region, the greater the chances to develop compensatory mechanisms. The essential

Table 16-8. Schematic Recapitulation of Motor System Lesions

	Lower Motor Neurons	Cerebellum	Subcortical Nuclei	Sensory Motor Cortex
Muscles	Atrophy, fibrillations, and fasciculation			No significant atrophy
Voluntary movements	Impaired or abolished	Impaired	Impaired	Impaired or abolished
Muscle tone	Hypotonus (flaccid)	Range: hypotonus (most commonly)	Range: hypertonus (most commonly)	Predominant hypertonus (spastic)
Myotatic reflexes	Reduced or abolished	Reduced; pendular reflexes may appear	Normal or enhanced; most frequently lead pipe or cogwheel	Predominant clasp-knife; clonus
Dyskinesias	Hypo- or akinesia	Hypokinesia and hyperkinesia (intention tremor)	Hypokinesia and hyperkinesia, chorea; athetosis, dystonia, hemiballism, tremor at rest may appear in parkinsonism	Hypokinesia
Muscle strength	Diminished or abolished	Diminished	Altered (most commonly)	Diminished or abolished
Muscle power	Diminished or abolished	Diminished	Diminished	Diminished or abolished

points to keep in perspective in a sensorimotor cortical lesion are explained below.

1. The initial state following the lesion is flaccid paralysis of the innervated region.
2. Some time after the lesion has come about, one may find by palpation that some muscle groups are flabby and hypotonic while others are hypertonic. This is due to the suppression of the regulatory control exerted over the motor neuron groups by the corticospinal tracts. This lack of control leaves the motor neuron groups at the mercy of brain stem influences and spinal cord inputs. The resulting imbalance of tone between antagonist groups of muscles causes abnormal postural patterns to develop. If the whole cortex is affected, the posture of the body is characterized as illustrated in Figure 16-4 by extended lower limbs and semiflexed up-per limbs. This posture is characteristic for **decorticate rigidity.** If one rotates the head of a person in such a condition to the right, the right upper limb is caused to extend and the left upper limb to flex. This phenomenon is inter-

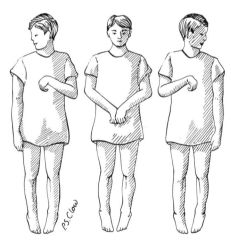

Fig. 16-4. Decorticate rigidity.

preted to be the release of the reflex mechanism for the performance of automatic walking established between the brain stem and spinal cord. Decortication releases the action of this circuitry. Rotation of the head stimulates mostly upper neck joint receptors, while it also may affect receptors of the utricle and saccule and those of the neck muscles. Such stimulation causes signals to be sent to the tectum and the cerebellum, from where discharges reach the spinal cord.

3. The imbalance of tone between antagonist muscle groups produces in the dominant hypertonic muscle groups a state of spasticity, characterized by exaggerated hyperreflexive reactions to passive sudden stretch. This reaction can be tested in two ways. One is by a brisk and lightly sustained stretching of the muscles, which triggers a reaction consisting of rhythmic muscle contractions known as **clonus.** The other is by a brisk and continuous stretching of the muscles, which triggers a reaction characterized by two phases: first an increased muscular resistance to the stretch, followed quickly by a suppression of the resistance. This is called a **clasp-knife phenomenon** of spastic muscles, as it resembles the opening of a pocket-knife blade.

   The first step of the reaction, i.e., the increased resistance, is due to an increased activity of the myotatic stretch reflex. The second step, i.e., the fading of the resistance, is due to exaggerated inhibition of the myotatic reflex by Golgi tendon organs (Ib) and by group II afferents.

4. Another elicitable sign due to the release of the corticospinal regulatory motor control is Babinski's sign.

In summary, a lesion of the sensorimotor cortex may produce a release of regulatory motor control characterized by paralysis, first flaccid (hypotonic), followed by imbalanced tone of muscle groups. The hypertonic groups display a state of spasticity, detectable through their strong hyperreflexive responses to passive movements like myotatic reflex, clasp-knife phenomenon, and clonus. Babinski's sign may be elicitable.

Decerebrate Rigidity

If a transection is made at the level of the mesencephalon that functionally disconnects the cerebrum from the brain stem **(decerebration** or **encèphale isolé),** a syndromic state called **decerebrate rigidity** appears, the main characteristic of which is a pronounced increase in muscular tone in the extensor (antigravity) muscles, as shown in Figure 16-5.

When tested, the myotatic reflex responses are found to be markedly increased. The lengthening reaction (clasp-knife phenomenon) appears in response to passive stretching of the muscles.

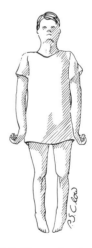

Fig. 16-5. Decerebrate rigidity.

If in the transection the red nucleus is destroyed also, the signs of decerebrate rigidity become more obvious, because the stimulatory influence of the red nucleus over flexor muscles is eliminated.

If in this decerebrate state the proprioceptive path spinocerebellum—interpositus to lateral vestibular nucleus is interrupted by the destruction of the nucleus interpositus, which exerts an inhibitory influence on the lateral vestibular nucleus, the extensor rigidity becomes more pronounced with still more exaggerated tilting of the head, a posture known as **opisthotonus** (Gr. *opisthen* behind; *tonos* tone), i.e., increased tone in the back.

The enhanced tonic activity of the vestibular nucleus over the γ motor neurons exerts through the spindles a tonic hyperactivity on α motor neurons, hence known as γ **rigidity.** There is also a relative increase of tonic stimulation from the vestibular nucleus on α motor neurons of extensor muscles over flexors. If the vestibular nucleus is destroyed, the extensor hyperactivity disappears.

Syndromic States of Internal Capsule Lesions

In comprehensive textbooks of clinical neuroanatomy it is usual to find a stereotyped description of a syndrome caused by lesions of the internal capsule. This syndrome has been tagged with the very misleading term **pyramidal syndrome,** based on the old erroneous conception that the fibers composing the pyramidal tract are the most important (if not the only) ones lesioned.

Recently, a more correct term has been introduced—the **internal capsule syndrome.** Although this term certainly is an improvement, it still presents inconsistencies.

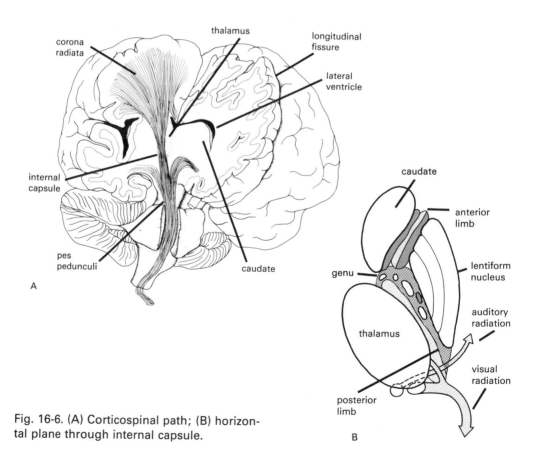

Fig. 16-6. (A) Corticospinal path; (B) horizontal plane through internal capsule.

1. The signs appearing after the lesion has occurred keep changing as time progresses.
2. The internal capsule is a large structure and varies with regard to its fiber components in its different regions and levels (Fig. 16-6), which has a decisive bearing on which types of signs will appear in the patient. For instance, the lesion may affect one limb (monoplegia) or one half of the body (hemiplegia). If the lesion involves the lower portion of the capsule, the fibers of the optic radiation may become affected, resulting in defects in vision, etc.
3. "Syndrome" ought to refer to a specific set of signs and it does not in this case. The term **syndromic states of internal capsule lesions** is generally used to side-step this dilemma in the nomenclature. Similarly, for other specific situations, other distinctive terms are used.

The most frequent causes of internal capsule lesions are vascular (hemorrhage, thrombosis, emboli), affecting the vessels irrigating the internal capsule, the vessel branches of the middle cerebral artery being the ones most often affected. Such vascular lesions belong to the general group of cerebral vascular lesions known as cerebral stroke lesions.

Internal Capsule Hemiplegic States

The most frequent signs brought on by sudden vascular lesions of the internal capsule usually affect contralaterally the limbs, lower face, tongue, and a few other structures. These signs add up to **hemiplegia** (Gr. *hemi* half, right or left; *plegia* paralysis or paresis).

Initial Stage or Shock Stage

In the **initial** or **shock stage of internal capsule hemiplegia** the patient may concurrently become unconscious, while all his/her body muscles become flaccid and his/her muscle reflexes abolished.

Unilateral internal capsule lesions do not cause loss of consciousness, nor do other unilateral subcortical or cortical hemisphere lesions causing only hemiplegia.

If the patient does not lose consciousness, the face, arm, and leg contralateral to the affected capsule lose muscle tone, related reflexes become markedly diminished or even abolished, and Babinski's sign may be elicited.

Compensatory Stage

If the patient recovers from the shock stage, the following syndrome develops on the affected side.

The abdominal reflexes remain absent. Five to 10 hours after the stroke one may obtain a plantar dorsiflexion response (i.e., Babinski's sign, if it was not previously elicitable).

One to 3 days later, the myotatic reflexes may be elicited, first becoming brisker than in the unaffected, normal side and finally hyperreflexive. Sometimes this hyperreflexive state may not develop within the usual period of a few days but after weeks or months.

As verified by palpation, the muscles at rest may be flabby or hypertonic, depending on the inputs received by the affected body part since the occurrence of the lesion. For instance, when the patient is in bed, the continuous weight of a heavy blanket on the tip of his/her toes will render the toe muscles hypertonic with hyperactive muscle spindle activity.

A description similar to the one given for sensorimotor cortical lesions affecting the muscles applies to internal capsule lesions, like muscle spasticity, clasp-knife phenomenon and clonus.

The passive resistance to stretching is more obvious in the lower limb when flexing it, because the hypertonus predomi-

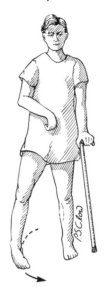

Fig. 16-7. Hemiparetic posture and walk.

nates in the extensor muscles. The hip is adducted, the knee is extended, and plantar flexion is present.

The passive resistance to stretching is more obvious in the upper limb when extending it, because the hypertonus predominates in the flexor muscles. The shoulder is adducted, the elbow flexed, the hand pronated, and fingers flexed.

If the patient is kept with the lower limbs flexed, extension hypertonus and hyperactivity of extensor muscles may be avoided. The paralysis or paresis affects the limb and, more particularly, the hand and foot. Isolated, voluntary movement of one finger or toe is impossible. The muscles involved in the majority of skilled motor movements are affected to the largest degree. The trunk muscles are less affected (because of their bilateral innervation and lesser dependence on cortical control).

There may be, more or less, retention or return of voluntary movement, starting in the proximal muscles. Also the regaining of control of voluntary muscle activity movement is more pronounced in the lower than the upper limb (Fig. 16-7).

The course of recovery depends on the particular physiotherapeutic method employed as well as other individual factors (age, level of cooperation, determination, etc.).

Suggested Readings

Adam J, Marsden CD, Merton PA, Morton HB: The effect of lesions in the internal capsule and the sensorimotor cortex on servo action in the human hand, J Physiol (London) 254:27–28P, 1976.

Barr ML, Kiernan JA: The Human Nervous System. Fourth Edition. Harper and Row, Philadelphia, pp. 331–344, 1983.

Brooks VB, Ed.: Motor Control. Handbook of Physiology. Second Edition. Section I: The Nervous System, Vol. 2. American Physiological Society, Bethesda, 1981.

Carpenter MB: Human Neuroanatomy. Seventh Edition. Williams and Wilkins, Baltimore, pp. 496–520, 1976.

Davis HL, Kiernan JA: Effect of nerve extract on denervated or immobilized muscles, Exp Neurol 72:582–591, 1981.

Dray A: The physiology and pharmacology of mammalian basal ganglia, Progr Neurobiol 14:221–235, 1980.

Hardy TL, Bertrand G, Thompson CJ: The position and organization of motor fibers in the internal capsule found during stereotactic surgery, Appl Neurophysiol 42:160–170, 1979.

Heimer L: The Human Brain and Spinal Cord, Springer-Verlag, New York, pp. 183–209, 1983.

House EL, Pansky B, Siegel A: A Systematic Approach to Neuroscience. Third Edition. McGraw-Hill, New York, pp. 350–397, 1979.

Kuypers HGJM: Anatomy of the descending pathways. In Handbook of Physiology, Sec. 1, The Nervous System, Vol. 2: Motor Control Part 2. American Physiological Society, pp. 597–666, 1981.

Kuypers HGJM, Martin GF, Eds.: Anatomy of descending pathways to the spinal cord, Progress in Brain Research, 57, Elsevier Excerpta Medica, Elsevier Science Publishers, New York, 1982.

Lundberg A: Control of spinal mechanisms from the brain. In Tower DB, Ed.: The Nervous System, Vol. 1: The Basic Neurosciences, Raven Press, New York, pp. 253–265, 1975.

Melvill-Jones G, Watt DGD: Muscular control of landing from unexpected falls in man, J Physiol (London) 219:729–737, 1971.

Pearson K: The control of walking, Sci Am 235(6):72–86, 1976.

Roland PE, Larsen B, Lassen NA, Skinhöj E: Supplementary motor area and other cortical areas in organization of voluntary movements in man, J Neurophysiol 43:118–136, 1980.

Ross ED: Localization of the pyramidal tract in the internal capsule by whole brain dissection, Neurology 30:59–64, 1980.

Szabo J: Strionigral and nigrostriatal connections, Appl Neurophysiol 42:9–12, 979.

17

Somatosensory System

Origin of Somatosensory Signals

The soma (Gr. body), in particular, the skin, muscles and joints, and, in general, the connective tissue (all of which by definition excludes the body viscera), is the source of somatosensory signals. Changes in all these body tissues translate into such signals. The nature of these changes depends on the types of stimuli imposed.

Types of Stimuli

Stimulus energy imposed on the somatic tissues includes **mechanical, thermal,** and **chemical** and activates the receptor endings in these tissues.

Stimulus Characteristics

Three stimulus characteristics have been of main concern in research: intensity, duration, and repetitiveness.

Receptor Endings

Receptor endings were defined as nerve endings that convert and transduce stimulus energy into electrical potentials, which in the form of impulses are conducted along the neurons and transmitted to other cells.

Types of Somatic Receptors

Somatic receptors are classified according to the categories described in Chapter 4.

Correlation Between Types of Stimuli and Types of Receptors

A simplistic concept was developed in the past in which a rigorous correlation of one type or shape of nerve ending exclusively with one type of stimulus and one type of sensation was construed without consideration for the many factors and phenomena that are involved in the stimulus-sensation process. This correlation is now known in the literature as **receptor specificity,** which implies that each receptor is specifically sensitive to only one type of stimulus and produces exclusively one type of sensation.

In defiance of the concept of receptor specificity, the **pattern of stimulus** concept was presented. Its passionate developers denied the receptor specificity theory any value and emphasized, also in a single-minded manner, that the type of sensation generated by any type of stimulus is exclusively dependent on the characteristics of the stimulus.

The debate concerning these two concepts has been bringing new insights into the complex stimulus-sensation process little by little for many years. Both concepts have meritorious points per se.

Receptor Specificity and Sensation Specificity

Receptors may pick up one only, several, or many types of stimuli.

The present concept of **receptor specificity** relates only to the intrinsic specificity of the receptors to best sense a specific type of stimulus and does not address itself to the kind of sensation triggered.

The present concept of **sensation specificity** relates to many complex factors, like the characteristics of the stimulus, the characteristics of the receptor, the location of the receptor, the path traveled by the signal, and the status quo of the pathway.

Considerations on the Stimulus-Receptor Coupling Efficiency

The transduction of each type of stimulus energy into sensory signal involves primarily three factors: the characteristics of the stimulus (intensity, duration, repetitiveness, etc.), the characteristics of the receptor (physical and chemical), and the location of the receptor, i.e., its medium, which may interact with or modify the stimulus.

Receptor Response: Electrical Impulses, Sensory Signals

Regardless of the stimulus-receptor coupling efficiency, each receptor has a particular capacity for adaptation to the stimulus ranging from none at all to very expedient. This peculiarity of the receptor response lies behind the terms **receptor adaptation,** and **receptor fatigue.** Non-adapting receptors continue to produce impulses as long as the stimulus persists. This activity serves to keep the nervous system informed of the status of the body.

Very fast adapting receptors adapt rapidly and respond primarily to a change in stimulus intensity. For instance, they may discharge signals only at the onset of the stimulus, discharge no signals if the stimulus remains constant, and discharge again only when the stimulus is withdrawn. This pattern of discharge is called **on-off receptor response.** It serves to notify the nervous system of the changes of the body. This range of coding information in the nervous system is very useful for the evaluation of the characteristics of the stimuli.

Processing of Sensory Signals Within the Central Nervous System

As soon as signals of different sensory modalities reach the central nervous system (CNS) through afferent fibers, they spread through their terminals. They then become modified within the different CNS regions in a complex manner. The higher the number of links by which the signals are processed the more complex is the modification of the signals.

The laminae of Rexed cannot be related to any particular sensory modality, with the exception, perhaps, of lamina I for noxious signals.

Perception of Sensory Signals

It is a familiar fact that the mind may utilize the sensorial system within extremes which oscillate from a very objective replication of information data to a greatly distorted interpretative rendition, or even a totally subjective inventive recreation of facts.

Many steps are involved in the transfer of information of sensory signals into perceptual interpretation. In this chapter it is convenient to deal with a few of those steps, showing as an analytical example what normally goes on most of the times when we are stimulated.

Combinations of Receptor Stimulation

An analysis of receptor stimulation must take into regard **time** and **space dimensions.**

The time dimension is fundamental in the outcome of signal processing. For the time being, it is sufficient for the beginner to merely keep this dimension in mind.

At any given time a region, i.e., space, of the body may be stimulated by one or several types of stimuli. Considering the simple case of one type, e.g., a mechanical stimulus affecting the skin, there are various conceivable possibilities of receptor stimulation.

Several receptors of the same type (shape), all belonging to the same neuron, may become stimulated.

Several receptors of the same type (shape), belonging to different neurons, may become stimulated.

Several receptors of different types, belonging to different neurons, may become stimulated.

The processing of the signals generated in every case may be handled in a different way in each instant. Generally, it can be said that the more receptors become stimulated, the more intense the signals become. The intensity of a stimulus can be detected by two mechanisms: by **frequency code,** which focuses on the increase in the number of action potentials in a neuron as the number of its stimulated receptors increases, and by **population code,** which pays heed to the increase in the number of active neurons stimulated.

Convergence and Divergence of Signals Within the CNS

As illustrated in Figure 17-1, the primary sensory neurons establish synapses with a number of second afferent neurons. This is known as **divergence** or **spread of** the signals. As also illustrated in Figure 17-1, a second afferent neuron receives one or several synapses from different primary sensory neurons. This is known as **convergence of the signals.**

Reciprocal Inhibition

In Figure 17-2 neuronal synaptic chains are shown where neuron a excites a' but inhibits b' through an interneuron, and neuron b excites b' while in turn inhibiting a' through an interneuron. This arrangement is called **reciprocal inhibition.** Neurons a' and b' are antagonists (to each other), which is a manner of signal discrimination by creating contrast.

Recurrent Inhibition

As illustrated in Figure 17-2, by recurrent axonal branches acting upon interneurons, neuron b', when stimulated, may inhibit the activity of adjacent neurons a' and c'. This limits the spread of excitation and is called **recurrent inhibition,** which is also a manner of signal discrimination by creating contrast.

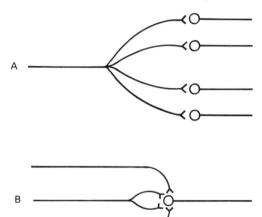

Fig. 17-1. Excitatory processes. (A) Divergence; (B) convergence.

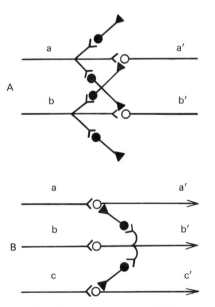

Fig. 17-2. Inhibitory processes. (A) Reciprocal inhibition; (B) recurrent inhibition.

Importance and Utility of These Inhibitory and Excitatory Processes

Viewing these inhibitory and excitatory processes not just as physical but as biophysical phenomena, one must call to mind the segmental pattern of organization and the tissue pattern of organization.

These two regional patterns of organization of the receptors and the systematic organization of pathways from the body to the brain permit the edification of an image of the body in the brain.

The highest centers of the brain establish priorities of information in the mapping process. For instance, the buccal and hand regions are very important for survival as compared to those of the limbs or trunk. The amplification in the cerebral cortex of each particular body region is executed along the specific pathways by the above-mentioned processes (divergence, convergence, inhibition, etc.).

Control of Higher Centers in Sensory Transmission

There is another important factor when considering how the brain manages this image of the body. Even if the process of body mapping in the cerebral cortex follows a set of priorities regarding the various aspects of sensation, the brain may need to modify these standard priorities of information arriving to the brain. In order to be able to conjure up the image of a particular spot in the body more accurately, or to establish any other changes in its priorities (like reducing or increasing the sensation of pain), the brain sends, through descending fibers, signals to the different sensory synaptic relay stations in each specific sensory path to modulate the activity as required.

Examples of descending pathways from primary sensory cortex that modulate the ascending afferent paths are corticothalamic (to ventralis posterior of thalamus), corticobulbar (to trigeminal, gracile, and cuneate nuclei), and corticospinal (to posterior horn).

Another example of a descending path particularly concerned with modulation of nociceptive information is the raphespinal tract (Fig. 17-3).

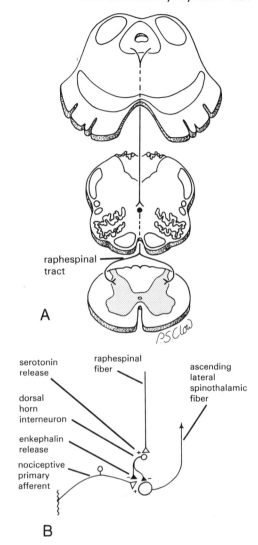

Fig. 17-3. (A) Raphespinal tract; (B) raphespinal fiber ending.

The raphespinal tract releases serotonin which activates enkephalinergic interneurons. These in turn inhibit the synaptic transmission of noxious signals.

These feed-back modulatory paths from higher centers to lower afferent synaptic stations afford freedom to the brain to make decisions as a unit regarding which informational priorities must be followed at a particular time. This central control of sensory transmission is the seat of great power. The information you permit to be processed in your brain may formulate your destiny.

Neuronal Receptive Field

The **receptive field** that each afferent neuron in the CNS has, is defined as the region of the body upon which stimulation excites or inhibits the activity of that neuron. This field can be modulated by increasing or reducing the excitation and by increasing or reducing the inhibition.

The smaller the receptive field of a neuron, the more topographically discriminative the information is that it processes. Conversely, nondiscriminative, diffuse information is processed by a large neuronal receptive field (Fig. 17-4).

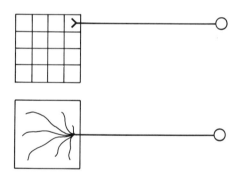

Fig. 17-4. Receptive fields.

Table 17-1. Characteristics of Two Submodalities of Pain Perception

Sharp Pain	Diffuse Pain
More accurately localized	Less accurately localized
Fast conduction (Aδ fibers)	Slow conduction (C fibers)
Short duration, closely related to the duration of the stimulus	May persist for some time after the removal of the stimulus.

Sensations

Sensory signals reaching the thalamocortical loops may produce **sensations.**

The various modalities of sensation within the somesthetic system are pain; warm and cold (temperature); light, crude, nondiscriminative touch; discriminative, refined touch; pressure; body position; body movement (kinesthesia); flutter and vibration; two-point discrimination touch; and stereognosis.

Pain

Pain is an unpleasant and warning sensation able to recruit more efficiently than any other modality of sensation the affective, intellectual, and emotional domains of the brain.

Pain Submodalities

Fitting adjectives for pain are burning, aching, stinging, searing, etc. One could list as many submodalities of pain as the number of accurately descriptive adjectives to cover the many subtleties of painful sensations.

Apart from this classification of pain submodalities by adjectives, it is important to recognize the difference between two submodalities of pain perception labeled as **sharp** and **diffuse (dull),** respectively. The more sharply the regional boundaries of pain are sensed (i.e., the more accurately its body source can be recognized), the more obviously it belongs to the submodality classified as sharp pain sensation. The reverse can be said for diffuse pain.

A list of attributes found within these two pain submodalities is presented in Table 17-1.

Generally, it is misleading to interchange "intense" or "severe" with the submodality "sharp," even if the correlation between intensity and sharpness is sufficiently strong to seem to equate them.

The receptors picking up noxious signals are principally chemoreceptors of a free nerve ending type, although other types of receptors also may pick up such signals. They are responsive to noxious substances of the kinds generated after cell injury, e.g., histamine and bradykinin, and release neurotransmitters, for example substance P.

Spinoreticulothalamic Path

Ontogenetically, the **spinoreticulothalamic** is the most primitive of all paths. It is a multisynaptic tract, linked to the neuronal system concerned with most vital functions. The noxious signals ascending through the reticular system reach the intralaminar thalamic nuclei. From there they diverge and spread to other thalamic nuclei, to subcortical nuclei, and to hypothalamus, recruiting and synchronizing the activity of neurons in these regions from which the signals in turn spread to cortical areas and the septal region where neuronal activity also becomes recruited and synchronized. The connection with the septal area for the arrival of noxious signals appears to support the view that the septal area is an important region for nociceptive awareness. Even if the somatosensory cortex is removed, the ensuing sensation is felt, whereas no pain is felt if the septal area is destroyed.

This multisynaptic nociceptive path is recognized as the most primitive path, poor in discrimination, slow in conduction, but with the strongest recruiting affective power. It has been correlated with the type of pain sensation identified as diffuse.

Anterolateral Spinothalamic Tract

The **anterolateral spinothalamic tract** gives off collaterals to the reticulothalamic path. It originates in the spinal cord in laminae I, V, VI, and VII, crosses to the opposite lateral funiculus, ascends, and ends primarily in a zone posterior to the ventralis posterior nucleus of the thalamus, the posterior region. Some endings spread to other intralaminar structures and the ventralis posterior nucleus. From these regions of the thalamus the signals may spread to other brain regions in general (as described for the spinoreticulothalamic path) or to the postcentral gyrus in particular.

The anterolateral spinothalamic tract is more accurate in discrimination, but has less recruiting affective power than the spinoreticulothalamic tract. It is related to the type of pain sensation labeled as sharp. In spite of the fact that its fibers (Aδ and C) conduct slowly, the signals traveling this path reach the thalamus faster than signals traveling the spinoreticulothalamic tract, principally because the anterolateral spinothalamic is an oligosynaptic tract. It is also old ontogenetically, but younger than the spinoreticulothalamic tract.

Surgical transection of the anterolateral white column (**chordotomy**) or the anterolateral spinothalamic tract (**tractotomy**) is a treatment of otherwise intractable pain.

Is There a Fast Conducting, Analytical, Nociceptive Path?

It may appear illogical that the nociceptive paths, being as they are concerned with pain, are slower than paths concerned with other modalities. To find an explanation for this, one may try to imagine the catastrophic consequences for the function of the mind if the fibers conducting unpleasant signals with neuronal recruiting power were the fastest in transmission. Fear would dominate any brain function and our behavior would be full of jumping patterns. Nevertheless, without having overriding priority, a warning signal in any case of bodily injury should travel quickly to the mind.

It appears that nature has resolved this problem by the development of an analytical nociceptive path, characterized by its ability to transmit to the brain cortex the warning, alerting signal component of nociceptors without imparting its unpleasant component. It is then up to the mind to decide what to do with it, whether to wait and expect the arrival of unpleasant sensations, to take quick action (either by blocking the noxious signals or by avoiding the source of the stimulus) or to disregard the warning. Such a role appears to be played together with other roles by the spinocervicothalamocortical path. This path is fast conducting and highly discriminative but has very little intrinsic neuronal recruiting power. Other brain circuits may link into this path and provide another route for the recruiting and spreading of signals. Further research to substantiate this view is required.

Warm and Cold Sensations

For a long time it was generally accepted that the signals generating sensations of cold and warmth travel through the anterolateral spinothalamic tract. More recent experimental work supports the view that there is a similar range of submodalities of temperature sensations as in pain and that related signals travel through paths with the same patterns of organization as those for the pain submodalities:

Spinoreticular—strong recruiting power and nondiscriminative, i.e., with very poor sense of regional localization; these signals are related to painful cold and painful warm sensations and relay in the posterior region of the thalamus.

Lateral spinothalamic—less recruiting power and limited sense of discriminative localization; these signals are related to painful cold and painful warm sensations as well as nonpainful cold and nonpainful warm sensations of restricted discriminative value.

Spinocervicothalamic tract—least recruiting power and more discriminative in localization.

Touch Sensation

Again, there are three identifiable submodalities of touch with similar patterns of pathways:

1. spinoreticular path—very poor in discriminative power;
2. anterolateral spinothalamic tract—intermediate in discriminative and in affective recruiting power; and
3. spinocervicothalamic and posterior column-medial lemniscus path—highly discriminative in power of localization, especially in the hands; poor in intrinsic affective recruiting power.

The anterolateral path is known in the literature as a vehicle for **light, crude, nondiscriminative touch.** The accompanying descriptive adjectives serve to underline the particular qualities of the touch.

The posterolateral path is known to serve for **discriminative, refined touch.** Many receptors of origin of this tactile sensation submodality are **Meissner corpuscles** and endings around the hair roots, although other receptors participate as well.

Touch sensation originates in the surface of the body.

Pressure Sensation

The **pressure receptor** signals are transmitted through both the anterolateral and posterolateral white columns, the posterolateral column path being the one providing for most for the discriminative pressure sensation. Many receptors of origin of this pressure sensation submodality are Pacinian corpuscles and Ruffini endings, although other receptors participate as well.

Body Movement Sense (Kinesthesia) and Body Position Sense

The main sources of information of the two modalities of sensation regarding

Table 17-2. Joint Receptors

Receptor	Adaptability	Information
Type I, Ruffini-like	Slow, tonic	Position
Type II, Pacini-like	Fast, phasic	Movement
Type III, Golgi-like	Very slow, tonic	Position maintenance
Type IV, free ending	Nonadaptive, tonic	Pain

body movement (kinesthesia) and **body position,** i.e., **proprioception,** are the receptor endings in muscle and joint structures (e.g., capsules, ligaments, muscle spindles, and tendons). Proprioceptive discrimination reaches the brain through the posterolateral white column.

The **receptors** in the joint for **body position** sense appear to be related mainly to a type with anatomical and physiological properties similar to the ones described by Ruffini in the dermis and therefore called **Ruffini-like endings,** or **type I joint receptors.** They are very slowly adapting receptors.

The **receptors** in the joint for **body movement** sense appear to be related mainly to a type with anatomical and physiological properties similar to the Pacinian corpuscles and are thus called **Pacinian-like** or **type II joint receptors.**

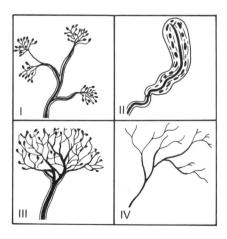

Fig. 17-5. Joint receptors.

Table 17-2 lists and Figure 17-5 illustrates four types of joint receptor endings.

Vibration Sense

Another term for **flutter** and **vibration sense** is **pallesthesia** (Gr. *pallein* to shake; *aisthesis* perception). It is a consequence of fast adapting receptors being stimulated repetitively. One may distinguish different types and submodalities according to their source (joints, subcutaneous tissue, etc.), traveling through the posterolateral and anterolateral white columns.

Two-Point Discriminative Touch

The **two-point discriminative touch** is not a sense per se but an ability of the nervous system to recognize each of two points independently when simultaneously touching the skin even if they are close to each other. This is possible through the posterolateral path by mechanisms like convergence and lateral inhibition (Fig. 17-6).

Stereognosis

Stereognosis is not a separate sense but an ability to recognize size, shape, and texture of objects. It requires the normal function and proper integration of several modalities of sensation in their most discriminative path (the posterolateral column).

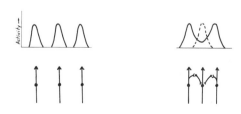

Fig. 17-6. Two-point discrimination.

Combination of Information from Different Signal Modalities

In every afferent path, blending of signals arriving from different receptors occurs in each relay station. The information transferred in the last link (i.e., the thalamocortical) is quite complex.

Evolutionary Trend of Sensory Pathways

It has been mentioned above that for each of a number of modalities of sensation there are several submodality paths, the list of which further research undoubtedly will enlarge. Table 17-3 presents a practical overview, in which the various submodalities hitherto identified are classified into two groups according to their structural or functional features.

One may pose questions like

Why has nature built up several parallel paths for each modality?
Why are they arranged in anterolateral and posterolateral groups?
What is the evolutionary trend in the development from the reticular, very affective, to the most discriminative path?

When pondering over these questions, one should bear in mind the following facts:

1. There are two major moving forces in any living system, namely: **survival** (principally aiming at maintaining homeostasis) and **expansion of life** (mainly striving to expand the interaction with the medium through analytical "intellectual" processes).
2. By grouping in the anterolateral column all the primitive information that is vital in respect to the different modalities of sensation, it can be processed independently and as a package throughout the paths. The blending of information throughout these paths with the various types of receptor endings appears to emphasize one role, i.e., nociception.
3. By grouping in the posterolateral column all the discriminative (analytical) information, imparted by different modalities of sensation, that can provide accurate knowledge of the interaction of man with the medium, the precise information signals can be processed independently as another distinct package throughout the path. The blending of information throughout these paths from the various types of receptors appears to emphasize one type, i.e., analytical information.
4. The independent and parallel processing is not a redundancy but enriches sensations in subtleties.

Table 17-3. Features of Submodalities of Sensation

Structural or Functional Feature	Nondiscriminative	Discriminative
Course	Anterolateral white column	Posterolateral white column
Synaptic relays	Mainly multisynaptic	Mainly oligosynaptic
Fiber size	Small and medium	Medium and large
Conduction	Slow	Fast
Main functional characteristic	Strong recruiting power of affective domain; poor power for analytical information; poor topographical discrimination	Strong power for analytical build-up; strong analytical information; conditioned recruiting power of affective domain; accurate discrimination

The parallel processing within the recruiting and discriminative groups is another efficient method that permits multiple forms of signal modulation.

One must realize that a total splitting and separation of sequential processing of both groups (survival and expansion of life) would be dangerous. It is for this reason that connections are established in each relay station along these two groups of paths, making any necessary overlapping possible.

Thalamic and Thalamocortical Loops

The thalamic nuclei establish loops with each other and with cortical areas.

In the following paragraphs a simplified pattern is outlined.

Intralaminar Nuclei

Input—nondiscriminative, nonanalytical information.

Main connection—with the hypothalamus, subcortical nuclei, and various thalamic nuclei. From these areas the signals may diffuse to various cortical areas in general and to the septal area in particular.

Ventralis Posterior

Main input—discriminative, analytical information.

Main connection—with primary somatosensory cortex, i.e., Brodmann's areas 1, 2, and 3.

Lateral Geniculate

Main input—visual analytical information.
Main connection—with calcarine cortex.

Medial Geniculate

Main input—auditory analytical information.

Main connection—with auditory cortex.

Pulvinar, Lateral Dorsal, and Lateral Posterior Nuclei

Main input—somatic and exteroceptive information.

Main connection—with associative sensory cortex in parietal, temporal, and occipital lobes.

Ventral Lateral and Ventral Anterior Nuclei

Main input—information from motor system.

Main connection—with the corticosubcorticocortical and the corticocerebellocortical loops.

Dorsomedial Nucleus

Main input—discriminative and nondiscriminative information related to somatic, visceral, and special senses.

Main connection—with other thalamic nuclei and with the anterior frontal lobe region.

Reticular Thalamic Nucleus

A function attributed to the reticular thalamic nucleus is to filter the ongoing signals between the thalamus and the cerebral hemispheres.

Anterior Nucleus

The anterior nucleus of the thalamus is considered to have an important role in memory processes, having as a link interconnections with the mammillary bodies and the cingulate gyrus.

The student must keep in mind that the

thalamic connections described above in a simplified manner are in reality more complex because of an overlapping between these groups.

One can do well to reflect on the tremendously expansive phenomenon occurring with regard to the discriminative, analytical signals from the level of the thalamus to the cerebral cortex.

Summary of Thalamocortical Connections

In a summary concerning the thalamocortical connections it is convenient to emphasize that most of the thalamus is specialized in processing discriminative information, while the intralaminar nuclei are concerned with nondiscriminative information, have great recruiting capacity and influence the activity of the whole cerebrum.

Lesions of Posterolateral White Column

Destruction of the posterolateral white column produces from the level of the lesion and below loss of the following discriminative modalities:

touch (two-point discrimination)
pressure sensation
position and movement sense—sensory ataxia
vibration sense

This sensory ataxia may not be noticeable due to the patient's use of visual cues to maintain his/her balance.

To distinguish this type of ataxia (sensory) from cerebellar ataxia, **Romberg's** test is performed. It consists of asking the patient to close his/her eyes when in a standing position. In a positive Romberg's test the patient will start (or increase the) swaying, because he/she has lost the visual clues essential to remain steady to compensate for sensory ataxia. In cerebellar ataxia there is very little or no increase of unsteadiness when closing the eyes.

An example of a disease affecting the dorsal roots and their corresponding fasciculi in the posterior white columns is found in **tertiary syphilis,** a neurosyphilitic affliction known as **tabes dorsalis.**

The student must realize that a disease is not a fixed entity but is a dynamic process involving a varying number of regions with a varying degree of severity.

In tabes dorsalis pervading mostly the lumbosacral enlargement, the above described signs affecting the lower limbs may be joined by several others, e.g.:

1. mild cutaneous stimuli like light stroking of the legs triggers radiating pain; this is called **dysesthesia,** a painful sensation triggered by a stimulus that does not ordinarily produce pain;
2. bilateral loss of knee and ankle jerks and hypotonia of lower limb musculature; and
3. urine retention.

These additional signs indicate further lesion(s) involving the posterior roots and ganglia with sparing and irritation of the small nociceptic neurons.

The disease may advance further and destroy also the small neurons, in which case a loss of pain and temperature sensation will result.

This variability of signs recorded within tabes dorsalis is illustrative of a most basic principle in learning to clinically evaluate disorders of the nervous system. Many clinical books on the subject describe in brief terms what most commonly happens. The student is admonished not to memorize such descriptions, the usefulness of

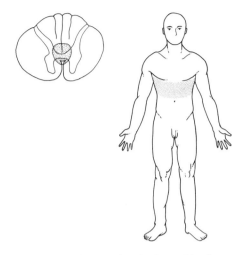

Fig. 17-7. Internal spinal cord lesion.

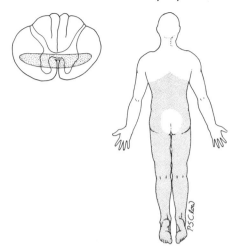

Fig. 17-8. Large internal spinal cord lesion.

which, in real clinical practice, proves to be very insufficient. If the student instead learns the potential ranges on the basis of normal structure and function, he/she stands a much better chance to acquire the knowledge needed to make the learning of clinical neurosciences and the gaining of experience through clinical practice a rewarding and useful enterprise.

The following are other examples of variations in signs caused by a lesion involving a few segments, e.g., T2–5.

The lesion may affect the spinal cord core only (Fig. 17-7). It produces detectable loss of pain (analgesia) and temperature sensation (thermoanesthesia) bilaterally (jacket-type anesthesia). This pattern of signs is known as a **commissural syndrome.** There are various etiologies producing such lesions, e.g., trauma (hematomyelia), neoplasm, syringomyela, etc. The differential diagnosis is based on a number of factors like the patient's clinical history, findings made using spinal cord imaging techniques, etc. The event where a patient loses one type of sensation but not the other is called **sensory dissociation of modalities.** This restricted spinal cord core lesion may expand along the length of the cord and/

or toward the periphery of the affected segments.

The lesion may extend as illustrated in Figure 17-8. It produces a loss of pain and temperature sensation from one or two segments below the upper border of the lesion downward except the sacral level. This is called **sacral sparing.** The signs appearing after lesions of the (anterolateral) spinothalamic tract are known as the **spinothalamic tract syndrome.** Some muscular deficiency related to the affected segments appears if several segments are involved because of the separation of ventral from intermediate and dorsal horn cells.

Other Patterns of Lesions Affecting the Spinal Cord

The lesion may affect the whole segment and is then a matter of a total transection.

The lesion may affect one or several segments on one side of the spinal cord and provokes then the Brown-Séquard's syndrome.

Spinal Cord Trauma

Traumatic lesions of the spinal cord may partially damage one or several segments. The most common result is an increasing gradient of degeneration starting in the core cord and progressing until it transects the cord completely. Most important are reports in the literature on preventive treatment of cases involving total transections. The degeneration following injury may take as long as 12 to 24 hours to become established. Treatment within this posttraumatic period with cerebrospinal fluid (CSF) dialysis of the region affected may halt the ongoing degenerative process.

Lesions at the Brain Stem Level Involving the Somatosensory System

Lesions at the brain stem level involving the somatosensory system may cause a variety of signs to appear, depending on the region(s) involved. A case is quoted to exemplify the **head-body sides dissociation** or **sensory dissociation of regions,** e.g., left side of the body and right side of the face (Fig. 13-12). The lesion affects the anterolateral spinothalamic and posterior white column-medial lemniscus, carrying signals from the left side of the body, and the right spinal trigeminal nucleus, receiving nociceptive signals from the right side of the face. The loss of sensory information from the left side of the body and of pain and temperature information from the right side of the face will be detectable.

Thalamic Lesions Affecting the Somatosensory System: Thalamic Syndrome

The term **thalamic syndrome** implies that the somatosensory system at the thalamic level is affected. It does not preclude the involvement of other sensory modalities like visual or auditory. The main char-acteristic of this syndrome is that if it involves one side of the thalamus, it causes complete loss contralaterally of somatosensory modalities in the face, trunk, and limbs. It is common in lesions of the thalamus to find that small neurons of the intralaminar nuclei survive the lesion and that the threshold for touch, pain, and temperature sensation becomes raised. However, when the threshold is reached, the sensations are exaggerated, perverted, and most disagreeable **(dysesthesia).**

Suprathalamic Lesions of the Somatosensory System

Lesions in the somatosensory pathways from the thalamus to the cortex or in the somatosensory cortex itself produce a contralateral sensory loss of discriminative sensory perceptions in congruence with the region lesioned and affecting nondiscriminative sensations (e.g., pain and temperature) very insignificantly.

Note: Signals producing the sensations of vibration spread from the thalamus to the somatosensory cortex, and through the intralaminar nuclei to other brain areas.

Clinical Examination of the Somatosensory System

Four aspects must be taken into account in sensory examinations: modalities and submodalities of sensation (type and quality), sensory loss (quantity), body regions affected (topography), and state of the associative and integrative sensory functions, e.g., stereognosis.

When attempting to evaluate the somatosensory system, one must be concerned not only with the topography and the different modalities but also with their submodalities, discriminative, and nondiscriminative, which allow for a quantitative and qualitative evaluation of each modality and also of the general discriminatory and affective states of the nervous system.

Suggested Readings

Barr ML, Kiernan JA: The Human Nervous System. Fourth Edition. Harper and Row, Philadelphia, pp. 275–293, 1983.

Beers RF, Bassett EF, Eds.: Mechanisms of Pain and Analgesic Compounds: Miles International Symposium Series, No. 11, Raven Press, New York, 1979.

Boivie JJG, Perl ER: Neural substrates of somatic sensation. In Hunt CC, Ed.: MTP International Review of Science, Physiology Series One, Vol. 3, Butterworths, London, pp. 303–411, 1975.

Cervero F, Iggo A: The substantia gelatinosa of the spinal cord. A critical review, Brain 103:717–772, 1980.

Christensen BN, Perl ER: Spinal neurons specifically excited by noxious or thermal stimuli: Marginal zone of the dorsal horn, J Neurophysiol 33:293–307, 1970.

Gordon G, Ed.: Active Touch. The Mechanism of Recognition of Objects by Manipulation. A Multi-disciplinary Approach, Pergamon Press, Oxford, 1978.

Hansebout RR, Tanner JA, Romero-Sierra C: Current status of spinal cord cooling in the treatment of acute spinal cord injury, Spine 9:508–511, 1984.

Heimer L: The Human Brain and Spinal Cord, Springer-Verlag, New York, pp. 165–182, 1983.

Jones EG, Powell TPS: Anatomical organization of the somatosensory cortex. In Iggo A, Ed.: Handbook of Sensory Physiology, Vol. 2, The Somatosensory System, Springer-Verlag, New York, pp. 579-620, 1973.

Kerr FWL, Wilson PR: Pain, Ann Rev Neurosci 1:83–102, 1978.

Nathan PW: The gate-control theory of pain: A critical review, Brain 99:123–158, 1976.

Rymer WZ, d'Almeida A: Joint position sense. The effects of muscle contraction, Brain 103:1–22, 1980.

18

Special Senses I

The Eye

The **eye** develops from the diencephalon as a vesicular outgrowth.

The **retina** (Fig. 18-1) is a collapsed vesicle or **optic cup** of two layers. The outer (more posterior) of these layers forms its pigment epithelium, while the inner (more anterior) forms its neural complex layer.

The optic cup is surrounded externally by the **choroid** and **sclera** (Fig. 18-2).

The anterior boundary of the retina with the ciliary region is called the **ora serrata** and forms the peripheral limit of vision of the retina.

Visual Paths

Light passing through the **cornea, lens,** and **neural layers** strikes the **pigment layer of the retina** (posterior layer), which it stimulates. The pigment layer is connected to the neural layers, which in turn become stimulated. Neurons of the retina send axons toward a region of the cup, where they converge in an area known as

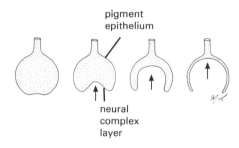

pigment
epithelium

neural
complex
layer

Fig. 18-1. Retina.

the **optic papilla** or **optic disc** and then continue posteriorly as a large bundle, namely, the **optic nerve** and **tract,** toward the brain to reach

1. various parts of the midbrain; the fibers form a reflex path to stimulate the motor nuclei of the eye in the brain stem;
2. the posterior region of the thalamus;
3. the lateral geniculate body of the thalamus; discriminative visual information is carried here, i.e., an amplification of the signals is accomplished by neurons of the lateral geniculate bodies projecting their axons as the geniculocalcarine tract to the calcarine cortex (visual cortex, area 17); and
4. the hypothalamus, through the retino-

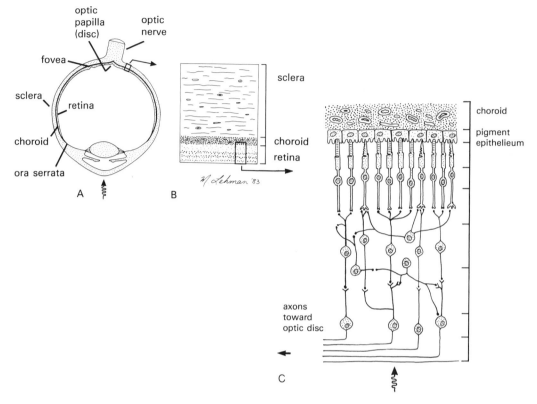

Fig. 18-2. Eye components of visual path. (A) Eye; (B) layers of eye; (C) retina.

hypothalamic tract. This tract is formed by collateral branches of the axons of the optic nerve, given off at the level of the optic chiasm to enter the hypothalamus. It seems that the visual input of these collaterals contributes to the circadian rhythm and hypothalamic secretory rhythms.

A View of the Retina with the Ophthalmoscope

Four main features of the retina can be observed when viewing the **fundus** (L. bottom) of the eye with the use of an ophthalmoscope:

Capillary Net

The heightened reddish color results from the capillary net of the central artery of the retina coming within the optic nerve

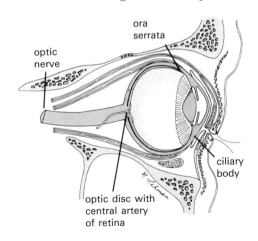

Fig. 18-3. Structures of the eye.

as a branch of the ophthalmic artery (Fig. 18-3).

Optic Papilla or Optic Disc

The **optic papilla** or **optic disc** is seen as a pale pink disc formed by the convergence of nerve fibers. The central artery irradiates from the disc to irrigate the retina. The optic papilla is responsible for the blind spot as it contains only nerve fibers and the artery. Its position is slightly medial to the posterior pole of the eyeball.

Fovea

The **fovea** is a dark spot positioned lateral to the optic papilla. It is devoid of vessels, which permits the observer to detect the dark pigment of the choroid. This spot is specialized in visual acuity and marks the center region of vision of the retina.

Macula

Surrounding the fovea is a broader spot, the macula, which is difficult to detect in normal light. Using red-free light, one can observe a yellow color, which is due to the presence of a yellow pigment. More specifically, this spot is hence known as **macula lutea** (L. yellow spot or stain).

Circuitry of the Retina

The circuitry of the retina (Fig. 18-4) is as follows: pigment cells to the photoreceptor cells (rod and cone cells) to the bipolar cells to the ganglion cells, whose axons form the optic nerve.

Modulation of the signals in these transmission lines is handled by a string of cells of three types, i.e., **amacrine, interplexiform,** and **horizontal cells.** Stimuli picked up by amacrine cells from synaptic activity between bipolar and ganglion cells modify the interplexiform cells, which in turn modify bipolar cell activity and the synaptic coupling of photoreceptors with bipolar cells through the horizontal cells.

This feed-back modulatory role of the retinal interneurons in the transmission of photoreceptor signals to the brain enriches

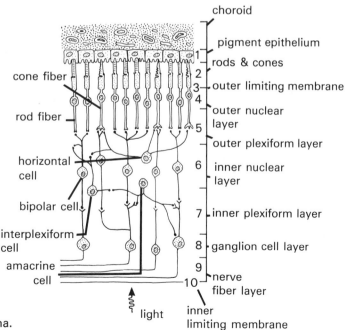

Fig. 18-4. Structure of the retina.

its information code values in respect to borders and contours, intensity changes of stimuli, etc.

In Figure 18-4 one can observe that the transmission line of cones is more specific than the rods, a fact which renders the cones better equipped for discriminative information.

Organization of Photoreceptors—Rods and Cones

Although similar, the **rods** and **cones** show some important differences.

Shape—as illustrated in Figure 18-5;
Number—7 million cones versus 130 million rods (a ratio of nearly 1 to 20);
Connectivity—one cone is related to one pigment cell and one bipolar cell, whereas several rods are related to one pigment cell and one bipolar cell;

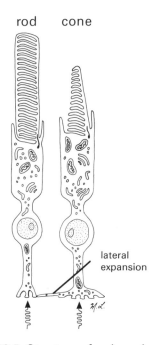

Fig. 18-5. Structure of rods and cones.

Distribution and function—rods are lacking in the fovea, their population increasing from the fovea toward the ora serrata. This population distribution makes the rods poor in information regarding central vision, i.e., vision in the center of the retina, but very able in peripheral vision. An opposite pattern of population distribution in the retina is presented by the cones, which are important in central vision. Their maximum concentration is in the fovea, high in the macular area, and diminishing toward the ora serrata (periphery).

The rods are very sensitive to light, even to dim light (night vision). The cones are sensitive to bright light and color but not to dim light.

Direction of Movement in Vision

Among the different mechanisms involved in code direction of movement in the visual field one such mechanism is based on the connections through lateral expansions between cones and rods (Fig. 18-5).

Outer Segment of Photoreceptors

The outer segments of photoreceptors are filled with hundreds of flattened double membrane saccules (discs), which are stacked along the length of the outer segments. The photosensitive chemical compound is situated in the membrane of the saccules. This compound in the rods consists chemically of a pigment, **rhodopsin,** a loose combination of a protein with **retinal,** which is a derivative of vitamin A. The rhodopsin molecules change their configuration when absorbing light and end up through other reactions with the pigment cells in membrane depolarization. Vitamin A deficiency causes blindness to dim light.

Retinal Detachment

On account of a number of reasons, e.g., a traumatic impact, the neural layer of the retina may become loosened from the pigment cell layer. This is called **retinal detachment** and produces blindness of that eye in which it occurs.

Fundus of the Eye—A Window to the Brain

By exploring the **fundus** of the eye, one may collect important information, not only of intrinsic concern regarding the retina, but also of pathologies affecting the brain, like intracranial pressure, expressed by **edema of the papilla (papilledema).**

Visual Reflex Path

In the visual reflex path the light signals are conducted from the eye directly through the optic nerve and tract to the midbrain where the path establishes connections with the pretectal area, cranial nerve motor nuclei, the reticular formation, and the tectum of the midbrain. It provides an avenue for visual motor reflexes, i.e., closing of the eyelids, pupillary and ciliary body adjustments, etc.

Visual Conscious Path

With visual information a precise image of the **field of vision** is built up in the primary sensory visual cortex. This is accomplished by topographically linking point by point the three regions, namely, the retina, the lateral geniculate body, and area 17.

Due to the large number in population of photoreceptors (137 million), optic nerve fibers (1 million), lateral geniculate body cells, geniculocalcarine fibers, and calcarine cells, together with their connectivity patterns, a very impressive image for discriminative information is built up.

Retinal Image

The retina inverts (shifts up-down) and reverses (shifts right-left) the **field of vision,** just as a camera does with an image.

The division of the retina by two perpendicular lines gives four retinal quadrants, i.e., upper and lower left and upper and lower right.

Binocular Vision

In **binocular vision** the superposition of two images is a requirement for three-dimensional vision. This is accomplished by pairing the left retinal quadrants on the left geniculate body (Fig. 18-6). It requires the decussation of fibers and the formation of the chiasm.

The level of the chiasm marks the limits of the optic nerve and optic tract.

The optic nerve carries information from the corresponding eye. The optic tract carries information from the opposite field of vision, i.e., right optic tract and right geniculate body (left field of vision) and left optic tract and left geniculate body (right field of vision).

The mapping of the signals in the geniculate body accomplishes two main objectives: (1) it enhances the macular field of vision; and (2) the medial portion receives the lower quadrants of the opposite field of vision and transfers them to the calcarine cortex, above the calcarine sulcus. The lateral portion of the geniculate receives the upper quadrants of the opposite field of vision and transfers them to the calcarine cortex, below the calcarine sulcus.

Calcarine Sulcus

Three principal facts are emphasized about the **calcarine sulcus.**

One third of the calcarine cortex is concerned with fibers of the macula. This is a great amplification for visual acuity.

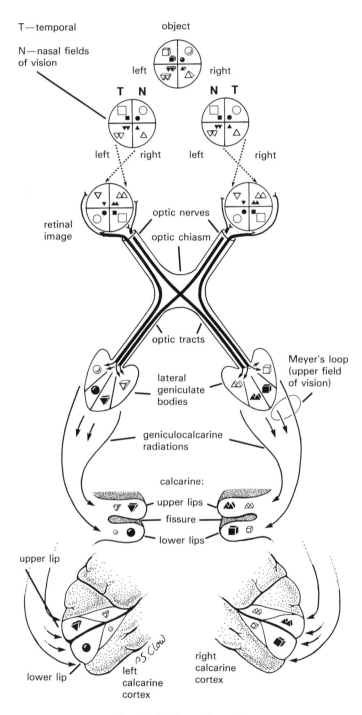

Fig. 18-6. Binocular vision.

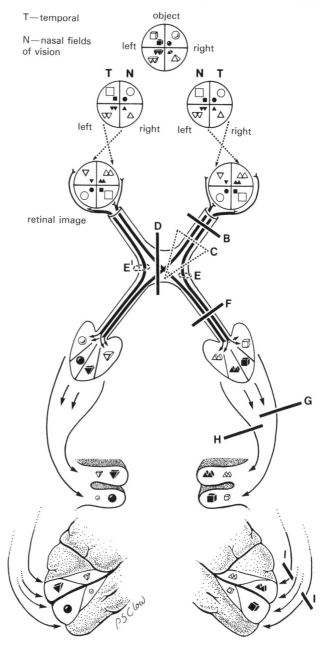

Fig. 18-7. (A) Lesions of visual path (Figure continues).

Each calcarine cortex receives information from the opposite field of vision: right receives from left and left receives from right.

The upper calcarine cortex images the lower quadrant field of vision and the lower calcarine cortex images the upper quadrant field of vision.

Visual Defects Due to Lesions of the Pathways

In Figures 18-7A and 18-7B a number of lesions are presented with related clinical terms.

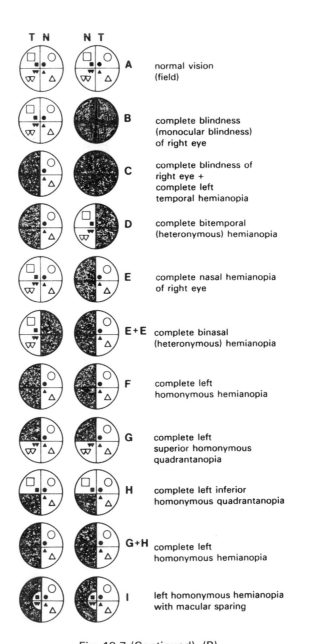

A	normal vision (field)
B	complete blindness (monocular blindness) of right eye
C	complete blindness of right eye + complete left temporal hemianopia
D	complete bitemporal (heteronymous) hemianopia
E	complete nasal hemianopia of right eye
E+E	complete binasal (heteronymous) hemianopia
F	complete left homonymous hemianopia
G	complete left superior homonymous quadrantanopia
H	complete left inferior homonymous quadrantanopia
G+H	complete left homonymous hemianopia
I	left homonymous hemianopia with macular sparing

Fig. 18-7 (Continued). (B).

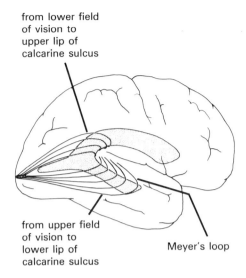

from lower field
of vision to
upper lip of
calcarine sulcus

from upper field
of vision to
lower lip of
calcarine sulcus

Meyer's loop

Fig. 18-8. Geniculocalcarine fibers.

Conscious Eye Movements

Area 17 projects fibers to the frontal eye fields, which in turn send fibers to motor areas 4 and 6, which relay in brain stem interneurons and motor nuclei of the eye and trigger voluntary eye movements.

Olfactory System

The **olfactory system** picks up stimuli produced by dissolved chemical substances in the fluid mucus coating the olfactory epithelium. The sensory olfactory receptors are bipolar neurons with long cilia embedded in this mucous coat.

Note: The student will notice that the clinical terminology employs **nasal** and **temporal** (N and T in Fig. 18-7). These terms relate to the nose and temporal region, respectively.

Further Thalamocortical Processing of Visual Sensations

Table 18-1 presents a number of loops which are established to enhance discrimination of visual stimuli.

Areas 18 and 19 contribute information to the association cortex of multiple modalities, i.e., areas 37, 39, and 40, where complex discriminative sensory association functions are processed, for instance, stereognosis.

Table 18-1. Loops of the Visual Path

	Area 17	
	↗ ↕ ↖	
Lateral geniculate body	↔ Pulvinar ↔	Visual association areas 18 and 19

Components of the Olfactory Path

The **olfactory path** (Fig. 18-9) consists of bipolar neurons of the olfactory epithe-

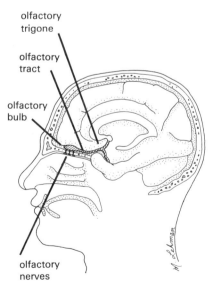

olfactory
trigone

olfactory
tract

olfactory
bulb

olfactory
nerves

Fig. 18-9. Olfactory path.

lium, olfactory nerves, olfactory bulb, olfactory tract, and olfactory trigone, which branches out into the medial, intermediate, and lateral olfactory striae.

Olfactory Epithelium

The olfactory epithelium is found in the upper part of the nasal cavity. Its components are the bipolar receptor neurons, surrounded by supporting cells, which are secretory, the **Bowman's glands,** and the **basal cells** (Fig. 18-10).

The basal cells are constantly dividing into cells which develop into bipolar olfactory neurons, replacing old ones. Bipolar receptor neurons have a life span of 2 months.

Bipolar Neurons

The peripheral process of a bipolar neuron is shaped like a bulb and projects the long cilia.

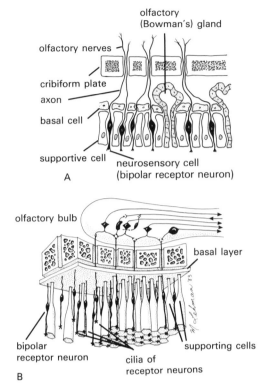

Fig. 18-10. (A) Cells of olfactory epithelium; (B) structure of olfactory epithelium.

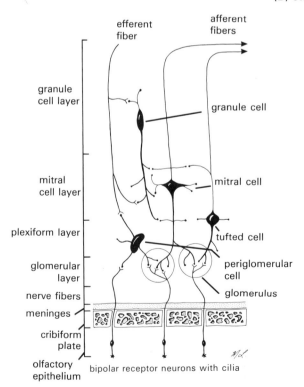

Fig. 18-11. Circuitry of olfactory bulb.

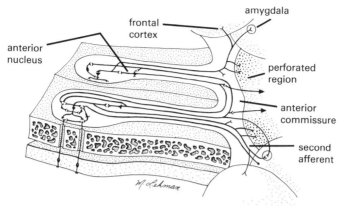

Fig. 18-12. Olfactory tract.

The central processes of bipolar receptor neurons (there are 25 million cells) are nonmyelinated axons (**fila olfactoria**) grouped together in about 20 bundles known as olfactory nerves. These nerves pass through the foramina of the cribiform plate of the ethmoid bone, becoming surrounded by tubular sheaths of the meninges. This arrangement places the subarachnoid space in close contact with lymphatics of the nasal region, in which spread of nasal infections to the meninges and the brain may occur. Trauma of this region may produce **anosmia,** i.e., loss of the sense of smell. The olfactory nerves synapse within the olfactory bulb.

Olfactory Bulb

The **olfactory bulb** contains neurons called the **mitral** and **tufted cells,** whose axons transmit impulses toward the brain, and interneurons of two types, i.e., **periglomerular** and **granule cells** (the latter have no axons), modulating and controlling the activity of the mitral and tufted cells, in accordance with their various inputs (Fig. 18-11).

Olfactory Tract

The **olfactory tract** (Fig. 18-12) is made up of afferent fibers of the mitral and tufted cells coursing toward the brain. It also contains efferent fibers.

Olfactory Trigone

At its base, the **olfactory tract** spreads its fibers into the **olfactory trigone** (Fig. 18-13), which anteriorly limits the anterior perforated region.

Lateral Olfactory Stria

Most of the fibers of the olfactory tract course laterally, forming the **lateral olfactory stria** and spreading in the temporal cortex to reach the cortex of the uncus, the amygdala, the frontal cortex of the limen insulae, and the anterior part of the parahippocampal gyrus.

These frontal and temporal regions are together called the **lateral olfactory area** and the cortical regions the **primary olfactory cortical area.** They establish connections with the hippocampus, thalamus, hypothalamus, brain stem reticular formation, septal region, and other cortical areas.

Intermediate Olfactory Stria

The **intermediate olfactory stria,** consisting of a much smaller number of fibers than the lateral stria, ends in the immediate **olfactory tubercle,** an ill-defined area within the anterior perforated region. This tubercle receives inputs from the temporal lobe as well as other cerebral regions. Its role is a matter of debate.

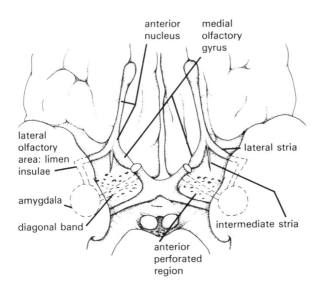

anterior nucleus

medial olfactory gyrus

lateral olfactory area: limen insulae

lateral stria

amygdala

diagonal band

intermediate stria

anterior perforated region

Fig. 18-13. Olfactory trigone.

Medial Olfactory Stria

The **medial olfactory stria** is in essence very short and lies masked by the prominent medial olfactory gyrus.

Medial Olfactory Gyrus

There is as yet no agreement about the connections and function of the **medial olfactory gyrus.** It is part of what is known as the **paraolfactory area.**

Anterior Olfactory Nucleus

The **anterior olfactory nucleus** is an ill-defined structure with components located in the olfactory tract and medial olfactory stria. It contains cells whose axons contribute to the forming of the medial olfactory stria and travel through the medial olfactory gyrus and the anterior commissure to end in the contralateral anterior olfactory nucleus and bulb.

The Term "Paraolfactory Area"

The term **paraolfactory** or **medial olfactory area** has been designated to the area of the brain also known as the **subcallosal area,** medial olfactory gyrus, and **septal area.** Paraolfactory area is a misleading term, because it suggests that olfaction is its main function. In reality, this region receives inputs from all types of sensory modalities, olfaction being only one of them. The olfactory signals reaching the septal area arrive through polysynaptic paths. No satisfactory scientific reason why particularly the olfactory element of this brain region should be stressed has yet been presented.

Control of Olfactory Signals

The regions of the brain receiving olfactory input send back centrifugal fibers to the olfactory bulb to modulate its activity.

Importance of the Olfactory System

Until the last decades, the importance of the human olfactory system in brain function had been underestimated. It now appears possible that the olfactory system is involved in functions other than those related to smell, e.g., food intake, reproductive and endocrine functions. For instance, some chemical constants of the air may impart sensory stimulation of vital informative value to the brain.

Olfactory Hallucinations

When a patient suffers from olfactory hallucinations, like the sensation of a disagreeable odor without normal cause, one may consider the primary olfactory region (temporal lobe) as a possible origin of this disturbance. If such hallucinations are accompanied by abnormal buccal movements and a dream-like state of mind, this is known as **uncinate fits** or the **uncinate syndrome.**

Taste System

Four taste sensations are considered basic, i.e.: sweet, sour, bitter, and salty. A method of testing this sense is illustrated in Figure 18-14. The receptor organs are the **taste buds** on the surface of two types of **papillae,** namely, the **fungiform** and the **vallate.** They have a wide distribution within the mouth. The highest concentration is in the posterior one-third of the tongue (with mostly vallate papillae) and the lowest in the anterior two-thirds of the tongue (with mostly fungiform papillae). There are some in the palate and, least of all, in the uvula.

Neuroepithelial sensory cells, surrounded by subtentacular cells, project

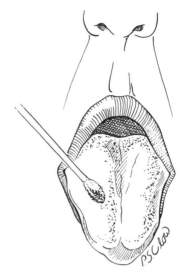

Fig. 18-14. Procedure for testing taste.

cilia to pick up chemical stimuli, which are transmitted to the nerve endings (Fig. 18-15).

The neuroepithelial sensory cells have a very short life span and are replaced by new cells differentiated from the basal cells.

The taste nerve endings belong to three cranial nerves, namely, the facial—anterior two-thirds of tongue and palate; the glossopharyngeal—posterior one-third of tongue; and the vagus—uvula and its posterior region; in adults the papillae in this region atrophy and they hence merit no elaboration.

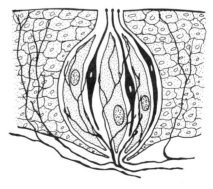

Fig. 18-15. Taste bud.

Taste Pathways

The **taste signals** travel from the sensory receptors to the rostral region of the solitary nucleus through the solitary tract.

Taste Pathway from Solitary Nucleus to Cerebrum

Diffuse Path

In the **diffuse path,** signals ascend in the reticular formation through the central tegmental tract and reach the hypothalamus and intralaminar nuclei of the thalamus.

Discriminative Path

In the **discriminative path,** signals travel along specific fibers distributed within the trigeminal lemniscal path and reach the ventralis posteromedialis of the thalamus. The relayed signals reach area 43 of Brodmann.

The **association taste area** is located in the anterior region of the second sensorimotor cortex near the insular cortex.

The lack or loss of taste is called **ageusia.**

Suggested Readings

Amoore JE: Four primary odor modalities of man: experimental evidence and possible significance. In Denton DA, Coghlan JA, Eds.: Olfaction and Taste V, pp. 283–289, Academic Press, New York, 1975.

Barr ML, Kiernan JA: The Human Nervous System. Fourth Edition. Harper and Row, Philadelphia, Chapters 17 and 20, 1983.

Bender MB: Brain control of conjugate horizontal and vertical eye movements. A survey of the structural and functional correlates, Brain 103:23–69, 1980.

Boynton RM: Human Color Vision, Holt, Rinehart and Winston, New York, 1979.

Doty RL: Mammalian Olfaction, Reproductive Processes, and Behavior, Academic Press, New York, 1976.

Eslinger PJ, Damasio AR, Van Hoesen GW: Olfactory dysfunction in man: A review of anatomical and behavioral aspects, Brain and Cognition 1:259–285, 1982.

Heimer L, Van Hoesen GW, Rosene DL: The olfactory pathways and the anterior perforated substance in the primate brain, Int J Neurol 12:42–52, 1977.

Land EH: The retinex theory of color vision, Sci Am 237(6):108–128, 1977.

Pinching AJ: Clinical testing of olfaction reassessed, Brain 100:377–388, 1977.

Rodieck RW: Visual pathways, Ann Rev Neurosci 2:193–225, 1979.

Van Essen DC: Visual areas of the mammalian cerebral cortex, Ann Rev Neurosci 2:227–263, 1979.

Werblin FS: The control of sensitivity in the retina, Sci Am 228:70–79, 1973.

19

Special Senses II

Auditory System

In the **auditory apparatus** there are three main regions, namely, the **external, middle,** and **internal ear** (Fig. 19-1).

External Ear

The **external ear** consists of the **auricle (pinna)** and the **external acoustic meatus (external auditory canal).**

The **tympanic membrane (eardrum)** separates the external from the middle ear.

Middle Ear

The **middle ear** consists of the **middle ear (tympanic) cavity** or **canal** containing air and three **ossicles,** i.e., **malleus** (L. hammer), **incus** (L. anvil), and **stapes** (L. stirrup). The tympanic cavity is connected to the pharynx through the eustachian tube, which opens during swallowing, thus permitting air pressure in the tympanic cavity to equal that of the exterior.

Of the **middle ear muscles,** the **tensor tympani,** innervated by the trigeminal, at-taches to the malleus. The **stapedius muscle,** innervated by the facial, attaches to the stapes.

Between the middle and inner ear there is a bony partition with two windows, i.e., the **oval window (fenestra vestibuli)** and the **round window (fenestra cochleae).**

Inner Ear

The **inner ear** (Fig. 19-2), also called **labyrinth** on account of its bony configuration, has three components: the **semicircular canals,** the **vestibule,** and the **cochlea.**

The bony labyrinth contains the **membraneous labyrinth,** which is very similar in shape. Between the bony and membraneous labyrinths is some fluid called **perilymph** (L. *lympha* water). The fluid within the membraneous labyrinth is called **endolymph.**

The **membraneous semicircular ducts** (with endolymph) are situated within the semicircular canals (with perilymph).

The membraneous cochlear duct (with endolymph) is located within the cochlear canal (with perilymph).

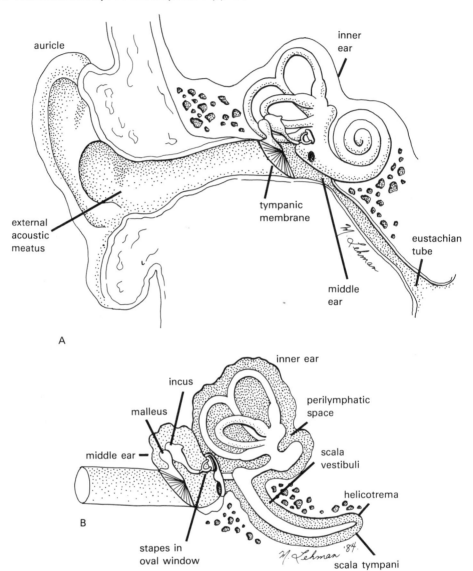

Fig. 19-1. (A) Hearing apparatus; (B) middle and inner ear.

The semicircular canals and most of the vestibule are concerned with equilibrium (vestibular system) and will be described later. For now we are concerned only with the auditory part, i.e., the cochlea and its basal region in the vestibule.

The Cochlea

The **cochlea** (Fig. 19-3) is shaped like a snail shell. The two and a half turns of the bony tube wrap around a bony core called the **modiolus,** which contains the **cochlear**

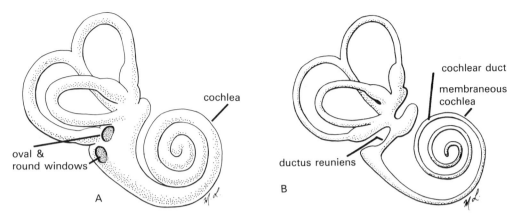

Fig. 19-2. (A) Bony labyrinth; (B) membraneous labyrinth.

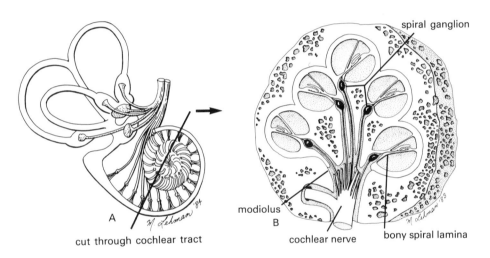

Fig. 19-3. (A) Innervation of labyrinth; (B) section through the cochlea.

or **spiral ganglion** consisting of bipolar cells.

The modiolus protrudes in the form of a bony ramp into the tube known as the bony **spiral lamina**. The **basilar membrane** extends from the edge of the spiral lamina to the lateral edge of the bony tube. This lateral attachment to the bone is reinforced by the **spiral ligament** (Fig. 19-4).

The **vestibular membrane** stretches from the spiral lamina to the bony wall. The bony spiral lamina, basilar membane, and vestibular membrane establish three compartments within the cavity of the cochlear canal. These three spiral compartments (Fig. 19-4) are the **scala media (cochlear duct** or **membraneous cochlea)**—within the basilar and vestibular membranes; the **scala vestibuli**—limited by the vestibular membrane and bone; and

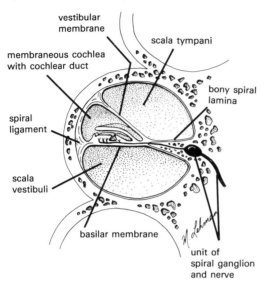

Fig. 19-4. Cross-section of the cochlear canal.

the **scala tympani**—limited by the basilar membrane and bone.

The tip of the membraneous cochlear duct ends near the tip of the bony cochlear canal, i.e., at the **cupula,** leaving a small aperture, the **helicotrema,** where the scala vestibuli communicates with the scala tympani.

The base end of the cochlear duct communicates through a small duct, **ductus reuniens,** with the saccule, which is one of the cavities of the membraneous vestibular apparatus.

Spiral Organ of Corti

The **spiral organ of Corti** is the sensory component of the cochlear duct. A number of cell components is illustrated in Figure 19-5. The endings of primary sensory neurons (bipolar ganglion cells) are in synaptic contact with the **sensory hair cells (auditory receptor cells).** The sensory hair cells bury their hair-like projections in the **tectorial membrane.**

Transduction of Sound into Auditory Sensory Signals

Sound is propagated as pressure waves, the frequency of which determines the

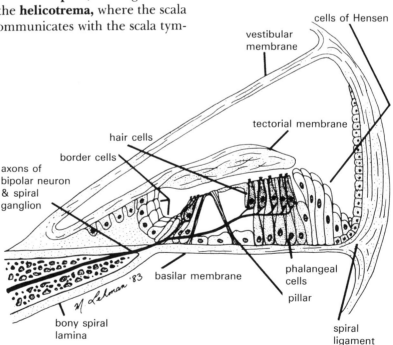

Fig. 19-5. Cochlear duct with organ of Corti.

pitch. This is expressed in cycles per second (c.p.s.); the higher the frequency, the higher the pitch. The audible frequencies for the human ear range between 20 and 20,000 c.p.s., with a gradual decrease in perception of high frequencies with aging.

The amplitude of the sound waves determines the intensity.

The external ear funnels the sound waves to the eardrum which vibrates. The malleus, attached to the eardrum, picks up the vibrations, which are transmitted mechanically through the incus to the stapes.

The foot-plate of the stapes is attached to the oval window by the annular ligament. The three ossicles act as an amplifier (mechanical transformer) by channeling the energy of vibrations of the large eardrum to the much smaller foot-plate.

The vibrations of the foot-plate set in motion perilymphatic waves that travel through the scala vestibuli to the helicotrema to the scala tympani and fade in the membrane of the round window.

The perilymphatic waves set in motion the endolymph and the basilar membrane. The resulting oscillations tilt the hairs of the auditory receptor cells, and a stimulus is transmitted to the sensory nerve endings.

Optimal Vibration Frequencies Along the Basilar Membrane

The basilar membrane has an optimal gradient of vibration for high pitch sounds at its base and for low pitch sounds at its tip. This optimal distribution of resonant frequencies (from high to low) along the length of the basilar membrane is the basis of distribution of the stimulus along the organ of Corti.

To understand this optimal gradient of vibration of the basilar membrane one must keep in mind its proportional change in width. At the base, the bony spiral lamina is broad and the basilar membrane is narrow. At the tip, the bony spiral lamina is narrow and the basilar membrane is broad.

Bipolar Neurons of the Spiral (Cochlear) Ganglion

The spiral (cochlear) ganglion, coiled within the modiolus, sends the peripheral processes of the bipolar neurons (original dendrites) through the bony spiral lamina and establishes synaptic contact with the hair cells. The central processes (or axons) concentrate at the base of the modiolus and travel within the internal auditory meatus as a component of the vestibulocochlear nerve and reach the medullopontine junction, ending in the ventral and dorsal cochlear nucleus.

Thalamocortical Auditory Paths

The auditory paths within the brain stem were described in Chapter 14. At this point, the emphasis is placed on the auditory paths at thalamocortical levels.

Fibers carrying auditory information from the inferior colliculus and a few fibers from the lateral lemniscus that bypass the inferior colliculus traverse the inferior brachium to reach two regions of the thalamus: the posterior region of the thalamus, from where they may spread to other brain areas; and the medial geniculate body, which sends the auditory radiation in the sublentiform part of the internal capsule to end in the primary auditory cortex of the temporal lobe (areas 41 and 42 of Brodmann).

Association loops are established between the auditory association cortex (Wernicke's area), the primary auditory cortex, the medial geniculate body, and the pulvinar. Finally, the connections are furnished with the lateral cortex association of multiple sensibilities, i.e., areas 37, 39, and 40.

Central Controls of Auditory Sensory Input

The auditory signals can be modulated in various ways.

The modulation signals may travel through descending pathways from the auditory cortex to the different relay stations of the auditory path. The last link in this centrifugal pathway consists of fibers from the superior olivary nucleus, i.e., the olivocochlear fibers which selectively inhibit the hair cells and nerve endings of neurons that are not responding optimally to a particular frequency, most probably to reduce the noise and sharpen the auditory information by increasing the signal-to-noise ratio.

Another mechanism of dampening unwanted sounds is by contracting the stapedius and tensor tympani muscles, which reduces the vibrations of the stapes and eardrum. These inhibitory mechanisms can operate reflexly through fibers from the superior olivary nucleus, synapsing in the motor nuclei of the facial and trigeminal nerves.

Tests of Hearing

Of importance in testing sensory functions is to establish the **threshold** of hearing, i.e., how weak a stimulus can be detected. A simple test for threshold is performed by rubbing two fingers together close to each ear.

Hearing loss may be caused by

1. A lesion of the sensory organ of Corti or the auditory nerve. This is called **neurosensory loss** or **neurosensory deafness.**
2. Mechanical impediment to conduction of sound waves from the external ear, through the external auditory meatus and ossicles of the middle ear, e.g., blocked or damaged auditory canal, fixed ossicles, etc. This type of hearing loss is called **conduction deafness.** A common cause of this kind of impairment in adults is **otosclerosis,** characterized by progressive ossification of the annular ligament of the stapes, which impedes the stapes to vibrate to sound waves.

Rinne's Test

Rinne's test (Fig. 19-6) assesses the threshold of hearing. It can be used to differentiate between neurosensory and conduction deafness. It consists of holding a faintly vibrating tuning fork on the mastoid process until it is no longer heard by the patient, at which time the fork is held beside the external ear. Since air conduction should be more efficient than bone conduction, the sound can be heard again if the conductive system (external-middle ear) is intact (normal Rinne's test response). If the air conduction system is impaired, the patient will sense less or noth-

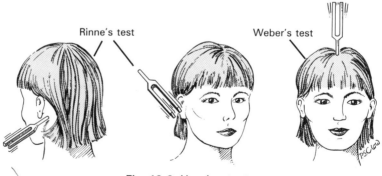

Fig. 19-6. Hearing tests.

ing when the fork is held beside the ear than when it is applied against the mastoid, because the bone, although poorly, permits the vibrations to be transmitted directly to the inner ear, bypassing the conduction channels of the external and middle ear. This is an abnormal Rinne's test response. In partial nerve deafness, the Rinne's test is normal, but both bone and air conduction are quantitatively decreased.

Weber's Test

Weber's test (Fig. 19-6) can also differentiate between neurosensory loss and conduction loss. It consists of placing a vibrating tuning fork on the midline of the forehead. In normal subjects it is heard equally well in both ears and the sound appears to arise in the midline.

In unilateral conduction deafness the sound appears to be louder in the diseased ear.

One can simulate the experience of the conduction loss by pressing a finger tip to one auditory canal. The side where the canal is blocked senses the vibrations better.

In unilateral sensory deafness the sound from the fork is heard better in the normal ear and the sound appears to arise on the healthy side.

Vestibular System

Vestibular Organ

The bony vestibular portion of the internal ear includes the **vestibule** and **semicircular canal.** The vestibule contains the membraneous **utricle** and **saccule.** The semicircular canals enclose the membraneous **semicircular ducts** (Fig. 19-7).

The membraneous utricle, saccule, and semicircular ducts are surrounded by perilymph and filled with endolymph.

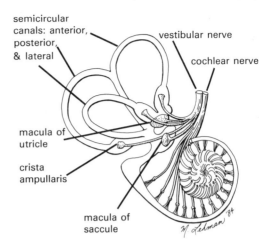

Fig. 19-7. Innervation of labyrinth.

Static Labyrinth

The utricle and saccule together form the portion of the vestibular organ specialized in giving information regarding the position (statics) and changes in position of the head, and this part is therefore known as the **static labyrinth.**

The utricle and saccule each contains a specialized area of sensory epithelium, called the **macula. The macula utriculi** lies at the base of the utricle. The **macula sacculi** is situated on the medial wall of the saccule. The positions of the maculae correspond to the horizontal and vertical planes of the head, respectively (Fig. 19-7).

The Maculae

Each macula (Fig. 19-8) contains **sensory hair cells.** These cells have, apart from the hairs, a **cilium.** The tips of the hairs and cilium are embedded in the gelatinous **otolithic membrane,** which contains fine concretions of calcium carbonate, the **otoliths (otoconia, statoliths, statoconia).** If the head is tilted, the gravitational force of the otolithic membrane and its otoliths affect the cilia, inhibiting some and exciting others, which stimulates the release of the

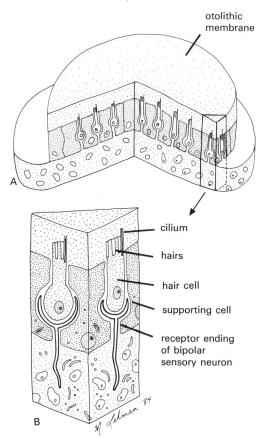

otolithic membrane

cilium

hairs

hair cell

supporting cell

receptor ending of bipolar sensory neuron

A

B

Fig. 19-8. Structure of macula utriculi (A) and hair cells (B).

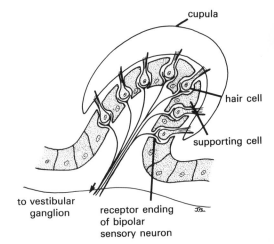

cupula

hair cell

supporting cell

to vestibular ganglion

receptor ending of bipolar sensory neuron

Fig. 19-9. Structure of the crista ampullaris.

the ampullae. The crista ampullaris contains sensory hair cells. Their hairs and cilium, embedded in gelatinous material, are together called the **cupula.**

The **cristae** are sensors of movement of the head. They respond specifically to rotational movement (also known as angular movement), especially when there is a change of speed, i.e., rotational acceleration or deceleration.

The stimuli picked up by the sensory hair cells are transmitted to the bipolar sensory neurons of the vestibular ganglion.

chemical transmitters in their synaptic contact with the nerve endings of the bipolar primary sensory neurons of the **vestibular ganglion (Scarpa's ganglion).**

Although the macula is mostly a static organ, quick tilting movements and **linear acceleration** or deceleration are also detected. Prolonged fluctuating stimulation of the macula produces motion sickness.

Kinetic Labyrinth

The **kinetic labyrinth** is made up of the **anterior, lateral,** and **posterior semicircular ducts.** Each duct has, at one end, an expansion or **ampulla** (L. jug).

The kinetic sensory organ, called **crista ampullaris** (Fig. 19-9), is situated within

Orientation of the Semicircular Ducts

The three semicircular ducts have a dis-

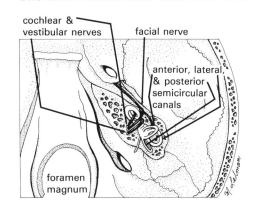

cochlear & vestibular nerves

facial nerve

anterior, lateral, & posterior semicircular canals

foramen magnum

Fig. 19-10. Orientation of semicircular ducts.

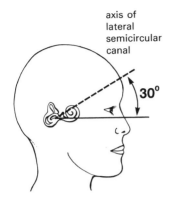

axis of
lateral
semicircular
canal

30°

Fig. 19-11. Orientation of the lateral duct.

Rule of Excitation

During a given movement, the response of a crista ampullaris is maximal when this movement is in the same plane as its semicircular duct. To best stimulate the crista ampullaris of the lateral semicircular duct during horizontal rotational movement, the head must be tilted 30° downward (Fig. 19-12).

Detection of Rotational Movement

The sensitive receptor organs pick up even subtle rotational movement like, for instance, normal head movement that accelerates slowly and does not last long.

When the head rotates to one side, the endolymph lags behind and stimulates the cupula in the opposite direction, i.e., the endolymph moves and stimulates the cupula in the opposite direction of a movement.

One may impose a strong stress to the receptors of rotational movement by spin-

tinct plane of orientation (Figs. 19-10 and 19-11). A certain correspondence in pairs of these planes exists between the left and the right semicircular ducts. The spatial plane pairs are the left posterior duct with the right anterior duct and the right posterior duct with the left anterior duct.

The lateral ducts are in the same plane. They are positioned at a 30° upward angle to the horizontal plane of the head as illustrated in Figure 19-11.

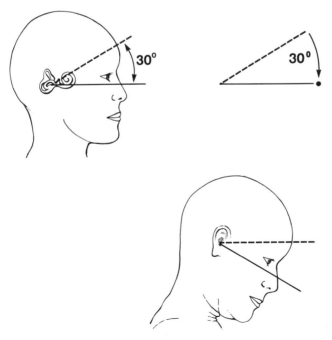

Fig. 19-12. Best position in testing effect of horizontal rotational movement.

ning the body, e.g., to the right, and then suddenly stopping. As a result, three phases can be distinguished:

1. Acceleration phase—the endolymph lags because of inertia during acceleration, making the cupula swing in the direction opposite to the movement of the head.
2. Constant velocity phase—there is no movement of the endolymph and no excitation of the cupula.
3. Stopping phase—when the movement is brought to a halt, the endolymph will continue by inertia to rotate to the right. This creates the illusion that the body is rotating in the opposite direction, i.e., to the left, and sensations of vertigo and nausea set in. Motor reflexes are triggered for body and eye displacement toward the right as well as slow eye movement to the right in a futile attempt to compensate for the illusion of falling to the left. This enhances the confusion of the mind, increases the reflex displacement of the body to the right, and ends by making one fall in that direction (right).

If one carefully observes the eyes of a person who has just stopped spinning around to the right, one will find that the eyes slowly displace to the right, move quickly to the left to recover the central position and then start again turning to the right (nystagmus).

In table form, the fast eye movements in a rotational test are in the acceleration phase—fast eye movement in the direction of rotation; and in the stopping phase—fast eye movement in the direction opposite to the rotation.

Caloric Irrigation Test

If the ear canal is irrigated with warm (usually 44°C) or cold water, convection currents of the endolymph are established, especially in the closest semicircular duct, namely, the lateral.

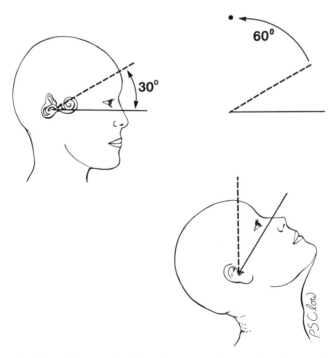

Fig. 19-13. Angle of head in caloric irrigation test when patient is standing or sitting up.

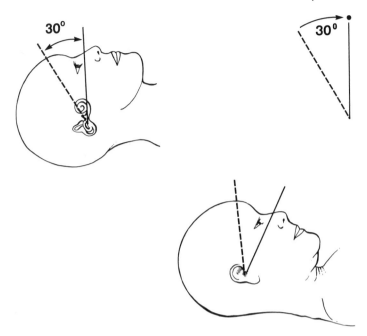

Fig. 19-14. Angle of head in caloric irrigation test when patient is in a horizontal position.

In a caloric irrigation test the patient holds the head in such a position that the lateral semicircular duct is vertical. In this manner the convection current effected by temperature will be reinforced by the gravitational force. To achieve a vertical position of the lateral semicircular canals in a standing or sitting position the head must be tilted 60° upward (Fig. 19-13). In a horizontal position the head must be tilted 30° downward (Fig. 19-14). When irrigating the right ear with cold water the endolymph becomes heavier and falls, on account of the fact that the endolymph is moving within the right lateral semicircular duct toward the right. It may produce symptoms of nausea and vertigo (sensation of rotation) toward the left, signs of postural deviations toward the right, and nystagmus, i.e., slow eye movements to the right and fast eye movements to the left.

The use of warm water in the test triggers the same signs and symptoms as cold water but with reversed direction (Table 19-1).

Table 19-1. Caloric Test

Cold water in ear—fast eye movement toward the opposite ear.
Warm water in ear—fast eye movement toward the irrigated ear.

Vertigo

Vertigo (the sensation of rotation either of the individual or of the environment) is a very common symptom in vestibular diseases affecting the labyrinth, vestibular nerve, or vestibular nuclei, although it may have other origins. A classical example of labyrinthine vertigo is **Ménière's disease,** which is due to edema of the labyrinth and which expresses itself in abrupt and severe attacks of vertigo. Nystagmus can also be present during the attacks.

Vestibular Ganglion

The vestibular ganglion is positioned at the bottom of the internal auditory meatus. The peripheral processes end in the vestibular nuclei.

The central pathways of the vestibular system were covered in Chapter 14.

Suggested Reading

Baloh RW, Honrubia V: Clinical Neurophysiology of the Vestibular System, FA Davis, Philadelphia, 1979.

Barr ML, Kiernan JA: The Human Nervous System. Fourth Edition. Harper and Row, Philadelphia, Chapters 21 and 22, 1983.

Brodal A, Pompeiano O, Eds.: Basic Aspects of Central Vestibular Mechanisms, Progress in Brain Research, Vol. 37, Elsevier, Amsterdam, 1972.

Celesia GG: Organization of auditory cortical areas in man, Brain 99:403–414, 1976.

Heimer L: The Human Brain and Spinal Cord, Springer-Verlag, New York, pp. 245–270, 1983.

Kelso JAS, Tuller B: Cognition and emotion. In Gazzaniga MS, Ed.: Handbook of Cognitive Neuroscience, Plenum Press, New York, 1984.

Königsmark BW, Ed.: Neuroanatomy of the Auditory System. Report on Workshop, Arch Otolaryng 98:397–413, 1973.

Miller JM, Towe AL: Audition: Structural and acoustical properties. In Ruch T, Patton HD, Eds.: Physiology and Biophysics, Twentieth Edition. WB Saunders, Philadelphia, pp. 339–434, 1979.

Möller AR, Boston P, Eds.: Basic Mechanisms in Hearing, Academic Press, New York, 1973.

Schubert ED: Hearing: Its Function and Dysfunction, Springer-Verlag, Wien, New York, 1980.

Smith CA: The inner ear: its embryological development and microstructure. In Tower DB, Ed.: The Nervous System, Vol. 3: Human Communication and Its Disorders, Raven Press, New York, pp. 1–18, 1975.

V
Integration

20

Visceral Nervous System

Vital Roles

The **visceral nervous system (VNS)** is concerned with **homeostasis,** i.e., the maintenance of an optimum internal environment. This involves the control of viscera, blood vessels, body fluids, and glands in many of their aspects, e.g., O_2–CO_2 body tissue concentration (respiration), reproductive functions, food demands, digestion and metabolism, body growth, temperature control, blood circulation, blood pressure, and chemical constants. All these are examples of basic functions for the survival of the individual and the species.

In the past, visceral functions in the central nervous system (CNS) were viewed to be restricted to a very few regions of which the hypothalamus was considered to be of the highest level. Currently, the involvement in visceral functions of other regions of the telencephalon are recognized, and their various possible roles are the subject of investigation. This changed view favors the perspective of the brain as an integrative unit.

Two Distinctive Features

One main characteristic of the VNS is that it builds up much less brain cortical circuitry than the discriminative exteroceptive and proprioceptive systems. Notwithstanding, it can influence all cortical activities of the CNS, for instance, by sharing common key structures or by releasing hormones. One should keep in mind that CNS is a visceral organ.

Another particular characteristic of the VNS is the morphology of its pathways. Often they appear not to be as precisely circumscribed as is typical of the somatic system. With the help of new techniques, researchers are still mapping out the sensory and motor paths of this system within the CNS.

Components

The components of the VNS at different levels are the peripheral visceral nervous system (described in Chapter 10) and the central visceral nervous system. Visceral components of the spinal cord, brain stem, diencephalon, and cerebral hemispheres are dealt with in this chapter.

Spinal Cord Components

The peripheral visceral afferent fibers enter through the posterior root and distribute their branches in a diffuse manner through the **Lissauer's tract** to reach the substantia gelatinosa, interneurons, and the intermediate visceral region, which contains the intermediomedial and intermediolateral nuclei.

Some axons of the intermediomedial visceral nucleus synapse in the preganglionic neurons of the intermediolateral nucleus to establish visceral reflexes.

Through their connections with the substantia gelatinosa and interneurons, the peripheral visceral afferent fibers are able to influence the spinal cord activity of that region, like somatic motor reflexes.

There are three polysynaptic paths of the intermediate visceral region:

One path transmits information through the substantia gelatinosa centralis to other spinal cord segments and the brain.

A second one transmits information through the spinoreticular tract to the brain stem.

A third path transmits information through the anterolateral spinothalamic tract to the intralaminar nuclei of the thalamus.

More details related to the visceral motor system at the spinal cord level are presented in Chapter 10.

Brain Stem Components

Vital Centers

A description of the **vital centers** of the brain stem is presented in Chapter 14 in connection with some of the visceral sensory inputs from cranial nerves. The ascending visceral tracts from the spinal cord also influence these centers.

Area Postrema

The **area postrema** is a small prominence on the caudal region of the floor of the fourth ventricle. Lacking a **blood-brain barrier (BBB)**, it lies open to be influenced by the cerebrospinal fluid (CSF) composition. It receives ascending visceral fibers from the cord and connects with the nucleus solitarius. The stimulation of the area postrema produces vomiting.

Reticular Formation

The **reticular formation** is involved in the processing of somatic as well as visceral signals. It intermediates sensory and motor signals.

The reticular formation, composed of a number of nuclei throughout the brain stem tegmentum, extends axons even beyond the brain stem. Midbrain cells reach diencephalic and telencephalic structures. Cells of the pons and medulla oblongata reach the spinal cord. The midbrain, pons, and medulla oblongata reticular nuclei are interconnected.

For purposes of studying the VNS, the reticular formation offers two convenient views in the lateromedial and the rostrocaudal planes.

There is a **lateral reticular group** of nuclei in the brain stem, consisting of parvicellular structures (small cells). These receive synaptic stimuli mostly of an exteroceptive nature and transmit them to the **medial reticular group** of nuclei of

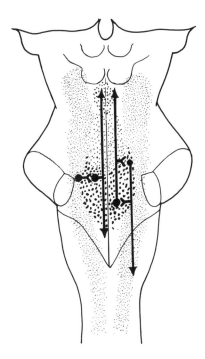

Fig. 20-1. Lateral (finely stipled) and medial (coarsely stipled) groups of reticular nuclei.

2. Their stimulation produces analgesia and sleepiness.
3. If lesioned, insomnia ensues.
4. The caudal raphe nuclei project fibers into the anterior and lateral funiculi of the spinal cord with endings in the anterior lateral and posterior horns and inferior olivary complex.
5. The rostral and caudal sets of nuclei project to the cerebellum and other nuclei of the reticular formation and locus ceruleus.
6. The rostral raphe nuclei project to locus ceruleus, other midbrain structures, intralaminar and midline nuclei, the habenula, hypothalamus, striatum, the amygdala, regions of the lamina terminalis, the anterior perforated region, the hippocampus, and neocortex. These ascending fibers are components of the dorsal longitudinal fasciculus of Schütz and the medial forebrain bundle.

Dorsal Longitudinal Fasciculus of Schütz

The **dorsal longitudinal fasciculus of Schütz** is seen as a bundle of nonmyelinated fibers in the periaqueductal gray matter of the midbrain. It links, among other structures, the hypothalamus with the midbrain reticular formation, from where signals can reach other visceral regions of the cerebrum, brain stem, and spinal cord.

Also part of the fasciculus are ascending fibers carrying nondiscriminative taste signals to intralaminar nuclei.

Locus Ceruleus

Locus ceruleus, which receives input from the raphe nuclei, is a nucleus located in the floor of the fourth ventricle at a rostral pontine level. It is very rich in **noradrenaline.** Its output reaches mostly the following structures: the spinal cord, infe-

magnocellular cells, which receive mostly synaptic stimuli of visceroceptive nature (Fig. 20-1).

The reticular formation also receives descending inputs from the diencephalon and telencephalon. There is scant scientific information about the precise output patterns through the different ascending and descending paths of the reticular formation, as the inputs are varied and complex.

Raphe Nuclei

The **raphe nuclei** can be grouped into rostral and caudal. They may be considered part of the reticular formation and feature the following main characteristics:

1. They are very rich in **serotonin,** i.e., **5-hydroxytryptamine,** a monoamine neurotransmitter.

rior olive, dorsal nucleus of vagus, cerebellum, colliculi, thalamus, hypothalamus, habenula, region of the lamina terminalis, hippocampus, amygdala, olfactory bulb, and brain cortex. It plays an important role as part of an activating system. The nerve endings are found intimately associated with cerebral arteries, suggesting their involvement in the regulation of cerebral blood flow.

Some of the fibers of the locus ceruleus are components of the **medial forebrain bundle.**

Substantia Nigra and Ventral Tegmental Area of Tsai

Two very important structures are the **substantia nigra** and the **ventral tegmental area of Tsai,** which abound in **dopamine,** a monoamine neurotransmitter.

The projection of the substantia nigra to the striatum and thalamus through the internal capsule is mentioned in Chapter 14. There are also projections to cortical areas.

The ventral tegmental area of Tsai projects through the medial forebrain bundle to the region of the lamina terminalis, cingulate gyrus, and orbitofrontal cortex.

It has been suggested that hyperactivity in these dopaminergic paths may produce schizophrenic states.

Medial Forebrain Bundle

The **medial forebrain bundle (medial telencephalic fasciculus)** is seen as a bundle of fibers coursing lateral to the hypothalamus from the region of the lamina terminalis to the midbrain. Beside the noradrenergic fibers from the locus ceruleus and dopaminergic fibers from the ventral tegmental area, other fibers contribute to this bundle, whose main origins are the orbitofrontal cortex, the cingulum, the primary olfactory area (olfactotegmental fibers), and the region of the lamina terminalis. These fibers synapse in the lateral hypothalamus, raphe nuclei, and the reticular formation of midbrain and pons,

from where the signals relay to reach other visceral nuclei.

Central Tegmental Tract

The **central tegmental tract** is a pathway from the midbrain to the inferior olivary complex. Its fibers originate in the tectum, red nucleus, periaqueductal gray, and other tegmental areas of the midbrain. These sources of fibers relay data received from cortex, cerebellum, and other sites. Forming part of this tract are ascending reticular fibers.

The coded signals traveling through this tract toward the inferior olivary complex integrate various complex functions.

The central tegmental tract courses medially to the fibers of the superior cerebellar peduncle at high pontine levels, takes a central tegmental position at a midpontine level, continues dorsally to the medial lemniscus in the caudal pons, and reaches dorsally the inferior olivary complex in the medulla oblongata (Fig. 20-2).

Visceral Diencephalon

Thalamus

The major division of the diencephalon, namely, the **thalamus,** encompasses some structures that intimately share somatic and visceral functions, i.e., intralaminar nuclei. These structures process nondiscriminative information and have connection with other thalamic nuclei which either process discriminative information or integrative information like the reticular thalamic anterior nucleus or the dorsomedial nucleus.

The midline nuclei process mostly visceral signals.

Subthalamus and Reticular Formation

Apart from these discrete visceral regions of the thalamus, the projections of the reticular formation and the subthala-

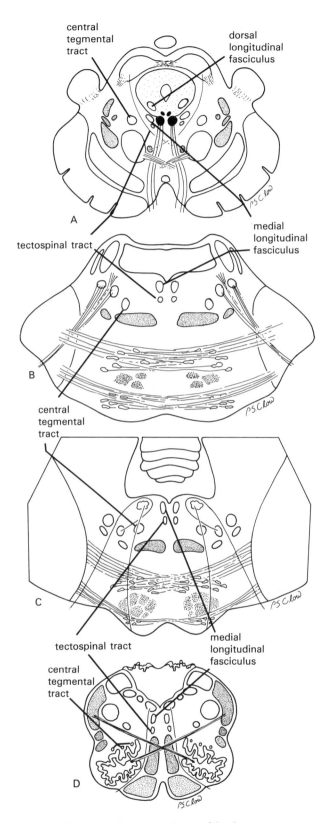

central
tegmental
tract

dorsal
longitudinal
fasciculus

A

medial
longitudinal
fasciculus

tectospinal tract

B

central
tegmental
tract

C

medial
longitudinal
fasciculus

tectospinal tract

central
tegmental
tract

D

Fig. 20-2. Cross-sections of brain stem.

mus also influence somatic and visceral activities.

Hypothalamus

The **hypothalamus** is mostly concerned with visceral functions. An account of the structure is given in Chapter 7.

There are two hypothalamohypophyseal **neuroendocrine systems** (Fig. 20-3): the **supraopticohypophyseal** or **hypothalamohypophyseal system,** which connects the supraoptic and paraventricular nuclei with the neurohypophysis; and the **tuberoinfundibular, tuberohypophyseal,** or **hypothalamoinfundibular portal system,**

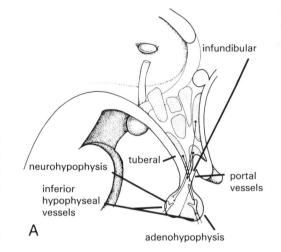

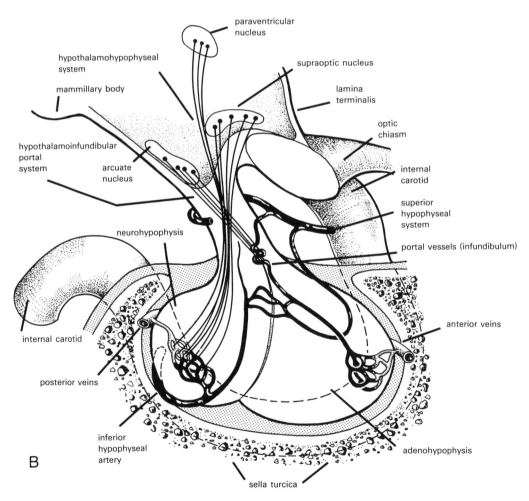

Fig. 20-3. (A) Hypothalamic neuroendocrine systems; (B) hypothalamohypophyseal systems.

which connects the hypothalamus with the adenohypophysis through a system of portal vessels.

Hypothalamohypophyseal System. The neurosecretory cells mostly of the supraoptic nucleus produce the **antidiuretic hormone (ADH).** This substance is transported through the axons to the neurohypophyseal capillary vessels.

ADH is released in response to a rise in osmotic pressure of the blood. The increment of this blood circulating hormone increases the resorption of water in the distal tubules of the kidneys. Interference with the production of ADH produces a hypothalamic syndrome called **diabetes insipidus,** characterized by an increased production of urine **(polyuria)** and excessive thirst **(polydipsia).**

The paraventricular nucleus secretes mostly **oxytocin,** which promotes the contraction of smooth muscles of the uterus and mammary glands.

Hypothalamoinfundibular Portal System. Nuclei situated in the tuberal region, mostly in the median eminence, send their axons to the infundibular region. The neurosecreted hormones reach the adenohypophysis by way of a vascular network called **pituitary portal vessels,** which transport the hormones to the adenohypophysis.

The neurosecretory cells of this **tuberoinfundibular system** produce hormones called **releasing** and **inhibiting factors (RF and IF).** Each pair of hormonal factors, RF and IF, respectively, excites and inhibits (controls) the productions of a specific hormone in the adenohypophysis. The hormones produced in the adenohypophysis are called **trophic** or **stimulating factors.** These hormones are **follicle stimulating (FSH)** and **luteinizing (LH)** in woman and **interstitial cell stimulating (ICSH)** in men; **luteotrophic (LTH)** or **prolactin; thyrotrophic** or **thyroid stimulating (TSH); adenocorticotrophic (ACTH);** and

growth or **somatotrophic (STH).**

The first four of these hormones are **gonadotrophic.** FSH promotes growth of ovarian follicles and spermatogenesis. LH promotes ovulation and converts the ruptured ovarian follicle into corpus luteum. ICSH stimulates interstitial cells of the testis to secrete **androgens.** LTH stimulates the corpus luteum to secrete **progesterone** and promotes secretion of milk in the lactating breast.

The arcuate nucleus has different neurotransmitter cells rich in substances such as **neuropeptides** and **dopamine,** which are projected to nearby structures, e.g., the median eminence.

The entire endocrine system is under the control of the hypothalamus, which in turn is regulated by many factors like the blood contents and environmental factors.

Lesions of the ventromedial nucleus result in **hyperphagia (overeating)** and **obesity** and is therefore sometimes referred to as a **satiety center.**

The associated hypothalamic signs of adiposity and underdevelopment of genitalia add up to Fröhlich's syndrome, or dystrophia adiposogenitalis.

Hypothalamohypophyseal tumors may encroach the optic chiasm, one optic tract, or compress the medial fibers of the optic tracts, etc. (Fig. 13-6), causing visual field defects.

Hypothalamic Control Centers. Experimental and clinical studies have been carried out in which correlations were established between stimulation or destruction of discrete regions of the hypothalamus and its functional consequences. It has created the basis for the conception of the hypothalamus as a set of centers with particular functions. A list of some of these centers is presented in Table 20-1.

With the purpose of emphasizing the complex function and interdependence of the whole hypothalamus as a unit, and without disregarding the specific functional involvement of each discrete region,

Table 20-1. Hypothalamic Functional Centers

Experiment	Region	Effect	Normal function
Lesion	Ventromedial	Voracious appetite and rage	Satiety center
Stimulation	Dorsomedial	Rage	
Lesion	Upper region of lateral	Loss of appetite	Hunger center
Lesion	Posterior and lateral	Loss of temperature maintenance	Temperature control center
Heating	Anterior	Peripheral vasodilation and sweating	Heat loss center
Destruction	Anterior	Hyperthermia	Heat loss center
Cooling	Posterior	Vasoconstriction, shivering, and increased metabolism	Heat generation and retention center

some more detailed information is presented below to exemplify the role of the hypothalamus in temperature control.

The capillary network of the **lamina terminalis,** a telencephalic structure, is well developed. Cells surrounding these capillaries are sensitive to a rise in temperature. The stimulated cells send their axons through the preoptic, anterior, lateral, and posterior hypothalamus and midbrain, synapsing via collateral and terminal endings in visceral (exciting) and reticular nuclei (inhibiting). Among the observable effects are vasodilation and sweating.

Peripheral **cold receptors** activate the brain stem reticular formation and the posterior hypothalamus, setting off an increase in metabolism, shivering, vasoconstriction, and piloerection.

The fever (**pyrexia**) of many diseases is caused by blood-borne substances, **pyrogens,** which stimulate mechanisms of body defense reactions like the sympathetic system in the confrontation with an adversary. The effects are very similar to the reactions of the body to cold, e.g., heat loss blocking mechanisms and shivering.

Hyperpyrexia is the term for high fever.

Connections of the Hypothalamus

The main paths and structures connecting with the hypothalamus are listed in Table 20-2.

Table 20-2. Main Connections of the Hypothalamus

Dorsal longitudinal fasciculus
Mammillotegmental
Mammillary peduncle
Mammillothalamic
Hypothalamothalamic
Medial forebrain bundle
Retinohypothalamic
Stria medullaris
Ventral amygdalar fibers
Hypothalamic autonomic nuclei

In essence, the hypothalamic connections link the hypothalamus with

1. the brain stem and spinal cord through reticular and visceral paths; interruption of the fibers that synapse with the sympathetic nuclei of the upper thoracic segments of the spinal cord produces **Horner's syndrome;**
2. the endocrine system;
3. other regions of the diencephalon; and
4. telencephalic visceral components.

These visceral pathways have potentials, ranging from subtle to very strong, to influence the somatic nervous system.

Epithalamus

The structures and connections of the epithalamus were described in Chapter 7. Further details follow.

Pineal Body

The **pineal body** or **gland** has **pinealocytes** and glial cells but no neurons. In the human, after the age of 16 years, granules of calcium and magnesium salts begin to deposit in the gland, which makes this structure a useful landmark in X-ray brain imaging.

The gland has an antigonadotrophic function. Experimental pinealectomy in animals produces genital hypertrophy. Administration of pineal extracts produces inhibition of the gonads. The activity of the pineal body is influenced by light.

Habenula

The habenular nuclei are an important visceral link between the region of the lamina terminalis (stria medullaris thalami) and the midbrain (habenulointerpeduncular fasciculus). From the interpeduncular nucleus connections are established with the autonomic nuclei and the reticular formation.

Two Extreme States of the Nervous System

The sympathetic and parasympathetic systems are coordinated and in balance, while each occupies its own domain. The state of defense (sympathetic) is characterized by fight-flight responses, and the state of confidence (parasympathetic) by relaxation responses and sleepiness.

Emotional Fainting Reactions

A massive reaction of the orbitofrontal cortex to strong warning signals during a state of confidence may enhance this state (instead of shifting it to a state of defense) and weakness, dizziness, and fainting responses may result.

Circumventricular Organs

The original ependymal cells in the CNS, i.e., the neuroepithelial cells, have in early stages of development long processes that traverse the whole thickness of the neural tube. Later on the ependymal cells lose these extensions, with the exception of a few small areas of the ependyma, where the cells retain them. These cells are known as **tanycytes** and the discrete areas as **circumventricular organs.**

These circumventricular organs (Fig. 20-4) have, apart from being located in the wall of the ventricles and containing tanycytes, two other characteristics in common. They have well-developed capillary loops, to which the tanycytes are attached, and the BBB is absent. Substances injected into the blood stream quickly enter the intercellular space of the circumventricular organs.

The following structures contain the circumventricular organs: the pineal body, neurohypophysis, lamina terminalis, subfornical and subcommissural organs, and area postrema. The last of these structures is located in the fourth ventricle and the others in the third ventricle.

The **subcommissural organ** is situated in the lining of the posterior commissure. The **subfornical organ** is in the lining between the columns of the fornix at the level of the interventricular foramina.

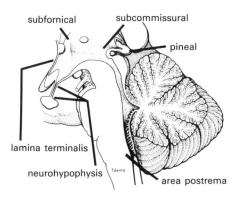

Fig. 20-4. Circumventricular organs.

Introduction to the Telencephalic Visceral Components

There are five particularly important concepts regarding the telencephalic VNS.

1. As knowledge progresses, involvement with visceral functions is attributed to the telencephalon to an increasing degree.
2. Greater overlapping connectivity is being discovered between what are considered visceral and somatic telencephalic regions.
3. The accomplishment of many visceral behavioral objectives (e.g., drinking, eating, sexual acts) requires intimate coordination of the visceral with the somatic system.
4. The region of the lamina terminalis appears to be an important link of visceral functions with other telencephalic functions.
5. The conception of the brain simply in a duality of roles, i.e., visceral or somatic, is an artificial one. Although useful as a premise for study, it is fraught with shortcomings.

Telencephalic Visceral Components

Because of their complex connections, none of the telencephalic structures must be considered as simple visceral centers. However, three areas can be viewed as visceral in their function, i.e., the region of the lamina terminalis, the amygdalar (amygdaloid) complex and neighboring cortex (i.e., the temporal pole), and some regions of the insula and the opercula.

The frontal cortex, particularly the inferomedial frontal cortex, has links with other visceral areas. This cortical region is believed to be concerned with processing the signal basis of thought of a subjective nature.

Also important to mention in this context is the **Papez' circuit,** which is shared by the somatic and visceral systems.

Region of the Lamina Terminalis

The **lamina terminalis** and its cell growth are telencephalic. The following regions are related to this structure: the preoptic region, septal area, anterior perforated substance, substantia innominata, and nucleus accumbens.

The **preoptic region** is situated posterior to the lamina terminalis (between the hypothalamus and lamina terminalis). Some textbooks view this region as part of the hypothalamus.

The **septal area,** also known as **precommissural septum** or **septum verum,** is anterior to the lamina terminalis. Anteriorly, it is separated from the subcallosal area by the posterior paraolfactory sulcus.

Notes: (1) In the literature the terms "septal area" and "subcallosal area" are sometimes used interchangeably in reference to either structure. (2) Another distinct septal area is the structure better known as septum pellucidum.

A list of nuclei of the septal area is presented in Table 20-3. Laterally and posteriorly, the septal area is continuous with the substantia innominata, which lies above the anterior perforated substance and below the rostral region of the lentiform nucleus. The substantia innominata is continuous laterally with the amygdaloid complex.

The septal area has connections with all the other regions of the lamina terminalis.

Table 20-3. Septal Nuclei

Dorsal group
Dorsal septal nucleus
Ventral group
Lateral septal nucleus
Medial septal nucleus
Nucleus of Broca
Diagonal band
Caudal group
Nucleus of the anterior commissure
Nucleus of the stria terminalis

It also establishes connections with the amygdala and hippocampus through the diagonal band and the cingulate gyrus. Furthermore, it contributes to the medial forebrain bundle, establishing connections with the orbitofrontal cortex, hypothalamus, and midbrain structures. Other connections are established with the amygdala through the stria terminalis. Through the stria medullaris the septal area connects with the habenula and through the fornix further connections are made with the hippocampus.

The **nucleus of the substantia innominata,** or **basal nucleus of Meynert,** projects to the cerebral cortex. It is very rich in acetylcholine. Cell degeneration of this nucleus is common in Alzheimer's presenile dementia (Fig. 20-5).

The **nucleus accumbens** (Fig. 20-5) is situated at the junction of the caudate nucleus and putamen.

Amygdala

The dorsomedial portion of the **amygdala (amygdaloid body)** is known as the **corticomedial group of nuclei.** It receives secondary olfactory fibers and is considered part of the primary olfactory area. The ventrolateral portion is known as the **basolateral group of nuclei.** Apart from its

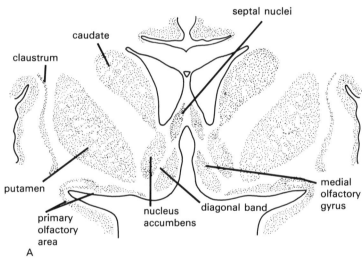

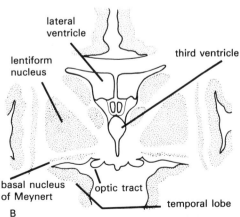

Fig. 20-5. Coronal section of brain through nucleus accumbens (A) and basal nucleus of Meynert (B).

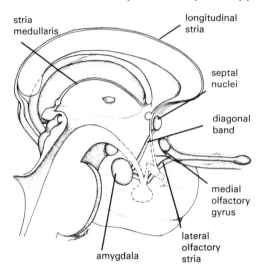

Fig. 20-6. Amygdala and olfactory system.

involvement in the primary olfactory area (Fig. 20-6) it has connections (Fig. 20-7) with

1. the dorsomedial nucleus of the thalamus through the ventral amygdalar fibers which join the inferior thalamic peduncle;
2. reticular nuclei of the brain stem through ventral amygdalar fibers which join the medial forebrain bundle;
3. the neighboring temporal cortex;

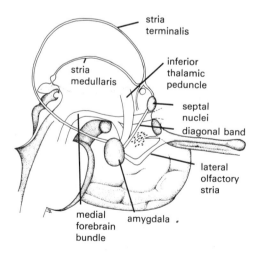

Fig. 20-7. Connections of amygdala.

4. the frontal cortex through the uncinate bundle and ventral amygdalar fibers;
5. the region of the lamina terminalis through the diagonal band;
6. the region of the lamina terminalis through the stria terminalis;
7. the hypothalamus through ventral amygdalar fibers;
8. the subiculum; and
9. the insular cortex.

Insular Cortex

The insular cortex receives communications from the intralaminar nuclei processing visceral information, including taste. It constitutes in part the seat of the somatosensory area II, which it shares with the surrounding parietal operculum and claustrum. It also has connections with the amygdala.

Claustrum

The connectivity and function of the **claustrum** is still a matter of debate. It has been claimed that it is connected with the insular cortex and the lentiform nucleus, the dorsomedial nucleus of the thalamus through the ansa peduncularis, and cortical areas in an arrangement similar to that of the connections of the cortex with the corpus striatum, suggesting that the claustrum is a visceral link of the corticosubcorticocortical loop, i.e., cortex → claustrum → thalamus → cortex.

Papez' Circuit

Two main elements form the **circuit of Papez** (Fig. 20-8), namely, the main loop and its various inputs and outputs.

The main loop consists of hippocampal formation → subiculum → fimbria → fornix → mammillary body → anterior nucleus of the thalamus → cingulate gyrus → hippocampal formation.

Data related to inputs and outputs of the Papez' circuit are still being gathered.

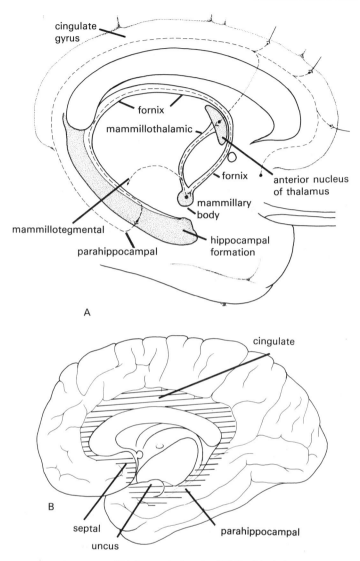

Fig. 20-8. (A) Papez' circuit; (B) limbic lobe.

The Limbic System Concept

The **limbic system** is a concept which has evolved from the interpretation by Broca in 1878 of the limbic lobe, which included the cingulate and parahippocampal gyri and the septal area (Fig. 20-8), and by Papez in 1937 with the description of the loop. Since the fifties, many scientists have contributed further data to expand this concept. Their principal premise was to use the concept as a unitary model to explain normal and pathological behavioral patterns. Many students have restricted the concept of the model and have identified it as the visceral brain without distinguishing it from the concept of the emotional brain (Fig. 20-9).

Input and output structures to the Papez' circuit are

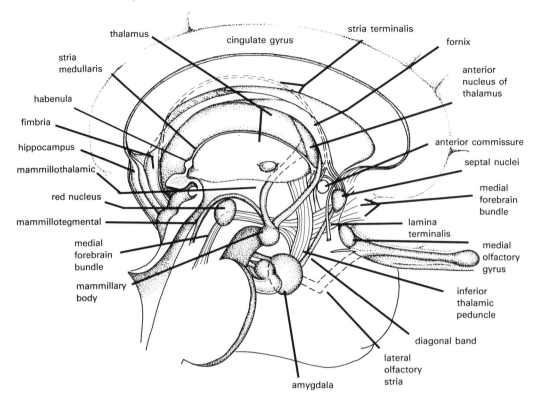

Fig. 20-9. Limbic system.

1. the frontal lobe through the uncinate bundle and the temporal lobe with the hippocampal formation;
2. the frontal, parietal, and occipital lobes through the cingulate gyrus with the hippocampal formation;
3. the temporal lobe with the hippocampal formation;
4. the region of the lamina terminalis together with all its connections (midbrain, hypothalamus, temporal lobe) through fiber connections with the fornix as well as with the cingulate gyrus;
5. the mammillary body with the midbrain tegmentum through the mammillotegmental tract; and
6. the olfactory system.

   It is obvious that the circuit of Papez is shared among other structures by the whole cerebral cortex. Nevertheless, the literature emphasizes in particular the following connections in the circuitry: (1) those of the anterior temporal lobe; (2) those of the region of the lamina terminalis; and (3) those of a visceral longitudinal axis composed of all the fiber paths connecting the midbrain with the hypothalamus and the region of the lamina terminalis (mesolimbic system) (Fig. 20-10).

   A present major problem related to the usage of this concept is the lack of conformity regarding its definition. Some scientists are abandoning the concept altogether and focus on more restricted and specific models instead. Other scientists continue in their efforts to improve the model of the limbic system.

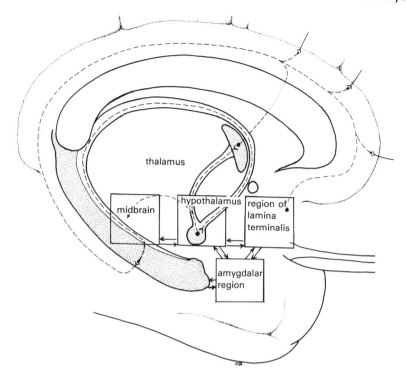

Fig. 20-10. Mesolimbic system.

Stimulation of the Cerebral Visceral Centers

The findings collected in the literature regarding the stimulation of the cerebral visceral centers can be grouped into three spectral categories of response: objective physiological reactions, subjective feelings, and behavioral changes.

Physiological Reactions

Most physiological reactions are of a visceral nature: salivation, changes in motility of the gastrointestinal tract, defecation, vomiting, respiratory arrest, alterations in blood pressure, shivering, piloerection, penile erection, temperature changes, etc.

Subjective Feelings

Within each of the cerebral visceral structures, **feelings** of aversion and pleasure have been reported to have a substrate. If an experimental or clinical subject is left to self-stimulate either pattern, appropriately, avoidance of or persistence in self-stimulation has resulted. These cerebral visceral substrates have thus been called **avoidance** and **reward centers,** respectively. They are located close to each other in each visceral brain region.

Behavioral Changes

Behavioral changes that have been observed oscillate from aggression to docility.

The link between the visceral brain regions and the three spectral categories of response to their stimulation has served as the basis to establish a direct correlation of these regions with feelings and behavioral patterns of affective states.

Distinction Between Subjective and Objective Sensations

The following generalizations are explicitly and implicitly recorded in the literature:

Subjective nondiscriminative sensations affect the homeostatic equilibrium of the organism (affective sensations).

In normal states, **objective discriminative sensations** do not affect the homeostatic equilibrium of the organism.

Most visceral sensations have a high content of subjectivity.

Visceral Pain—Referred Pain

The mind reads the nociceptive signals in accordance with the segmental somatic map and refers the source of visceral pain to the corresponding somatic segmental region of the wall of the trunk (Fig. 20-11 and Table 20-4).

Different hypotheses have been suggested to explain such phenomena of referred pain, e.g.:

1. The visceral and somatic nociceptive afferent fibers converge their synapses on the same pool of spinal cord neurons. Given the fact that the somatic pain experience is richer and more common than visceral pain, the mind misinterprets the signals and reads them to be somatic.

2. The visceral and somatic nociceptive path originating from each spinal cord

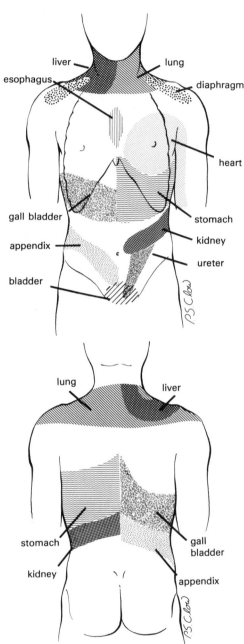

Fig. 20-11. Referred pain.

segment projects its impulses to (synapse with) the same group of cells in the ventral posterior nucleus of the thalamus, where there is a predominance of somatic information that topographically builds up the somatic body regions.

Table 20-4. Referred Pain

Pain of angina pectoris = upper left chest and down the inside of the left arm (T1–4).

Pain of gall bladder = right upper quadrant of abdomen and right infrascapular region (T6–8).

Diaphragm irritation = shoulder region (C3–5).

Stomach pain = epigastrium (T7–8).

Duodenal pain = anterior abdominal wall, just above the umbilicus (T9–10).

Pain of appendix = umbilicus (T10). The pain shifts to the lower right quadrant if the parietal peritoneum is affected.

Pain of renal pelvis and ureter = loin and inguinal region (T11 to L2).

Pain of esophagus = sternum (T4–5).

Pain of urinary bladder = pubic and suprapubic region (T11 to L2).

3. Stimulation of visceral nociceptors travels through afferent fibers within sympathetic nerves and reaches the corresponding intermediolateral sympathetic nuclei. Neurons of these nuclei constrict the vessels of their regional innervation of the thoracic wall (or limb) in a visceral hypoxic spasm which irritates somatic nociceptive terminals of the innervated region. This spasm triggers somatic nociceptive signals which reach the spinal cord and travel through the somatic nociceptive path (anterolateral spinothalamic tract) towards the brain cortex.

4. Afferent visceral nociceptors synapse on spinal cord interneurons which in turn overexcite the ventral somatic motor neurons that trigger somatic muscle spasms initiating somatic nociceptive signals.

Suggested Readings

Amaral DG, Sinnamon HM: The locus coeruleus: Neurobiology of a central noradrenergic nucleus, Progr Neurobiol 9:147–196, 1977.

Ben-Ari Y, Ed.: The Amygdaloid Complex, Elsevier/North-Holland Biomedical Press, Amsterdam, 1981.

Bloom FE: Neuropeptides, Sci Am 245(4):148–169, 1981.

Bystrzycka EK: Afferent projections to the dorsal and ventral respiratory nuclei in the medulla oblongata of the cat, studied by the horseradish peroxidase technique, Brain Res 185:59–66, 1980.

Cooper JR, Bloom FE, Roth RH: The Biochemical Basis of Neuropharmacology. Fourth Edition. Oxford University Press, New York, 1982.

Giesler GJ Jr, Liebeskind JC: Inhibition of visceral pain by electrical stimulation of the periaqueductal gray matter, Pain 2:43–48, 1976.

Girgis M: The rhinencephalon, Acta Anat 76:157–199, 1970.

Grossman SP: Behavioral functions of the septum: a re-analysis. In DeFrance JF, Ed.: The Septal Nuclei, Plenum Press, New York, pp. 361–422, 1976.

Hall E: The anatomy of the limbic system. In Mogenson GJ, Calaresu FR, Eds.: Neural Integration of Physiological Mechanisms and Behavior, University of Toronto Press, Toronto, pp. 68–94, 1975.

Heimer L: The Human Brain and Spinal Cord, Springer-Verlag, New York, Chapters 10, 15 and 17, 1983.

House EL, Pansky B, Siegel A: A Systematic Approach to Neuroscience. Third Edition. McGraw-Hill, New York, pp. 398–444, 1979.

Isaacson RL: The Limbic System. Second Edition. Plenum Press, New York, 1982.

Joseph SA, Knigge KM: The endocrine hypothalamus: recent anatomical studies. In Reichlin S, Baldessarini RJ, Martin JB, Eds.: The Hypothalamus, Raven Press, New York, pp. 15–47, 1978.

Livingstone KE, Escobar A: Anatomical bias of the limbic system concept: A proposed reorientation, Arch Neurol 24:17–21, 1971.

MacLean PD: Challenges of the Papez heritage. In Limbic Mechanisms. The Continuing Evolution of the Limbic System Concept, Plenum Press, New York, pp. 1–15, 1978.

Newman PP: Visceral Afferent Functions of the Nervous System, Edward Arnold, London, 1974.

Nygren L-G, Olson L: A new major projection from locus coeruleus, the main source of noradrenergic nerve terminals in the ventral and dorsal columns of the spinal cord, Brain Res 132:85–93, 1977.

Papez JW: A proposed mechanism for emotion, Arch Neurol Psychiatry 38:725–734, 1937.

Swanson LW, Mogenson GJ: Neural mechanisms for the functional coupling of autonomic, endocrine and somatomotor responses in adaptive behavior, Brain Res Rev 3:1–34, 1981.

21

Cerebral Cortex: Regional Structure and Function

Architecture

The nerve cells of the cortex or **pallium** are arranged in layers. A correlation between the number of cell layers and phylogenetic age has been established for each region of the cortex as shown in Table 21-1.

The archicortex and paleocortex are together known as **allocortex.** There is a region of the cortex whose **cytoarchitectonics** border between paleo- and neocortex. This is the **mesocortex** or **juxtaallocortex.**

The allocortex and mesocortex together are known as the **limbic lobe** (Fig. 21-1).

The neocortex or **isocortex** is composed of the **homotypical cortex** (Fig. 21-2), in which there are six distinct cellular layers, and the **heterotypical cortex** with two distinct types, i.e., the **granular cortex,** also known as **koniocortex** (Gr. *konios* dust) with cell layers II and IV well developed

Table 21-1. Phylogenetic Variances in Cerebral Cortex

Origin	Layers	Structure
Archicortex	Three	Hippocampal formation and dentate gyrus
Paleocortex	Transitional, between three and six	Pyriform cortex
Neocortex	Six	Most of cerebral cortex

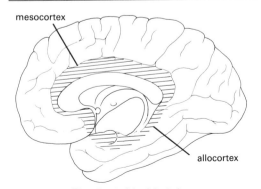

mesocortex

allocortex

Fig. 21-1. Limbic lobe.

355

Cortical Neurons

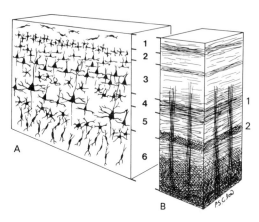

Fig. 21-2. Neocortex. (A) Cytoarchitecture: (1) molecular layer; (2) external granular layer; (3) external pyramidal layer; (4) internal granular layer; (5) internal pyramidal layer; (6) multiform layer. (B) Myeloarchitecture: (1) outer line of Baillarger; (2) inner line of Baillarger.

Cortical neurons have various shapes, some of which are transitional. They can be grouped into five main types.

Pyramidal Cells

A **pyramidal cell** has a dendritic process at its apex (apical dendrite) and several lateral dendritic processes. The axon, beside giving off some collateral branches within its cortical region, typically enters the white matter as one of the three fiber types, i.e., projection, association, or commissural fibers. The largest cortical neurons are found in area 4 and are known as **Betz's cells.**

Fusiform Cells

The cell bodies and dendrites of **fusiform cells** lend to them a spindle shape. Their axons also enter the underlying white matter.

Stellate Cells

Stellate cells are star-shaped, and are also known as **granular cells.** Their axons are short (Golgi type II) and target a nearby region. A variation of the stellate cell is the **basket cell,** so called because the axon ends as a basket around the soma of a neuron.

Cells of Martinotti

The main characteristic of the **cell of Martinotti** is that it projects its axon toward the surface of the cortex where it branches out in a horizontal plane.

Horizontal Cells of Cajal

Horizontal cells of Cajal are found in the most superficial layer, their dendrites and axons coursing horizontally along the surface of the cortex.

and identified as granular, and the **agranular cortex,** where cell layers II and IV are nearly agranular.

Examples of agranular cortex are the motor areas, or areas 4, 6, and 8 of Brodmann.

Examples of granular cortex are the primary sensory areas.

The categorizations above are based principally on the cytoarchitecture of the cortex. In addition, classifications founded on the fiber arrangement, or **myeloarchitecture,** are evidenced (Fig. 21-2).

Apart from the cyto- and myeloarchitectonic classifications, another system based on the patterns of the capillary vessels, i.e., **angioarchitectonic classification,** is gaining momentum.

In recent years the **chemoarchitectural mapping** or chemical composition of different regions of the cortex has been explored. This classification is increasingly regarded as an interesting conception to be developed further.

Two Patterns of Axonal Cell Arrangement

In reference to their axonal length, fibers are classified as **projection fibers** (long) and **local fibers** (short).

The pyramidal and fusiform cells project their long axons outside the cortex. They are known as **corticofugal fibers.** The stellate, Martinotti, and horizontal cells of Cajal maintain their axons within the cortex (intrinsic cortical connections).

Input to the Cortex

Fibers making axonal input to the cortex are known as **corticopetal fibers,** of which there are four types: (1) from diencephalic and more caudal regions projecting to the cortex (mostly from the thalamus); (2) intrinsic fiber input from nearby neurons; (3) associating fiber input through the white matter from other cortical regions of the same hemisphere; and (4) commissural fiber input from homologous regions of the other hemisphere through the appropriate commissure; the corpus callosum is by far the largest interhemispheric commissural bundle.

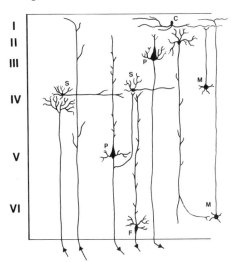

Fig. 21-3. Cerebrocortical input-output. C, horizontal cell of Cajal; F, fusiform cell; M, cell of Martinotti; P, pyramidal cell; S, stellate cell.

their respective cortical regions but also affect the regional cortical activity through collaterals (Fig. 21-3).

Columnar and Horizontal Organization of the Cortex

The intrinsic cortical circuitry is arranged in vertical and horizontal planes,

Input-Output of Cortical Layers

In a simplified view, all the cortical layers can be seen to receive a very rich input from many sources following rigid laws of synaptology.

Layers I, II, and IV are involved mostly in modulating the input-output of the cortex through enhancement and inhibition of local circuits. For instance, the main effect of the activity of basket cells appears to be the inhibition of other neurons.

Layers III, V, and VI not only are involved in sending output signals from

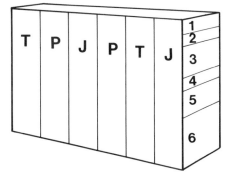

Fig. 21-4. Columnar and horizontal organization of cerebral cortex. T, touch; P, pressure; J, joint.

which are interdependent. This arrangement establishes the basis for analyzing the cortical circuits as working units according to local vertical or columnar units (**vertical planes**) and local horizontal units (**horizontal planes**) (Fig. 21-4). The number of cells composing each of these units, which count in the hundreds, varies in each cortical region and plane.

Recapitulation of Previously Mentioned Cortical Loops

Four main types of loops were mentioned in the chapters describing cortical regions.

Thalamocorticothalamic Loops

With respect to these loops it was emphasized how specific signals, e.g., visual, tactile, auditory, were transmitted in a very specific manner from the thalamus to the cortex and with a feedback from the cortex to the thalamus. This first connectivity was followed by successive and increasingly more complex associative thalamocorticothalamic loops and then by integrative thalamocorticothalamic loops.

Corticocortical Loops

Simultaneous with the establishment of connectivity between the thalamus and the cortex intercortical associative loops also are formed, e.g., between primary tactile, visual, and auditory signals within the same hemispere or between homologous regions of the two hemispheres. All such corticocortical loops become integrated through proper interconnections in the anterior frontal cortex.

Corticosubcorticocortical Loops and Corticocerebellocortical Loops

At the same time as the connectivity described above for thalamocorticothalamic and corticocortical loops is formed, the corticosubcorticocortical and corticocerebellocortical loops are established. These are concerned with the coordination of sensory motor activities as they arise, preparing and conditioning new sensory motor activity. Corticosubcorticocortical loops are described on page 280 and corticocerebellocortical loops on page 268.

The Activity of the Cerebral Cortex as a Continuum

The attractive conceptual analysis of the cortex as a number of circuits within their own frame of stimulus-response must not preclude the conceptual synthesis of the cortex as a continuum. The responses are the substrate for new stimuli; future events are rooted in past events.

Generation of Brain Circuits

The establishment of synaptic contacts between neurons is the basic vehicle for the generation of brain circuits.

The first circuits appearing in ontogenetic development are based on simple primary sensory inputs and simple primary motor outputs. They establish at a very early age the foundations for more complex neuronal loops.

The Time Factor in Development and Function

Each modality of sensation has a very critical, precise timing for the development of its specific fundamental connectiv-

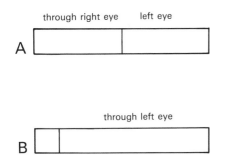

Fig. 21-5. Changes in calcarine cortex connectivity by sensory deprivation.

ity. If a sensory modality lags behind in relation to this critical time for the establishment of its basic connectivity, the subsequent loops and combinations of loops between all the sensory modalities and sensory motor loops will be formed and proceed to generate activity without the coparticipation of the undeveloped modality.

This factor of precise timing is rooted in genetic adjuncts and is dependent on environmental circumstances (nature and nurture). The spatial arrangement of neurons within the nervous system develops according to the inherited genetic plan, while the development of structure and function of brain cells and circuitry, rooted in genetic factors, depend also on operative environmental factors (Fig. 21-5).

In other words, genetic and environmental factors decide through neural space and time the structure and function of the nervous system.

Comments on Environmental Factors

One must realize how vast a territory is covered by the term "environmental factors." Already in uterine life innumerable environmental factors are in operation. During the first few years after birth the environment plays a particularly decisive role. Light, sound, tactile, and other stimuli are needed for the brain to properly develop the assemblage of primary sensory and primary motor neurons. Such assemblage is necessary for behavioral responses involving more than one sensory and one motor neuron.

When a stimulus from the environment triggers an appropriate response, it structurally links together sensory and motor neurons of the assemblies and becomes functionally an efficient phase sequence of impulses through the neural loop(s). These loops form the bases of behavior and interplay with the environment.

Note: The term "environment" includes both the outer and inner environments.

Language as an Example of Cortical Localization of Function

Broca described in 1861 the case of a patient who could understand language but who had lost his ability to speak. Postmortem gross examination of the brain

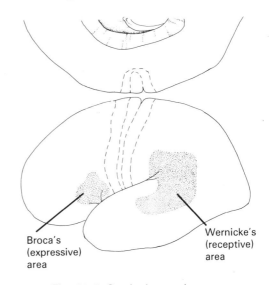

Fig. 21-6. Cortical speech areas.

surface showed a lesion in the posterior portion of the left frontal lobe and the region now known as **Broca's area** (motor speech area) (Fig. 21-6). In 1876 Wernicke described another cortical area, whose malfunction he found impaired comprehension of language; the patient could speak but not fully understand spoken language. This cortical area is composed principally of the posterior one-third of the superior temporal gyrus and was subsequently called **Wernicke's area** (sensory language area). Such impairments of the capacity to use words as symbols of ideas are called **aphasias.**

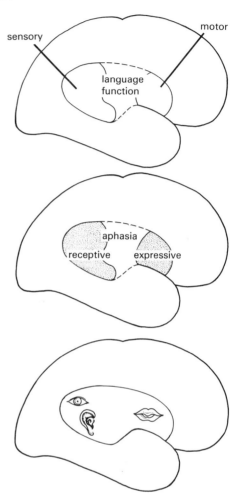

Fig. 21-7. Speech areas.

Aphasias

Aphasias result from lesions of cortical areas or their connections involved in language.

Reports of a long list and very complex classifications of aphasias have enriched the scientific literature in attempts to describe the particulars of language disturbances and correlate each type with discrete malfunctioning regions of the cortex. Classical clear-cut cases supporting such complex classifications of aphasias are not found in clinical practice. In all cases features are present which deviate from any one particular postulated syndrome and instead give evidence of several types of aphasias. This fact reinforces the view of the interdependence of many brain regions in the execution of complex brain functions. Nevertheless, to some degree, the basic general classification remains valid and useful as an outline of these disorders.

Main Types of Aphasias

The two most important groups of aphasias (Fig. 21-7) are shown in Table 21-2.

Dyslexia is a partial reduction of the

Table 21-2. Types of Aphasias

Group	Type
Expressive aphasias (motor)	Motor speech aphasia; Broca's aphasia (patient has nonfluent speech)
	Agraphia—loss of ability to write
Receptive aphasias (sensory)	Speech aphasia; Wernicke's aphasia (patient has impaired comprehension of language but has fluent speech)
	Alexia or visual aphasia—loss of ability to understand written language

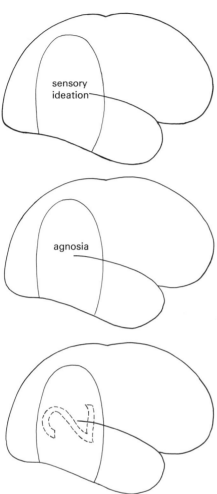

Fig. 21-8. Sensory ideation.

ability to understand written language.

Aphasia produced by the connection between Wernicke's and Broca's areas (arcuate fasciculus) is called **conduction aphasia.**

Global aphasia refers to total loss of language communication.

Based on clinical findings, it has been calculated that more than 90 percent of the population have a dominance of language function in the left hemisphere. Lesions in their right hemisphere produce minor signs of language disturbance.

Agnosias

As a counterterm of **gnosis** (Gr. knowledge), i.e., the understanding of sensory information, **agnosia** indicates an inability to comprehend the significance of sensory information. It mostly involves lesions of the association cortex (Fig. 21-8).

Types of Agnosias

Types and classifications of agnosias are abundant. Depending on which principal region of the association cortex is involved, they are classified as tactile, visual, auditory, and other agnosias.

A lesion that affects the posterior part of

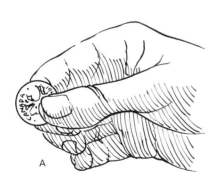

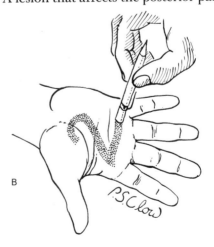

Fig. 21-9. (A) Stereognosis; (B) graphesthesia.

the parietal lobe and the upper part of the posterior temporal lobe in the right hemisphere produces **astereognosia,** i.e., an inability to grasp the understanding of the three dimensions of objects, even of one's own body image (Fig. 21-9).

Left and Right Hemispheral Dominance

It has been demonstrated that each hemisphere specializes and leads the other in a number of specific functions, e.g., the left hemisphere in speech, the right in three-dimensionality and the understanding of spatial dimensions.

The leading role in functions of each hemisphere does not mean total division of functions. Careful analysis of patients with lesions in one hemisphere uncovers, apart from the loss of its own dominant function, some deficiency of the dominant function of the opposite hemisphere.

In its leading specialization and functions, each hemisphere is aided and supported by the other. The transfer and coordination of function is carried out through commissural paths, especially the corpus callosum.

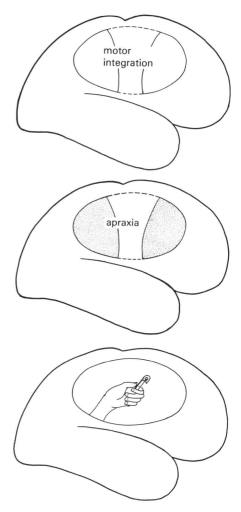

Fig. 21-10. Cortical motor skill areas.

Apraxias

Closely related to the agnosias and the aphasias is another group of disorders called **apraxias** (Gr. *a* not; *prassein* to do), which are characterized by an inability to perform complex learned movements despite the presence of normal muscle power, coordination, and sensation (Figs. 21-10 and 21-11).

Different types of apraxias have been described. One of them, **constructional apraxia,** is an inability to reproduce geometric figures or to spatially reconstruct visual images. Lesions of the parietal lobe have been found in this type of apraxia.

In some cases a patient's lack of ability to carry out skilled movements may be detected only when the clinician asks the patient to carry them out. The faulty response to the request may be indicative of a receptive phasic disturbance.

Note on the Term Agraphia

In the literature one may find **agraphias** classified within the aphasias (because it is a disturbance of language) and within the

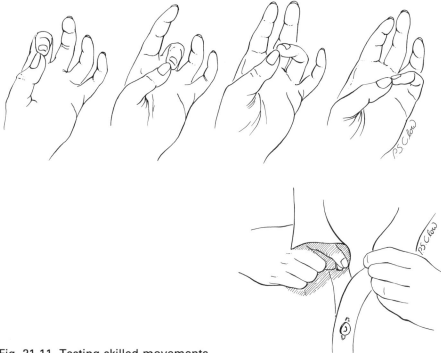

Fig. 21-11. Testing skilled movements.

apraxias (because it is a disturbance of learned skilled movements).

Note on the Term Anarthria

Anarthria (fr. Gr. *arthron* joint) means defective articulation of words, isolated or in speech. Amongst others, specific types may be **anarthria centralis** (due to a lesion in the precentral gyrus), and **anarthria literalis** (stuttering).

Learning and Memory

It was previously mentioned that environmental stimuli and experiences establish and modify neural connections and neural loops, which become increasingly more complex from early life on.

If one considers such structural events as the basis for learning and memory, any part of the nervous system is involved in memory.

One may analyze memory at different levels, e.g., memory of molecules, cells, circuits, sensations, feelings, ideas, thoughts, each involved in different information storage mechanisms. One may also study the phenomenon of memory, or the mechanisms of storage, as a short term event and as a long term event.

The capacity for remembering recent experienced events defines **short-term memory.**

The capacity for remembering events that have been experienced long ago defines **long-term memory.** Lack or loss of memory is called **amnesia.**

Retrieval processes, or the capacity to recall stored information, are intimately related to memory or storage processes.

Clinical findings establish the following facts:

1. Disturbances of one aspect or another of memory functions may be the result

of damage to almost any part of the brain.

2. Old learned experiences with long-term memory traces are less prone to be lost after damage to one or various brain regions than more recent or newly learned experiences with short-term memory traces.

3. In our effort to interact with new events we modify memory traces but retain the most imperative bits and pieces of information. The reconstruction (recall) of many past experiences becomes poorer and more distorted as time passes, but the experiences become more meaningful to us. This normal brain process of modifying its connectivities and functions expresses its plasticity.

4. Upon stimulation during surgical procedures of the temporal lobes, patients have vividly experienced past events or new sensations as familiar ones (déjà vu sensations).

5. Removal or lesions of both temporal lobes impairs the acquisition of new memories.

Hypotheses on Memory

Many hypotheses have been formulated in the past to explain memory, some of which ascribed its processes to specific brain regions. Those viewed to play the leading roles in memory functions are the brain regions involved in integrative functions. Some of these regions are described below.

The Hippocampus

It has been suggested that the hippocampus integrally codifies the activity of the brain.

The Papez Circuit

The disruption of the Papez circuit presents an obstacle for the processing of new signals in a manner similar to that in which old signals were processed. As a consequence, a proper association between new and old experiences is handicapped. Given the fact that many aspects of the processes involved in learning and memory of new events depend on their association with previously learned and memorized experiences, it follows that the acquisition of memory of new events will be hampered.

The Dorsomedial Thalamic Nucleus

Surgical destruction of the dorsomedial thalamic nucleus has been reported to produce memory deficits. One of the signs of Korsakoff's syndrome is amnesia. The dorsomedial thalamic nucleus is one of the structures most consistently lesioned in patients with this syndrome.

Other highly integrative areas like the anterior region of the temporal lobe (uncus, amygdala, anterior cingulate cortex and nearby lamina terminalis, and medial frontal cortex), if lesioned, greatly modify the memory processes.

Consciousness

Consciousness is awareness of the mind of one or many of its mental processes and cannot be localized to a specific brain region. It embraces all brain functions and thus permeates the whole nervous system.

A larger degree of alteration of consciousness has been found in connection with lesions of the axis: reticular formation—lamina terminalis—anterior frontal lobe than of other brain areas, pointing toward a strong relationship between consciousness and structures concerned with integrative functions.

Hitherto the highest function attributed to consciousness is the capability to develop insights into oneself and one's circumstances.

Consciousness may be reduced or lost for a variety of reasons, e.g., head injuries, intoxication, metabolic disturbances, or brain compression. The degree of loss of consciousness is medically expressed in the following terms: (1) confusion, disorientation; (2) drowsiness, lethargy, sleepiness; the patient can be awakened but tends to go back to sleep; (3) stupor, i.e., nearly complete unconsciousness; the patient may be able to respond briefly to commands; and (4) coma, i.e., absence of adaptive responses even to noxious stimuli.

One may notice that the degree of consciousness is measured by the reactive capacity to stimuli. Although this generally is a useful criterion, it does not preclude the possibility of some cases where there is retention of consciousness in combination with absence of adaptive responses.

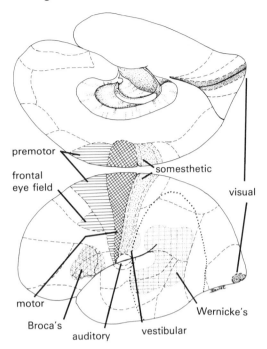

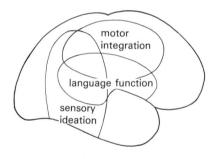

Fig. 21-12. Functional localization on the cerebral cortex.

Frontal Lobe Cortex

Some cortical regions of the frontal lobe have been described previously; they are illustrated in Figure 21-12 (primary motor area, premotor area, frontal eyefield, supplementary motor area, and motor speech area). The remaining cortical area of the frontal lobe anterior to these regions is known by the ill-conceived term **prefrontal cortex,** better named **anterior frontal cortex.**

Anterior Frontal Cortex

Patients with anterior frontal cortical injuries show in a number of cases a change in personality and behavior; higher mental faculties such as judgment, foresight, concern with ethical aspects, social principles, etc., become altered or even lost.

Phylogenetically, the anterior frontal cortex has developed the most of all the regions of the central nervous system (CNS).

The anterior frontal cortex, in contrast to other major cortical regions, does not receive primary sensory information. Nevertheless, it is strongly connected to all the associative regions of the neocortex. Besides these connections it has also others

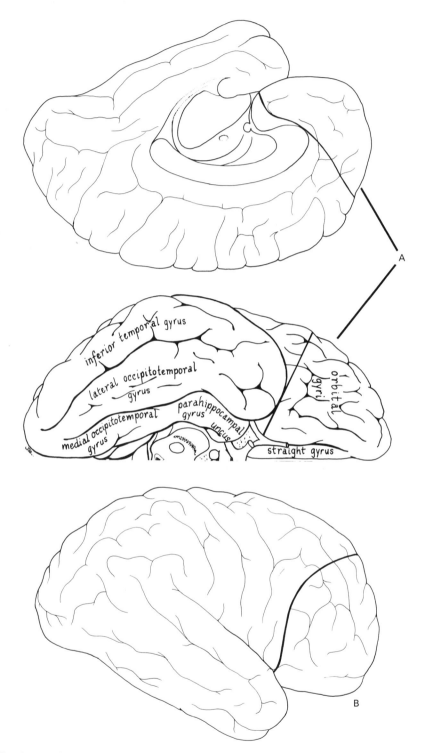

inferior temporal gyrus

lateral occipitotemporal gyrus

medial occipitotemporal gyrus

parahippocampal gyrus

uncus

orbital gyri

straight gyrus

A

B

Fig. 21-13. Anterior frontal cortex. (A) Inferomedial view; (B) dorsolateral view.

with the allocortex and mesocortex, subcortical brain regions, diencephalon, and brain stem. Its connectivity and functions give support to the concept of the anterior frontal cortex as a main integrator of functions.

Two Main Regions of the Anterior Frontal Cortex

Attempts to differentiate between minor parts of the anterior frontal cortex have produced meager results. However, based on the consequences of their lesions, the division of this cortex into inferomedial and dorsolateral regions (Fig. 21-13) appears to be justified.

Lesions of the **inferomedial frontal cortex** produce changes in ethical and social behavior.

Lesions of the **anterior dorsolateral frontal cortex** produce intellectual deficiencies.

Suggested Readings

Bach-y-Rita P: Brain plasticity as a basis for therapeutic procedures. In Bach-y-Rita P, Ed.: Recovery of Function. Theoretical Considerations for Brain Injury Rehabilitation, Huber, Bern, pp. 225–263, 1980.

Benson DF: Neurological correlates of aphasia and apraxia. In Matthews WB, Glaser GH, Eds.: Recent Advances in Clinical Neurology, No. 2, Churchill Livingstone, Edinburgh, pp. 163–175, 1978.

Berger B, Thierry AM, Tassin JP, Moyne MA: Dopaminergic innervation of the rat prefrontal cortex: a fluorescence histochemical study, Brain Res 106:133–145, 1976.

Brazier MAB, Petsche H, Eds: Architectonics of the Cerebral Cortex. Int. Brain Res. Org. (IBRO) Monogr. Ser., Vol. 3, Raven Press, New York, 1978.

Carpenter MB: Human Neuroanatomy. Seventh Edition. Williams and Wilkins, Baltimore, pp. 547–599, 1976.

Cofer CN, Ed.: The Structure of Human Memory, WH Freeman and Co., San Francisco, 1976.

Deutsch D, Deutsch JA, Eds.: Short-Term Memory, Academic Press, New York, 1975.

Eidelberg E, Stein DG, Eds.: Functional recovery after lesions of the nervous system, Neurosci Res Progr Bull 12:189–303, 1974.

Fleischhauer K: Cortical architectonics: the last 50 years and some problems of today. In Brazier MAB, Petsche H, Eds.: Architectonics of the Cerebral Cortex, IBRO 3, Raven Press, New York, pp. 99–117, 1978.

Globus GG, Maxwell G, Savodnik I, Eds.: Consciousness and the Brain. A Scientific and Philosophical Inquiry, Plenum Press, New York, 1976.

Harnad S, Doty RW, Goldstein L, Jaynes J, Krauthamer G, Eds.: Lateralization in the Nervous System, Academic Press, New York, 1977.

Horel JA: The neuroanatomy of amnesia. A critique of the hippocampal memory hypothesis, Brain 101:403–445, 1978.

Jones EG, Wise SP: Size, laminar and columnar distribution of efferent cells in the sensory-motor cortex of monkeys, J Comp Neurol 175:391–438, 1977.

Kandel ER: Cellular Basis of Behavior, WH Freeman and Co., San Francisco, Chapters 12 and 13, 1976.

Kinsbourne M, Ed.: Asymmetrical Function of the Brain, Cambridge University Press, Cambridge, 1978.

Kuffler SW, Nicholls JG: From Neuron to Brain, Sinauer Associates, Sunderland, Mass., 1976.

Marin-Padilla M, Stibitz GR: Three-dimensional reconstruction of the basket cell of the human motor cortex, Brain Res 70:511–514, 1974.

Mogenson GJ, Calaresu FR, Eds.: Neural Integration of Physiological Mechanisms and Behaviour, University of Toronto Press, Toronto, 1975.

Morley TP, Ed.: Current Controversies in Neurosurgery, WB Saunders, Philadelphia, 1976.

Springer SP, Deutsch G: Left Brain, Right Brain, WH Freeman and Co., San Francisco, 1981.

Szentagothai J: The 'module-concept' in cerebral cortex architecture, Brain Res 95:475–496, 1975.

22

Vascular Supply

An introduction to the vascular supply of the nervous system was presented in Chapter 3. This chapter intends to render a more detailed account.

Peripheral Nerves

Along the entire course of the peripheral nerves there is a well-developed and highly anastomotic plexus of small arterioles that derive from the neighboring vessels (Fig. 22-1).

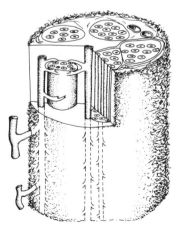

Fig. 22-1. Vascular supply of peripheral nerve.

Spinal Cord

There are two distinct sources of blood to the spinal cord, namely, spinal branches of the vertebral arteries and segmental spinal branches.

Spinal Branches of the Vertebral Arteries

Each vertebral artery gives off an **anterior** and a **posterior spinal branch.** The two anterior branches (left and right) fuse in the configuration of a Y and run caudally along the ventral median fissure as the **anterior spinal artery** (Fig. 22-2).

The two posterior branches course caudally along the line of attachment of the dorsal roots of the spinal nerves as the **posterior spinal arteries** (Fig. 22-2).

Segmental Spinal Branches

The **segmental spinal arteries** reach the inside of the vertebral canal through the intervertebral foramina. These arteries are branches of the following vessels: vertebral and ascending cervical or deep cervical ar-

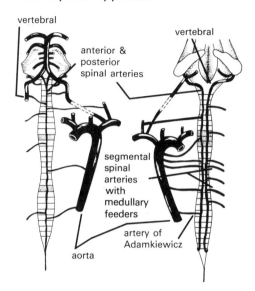

Fig. 22-2. Vascular supply of spinal cord.

teries—at cervical segments; posterior intercostal vessels—at thoracic segments, lumbar arteries—at low thoracic and lumbar segments; and sacral arteries—at sacral levels.

The segmental spinal arteries, in addition to supplying branches within the vertebral canal to the vertebrae, give rise to the anterior and posterior radicular arteries (Fig. 22-3).

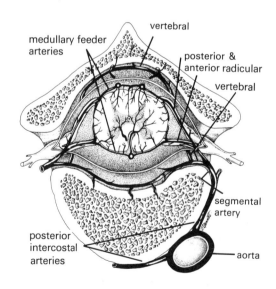

Fig. 22-3. Vascular supply of spinal cord.

Radicular Arteries

The **anterior radicular arteries** travel along the anterior roots.

The **posterior radicular arteries** travel along the posterior roots and anastomose with the posterior spinal arteries (Fig. 22-3).

All roots are supplied by the radicular arteries.

Medullary Feeder Branches

At certain vertebral levels, anterior and posterior medullary feeder branches arise from the segmental spinal arteries to join the longitudinally coursing anterior and posterior spinal arteries. There are about 8 **anterior medullary feeder arteries** (counting left and right sides) and about 12 **posterior medullary feeder arteries** (counting left and right sides). The largest of all these is the **great anterior medullary artery** or **artery of Adamkiewicz** (Fig. 22-2), which is a branch of the lumbar artery originating in the aorta. If this branch is lesioned, lumbosacral spinal cord ischemia is produced. The effects of deficiencies in vascular supply are most commonly ob-

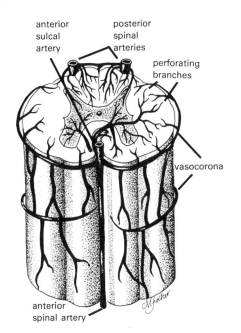

anterior sulcal artery

posterior spinal arteries

perforating branches

vasocorona

anterior spinal artery

Fig. 22-4. Vascular supply of spinal cord.

served in upper thoracic and lumbar segments (Fig. 22-2).

Vasocorona

The anterior and two posterior spinal arteries form a fine plexus of vessels around the spinal cord pial surface, from which short penetrating branches supply a narrow zone of white matter. This vascular plexus is called **vasocorona** (Fig. 22-4).

Sulcal Arteries

The **sulcal arteries** (Fig. 22-4) are penetrating branches of the anterior and posterior spinal arteries.

The **anterior sulcal arteries** alternate their direction in succession to the right and left.

The **anterior spinal arteries** and its **branches** (the **anterior sulcal arteries**) irrigate the anterior two-thirds of the spinal cord. The **posterior spinal arteries** and their penetrating branches supply the posterior one-third of the cord.

Lesions of the anterior spinal artery and

branches cause motor deficiencies and loss of pain and temperature sensation below the level of the lesion, whereas vibration and position sense remain intact, since the posterior one-third of the cord is unaffected.

Blood Supply of the Brain Stem

Medulla Oblongata

The **medulla oblongata** is irrigated by the vertebral artery and its branches. These branches are direct vertebral penetrating vessels, collaterals of the anterior and posterior spinal arteries, and the posteroinferior cerebellar artery.

Figures 22-5 and 22-6 illustrate the regional supply of these branches. The posteroinferior cerebellar artery is the largest branch of the vertebral arteries. With a winding and elaborate course it supplies part of the dorsolateral region of the medulla, the choroid plexus (with the choroidal arteries) of the fourth ventricle, and the posteroinferior region of the cerebellar hemisphere, inferior vermis, and central nuclei of cerebellum.

Occlusion of the posteroinferior cerebellar artery may produce the **lateral medullary** or **Wallenberg's syndrome** (Fig. 22-7), which is characterized by

contralateral impairment of pain and temperature sensation (anterolateral spinothalamic tract);

ipsilateral impairment of pain and temperature sensation in the face (descending trigeminal nucleus);

ipsilateral Horner's syndrome, i.e., miosis, ptosis, and decreased sweating (descending sympathetic fibers);

dysphagia and dysarthria (nucleus ambiguus);

vertigo, nausea, and nystagmus (vestibular nuclei); and

ipsilateral limb ataxia (inferior cerebellar peduncle).

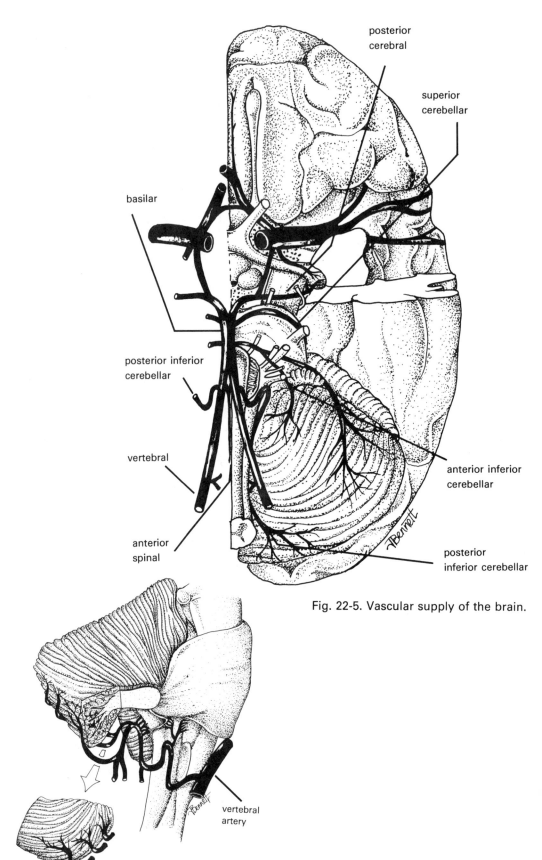

posterior
cerebral

superior
cerebellar

basilar

posterior inferior
cerebellar

vertebral

anterior
spinal

anterior inferior
cerebellar

posterior
inferior cerebellar

Fig. 22-5. Vascular supply of the brain.

vertebral
artery

Fig. 22-6. Posterior inferior cerebellar artery.

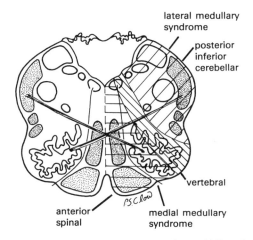

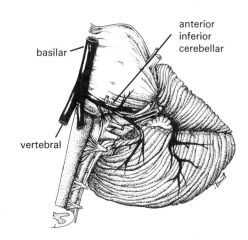

Fig. 22-7. Vascular supply of medulla oblongata.

Fig. 22-8. Anterior inferior cerebellar artery.

Note: Dysarthria is an impairment of articulation. Dysarthric speech is due to malfunction of speech muscles and their motor neurons.

Medial Medullary Syndrome

The **medial medullary syndrome** (Fig. 22-7) results from vascular occlusion of the anterior paramedian region and may include the following signs: ipsilateral paralysis of the tongue (hypoglossal nerve), contralateral paralysis of arm and leg (corticospinal tract), and contralateral impairment of discriminative touch and position sense (medial lemniscus).

Pons and Cerebellum

The pons and most of the cerebellum are irrigated by the **basilar artery** and its **branches** (Figs. 22-5, 22-8, and 22-10). These branches are the **pontine paramedian, anterior inferior cerebellar, internal auditory,** and **superior cerebellar arteries.**

The anterior inferior cerebellar artery (Fig. 22-8) splits in its lateral course into the superior and inferior branches, embracing the cranial nerves VII and VIII. The inferior branch may give off the internal auditory branch which continues with cranial nerve VIII. This internal auditory artery, also called **labyrinthine artery,** may come directly from the basilar artery. The upper branch follows the brachium pontis and turns onto the inferior surface of the cerebellum.

Some collaterals of the anterior inferior cerebellar artery irrigate the upper medulla oblongata.

Lateral Pontine Syndrome

Occlusion of the anterior inferior cerebellar artery underlies the **lateral pontine syndrome** (Fig. 22-9), which may include:

contralateral impairment of pain and temperature sensation in the trunk and extremities (anterolateral spinothalamic tract);

ipsilateral impairment of sensation in the face (trigeminal);

ipsilateral paralysis of conjugate gaze to the side of the lesion (abducens);

ipsilateral facial paralysis (facial);

ipsilateral cerebellar ataxia (middle cerebellar peduncle and cerebellar hemisphere); and

ipsilateral vertigo, nystagmus, and deafness (statoacoustic).

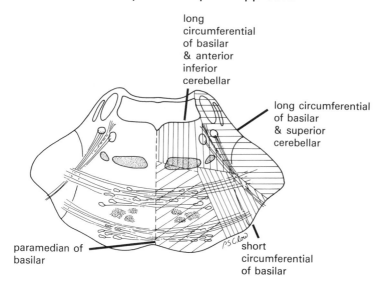

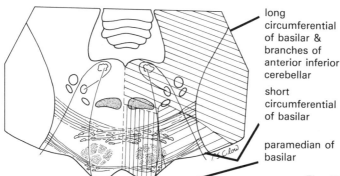

Fig. 22-9. Vascular supply of pons.

Medial Pontine Syndrome

In the **medial pontine syndrome** some or all of the paramedian arteries may become occluded. Depending on which vessels are involved and the extent to which they are affected, different signs may become manifest, e.g., contralateral paralysis of extremities (corticospinal tract), contralateral impairment of discriminative touch and position sense (medial lemniscus), ipsilateral inward deviation of the eye (abducens), and ipsilateral paralysis of the face (facial).

Superior Cerebellar Artery

The **superior cerebellar artery** (Fig. 22-10) courses laterally on the upper border of the pons, reaches the dorsal region and climbs over the superior surface of the cerebellum, supplying the cortex, medullary center, and nuclei. It gives off branches to the upper pons, basis pedunculi, the tegmentum of the midbrain, superior cerebellar peduncle, and the inferior colliculus.

Basilar Artery Syndrome

The **basilar artery syndrome** results from a total occlusion of the basilar artery. Typical signs are impaired sensation (sensory pathways), impaired movement and nystagmus (descending motor paths, cranial nerve motor nuclei, cerebellar structures), disturbance of consciousness, even coma (reticular formation), and death (vital centers) within hours or days.

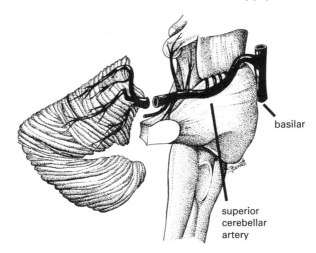

Fig. 22-10. Superior cerebellar artery.

Posterior Cerebral Artery

Most of the midbrain and diencephalon are irrigated by the **posterior cerebral arteries,** which are terminal branches of the basilar artery (Fig. 22-11).

The posterior cerebral artery (Figs. 22-11 to 22-16) ascends at the border of the interpeduncular fossa medial to cranial nerve III and turns laterally around the cerebral peduncle (Fig. 22-11). It then progresses to the cleft between the brain stem and the parahippocampal gyrus (Fig. 22-14) and continues dorsally until it lands under the splenium of the corpus callosum, where it turns posteriorly along the calcarine sulcus toward the occipital pole.

Branches to the Midbrain and Diencephalon

1. **Paramedian branches** (Fig. 22-15) travel through the posterior perforated substance. Large and long vessels penetrate as far as the aqueduct, supplying the medial part of the basis pedunculi, the medial part of the brachium conjunctivum, the red nucleus, and the motor nuclei of the cranial nerves III

and IV. Vascular occlusion of this region (Fig. 22-15) affecting the base of the midbrain produces the **mediobasal mesencephalic syndrome of Weber.** Predominant signs are contralateral hemiplegia (corticospinal tract) and ipsilateral paralysis of the oculomotor nerve, i.e., ipsilateral ptosis, dilation of pupil, absent light reflex, and outward and downward deviation of the eye. Vascular occlusion of this region affecting the tegmentum of midbrain produces **Benedikt's syndrome.** Predomi-

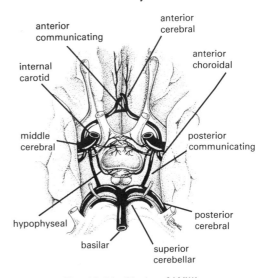

Fig. 22-11. Circle of Willis.

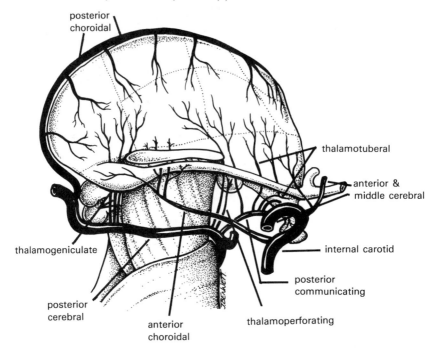

Fig. 22-12. Vascular supply of midbrain and diencephalon.

nant signs are cranial nerve III palsy, contralateral cerebellar ataxia (red nucleus and its cerebellar connections through the brachium conjunctivum), and tremor.

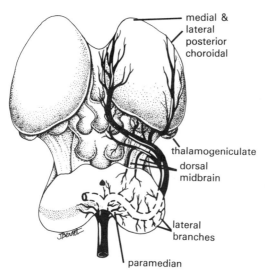

Fig. 22-13. Posterior cerebral artery. Blood supply to midbrain and diencephalon.

2. The **thalamoperforating branches** (Fig. 22-12) enter the ventral diencephalon just behind the mammillary bodies and irrigate the subthalamus and part of the thalamus.

3. The **dorsal midbrain branch** (Fig. 22-13) supplies the lateral portion of the basis pedunculi, tegmentum, brachium of the inferior colliculus, tectum, and superior and inferior colliculi.

4. The **thalamogeniculate arteries** (Figs. 22-12 and 22-13) irrigate the region of the inferoposterolateral thalamus, the geniculate bodies, and ventralis posterior nucleus.

5. The **lateral posterior choroidal artery** (Fig. 22-13) climbs onto the dorsolateral surface of the thalamus, giving off branches to the choroidal plexus of the lateral ventricle, irrigating also the thalamus.

6. The **medial posterior choroidal artery** (Fig. 22-13) courses near the midline below the corpus callosum, irrigating the epithalamus, dorsomedial thala-

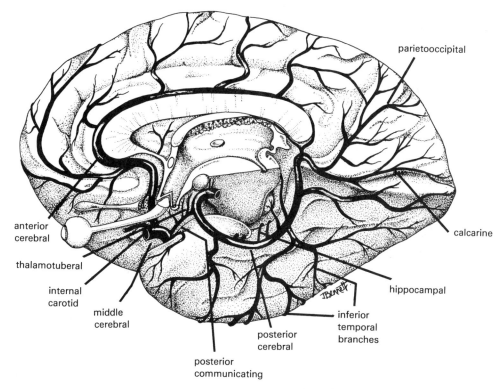

Fig. 22-14. Vascular supply of cerebrum.

parietooccipital

calcarine

anterior
cerebral

thalamotuberal

internal
carotid

middle
cerebral

posterior
communicating

posterior
cerebral

inferior
temporal
branches

hippocampal

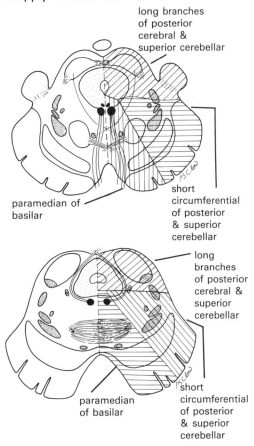

long branches
of posterior
cerebral &
superior cerebellar

paramedian of
basilar

short
circumferential
of posterior
& superior
cerebellar

long
branches
of posterior
cerebral &
superior
cerebellar

paramedian
of basilar

short
circumferential
of posterior
& superior
cerebellar

Fig. 22-15. Vascular supply of midbrain.

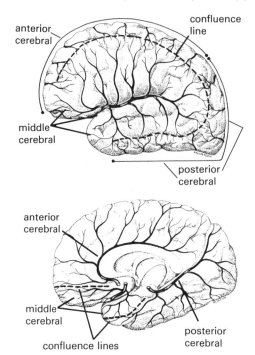

Fig. 22-16. Vascular supply of cerebral hemisphere.

mus, fornix, and choroid plexus of the third ventricle.

Occlusion of the vessels to the thalamus may produce a thalamic syndrome, whose main signs, all appearing contralaterally, are hemiparesis, impairment of discriminative sensibilities, disorders of movements, and sudden crisis of pain.

Branches to the Cerebral Hemisphere

The posterior cerebral artery sends branches to specific structures of the cerebral hemisphere.

Branches course to the hippocampal formation (Fig. 22-14).

Several slender and short vessels irrigate the uncus, the medial surface of the parahippocampal gyrus, and the hippocampal fissure, traveling along the dentate gyrus to the hippocampus proper.

The branches to the hippocampus proper are the longest and are prone to

become occluded by pressure (herniation) on the hippocampal formation of the free edge of the tentorium cerebelli. Pathologists call this most vulnerable part of the hippocampal formation **Sommer's sector** (Fig. 22-17).

Branches to the inferior surface of the **temporal** and **occipital lobes** or **inferior temporal branches** (Fig. 22-14) course laterally, crossing the parahippocampal gyrus, fan out profusely and reach the inferolateral border of the hemisphere, including the inferior region of the occipital pole. Their terminals appear in the inferolateral surface and posterior pole surface of the hemisphere where they form a watershed area (confluence line) with the terminals of the middle cerebral artery of that region (Fig. 22-16).

The **calcarine branch** (Fig. 22-14) courses in the calcarine fissure and irrigates the calcarine region of the visual cortex.

Occlusion of the vessels to the calcarine region causes blindness in the contralateral field of vision.

The **parietooccipital artery** (Fig. 22-14) normally runs along the parietooccipital

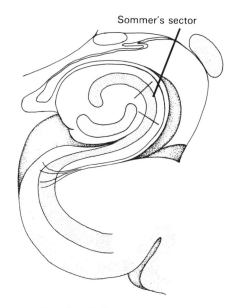

Fig. 22-17. Sommer's sector.

sulcus. It supplies that region and overlaps the superior border of the hemisphere. The terminal supplies part of the lateral surface of the occipital lobe, forming a watershed area (confluence line) with the terminals of the middle and anterior cerebral arteries (Fig. 22-16).

Internal Carotid Artery

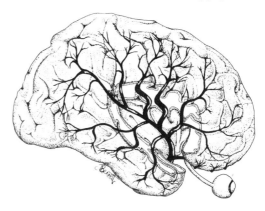

Fig. 22-19. Middle cerebral artery exposed to view.

Branches of the **internal carotid artery** are the **hypophyseal arteries** (Fig. 22-11), the **ophthalmic artery,** the **anterior choroidal artery** (Figs. 22-12 and 22-18), the **posterior communicating artery** (Figs. 22-11, 22-12, 22-14, and 22-18); and the **anterior** (Fig. 22-14) and **middle cerebral arteries** (Fig. 22-19).

Hypophyseal Arteries

The **hypophyseal arteries** (Fig. 20-3) originate from the cavernous (inferior hy-

pophyseal) and postclinoid (superior hypophyseal) portions of the internal carotid. They irrigate the pituitary, infundibular stem, and median eminence.

Ophthalmic Artery

The **ophthalmic artery** takes off as soon as the internal carotid enters the subarachnoid space. It proceeds toward the optic foramen and supplies the eye and other structures of the orbit as well as the paranasal sinuses and the frontal area of the scalp. It establishes several anastomatic connections with branches of the external carotid artery.

Anterior Choroidal Artery

The **anterior choroidal artery** (Figs. 22-12 and 22-18) originates from the distal part of the internal carotid or the beginning of the middle cerebral and irrigates many more areas than what its name implies. Its main course runs with the optic tract and it gives off branches to the uncus, amygdala, hippocampus, optic tract, lateral geniculate, optic radiation, posterior and sublenticular limbs of the internal capsule, subthalamus, putamen, and pallidum.

Owing to its long course and small cali-

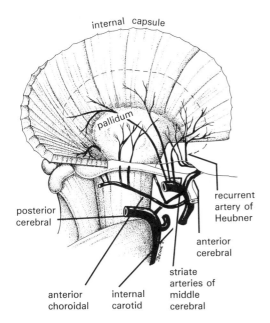

Fig. 22-18. Vascular supply to the core of the brain.

ber, the anterior choroidal artery is prone to thrombosis.

Posterior Communicating Artery

The **thalamotuberal vessels** (Figs. 22-12 and 22-14) are the main branches of the posterior communicating artery. They irrigate all but the most anterior regions of the hypothalamus, subthalamus, and a small portion of the surrounding thalamus. They also contribute to the irrigation of the genu of the internal capsule.

Anterior Cerebral Artery

The **anterior cerebral artery** (Figs. 22-11, 22-14, and 22-20) branches off from the internal carotid artery and courses medially and anteriorly between the optic nerve below and the anterior perforated area above. On the medial surface of the hemisphere it courses to the genu of the corpus callosum and continues along the surface of the callosum as the **pericallosal artery** toward the splenium, giving off a large branch, the **callosomarginal artery.**

Core or Central Branches

The **core** or **central branches** (Figs. 22-12 and 22-20) irrigate the optic chiasm and the regions of the lamina terminalis (preoptic region, septal area, septum pellucidum, etc.). A long branch, the **recurrent artery of Heubner,** also called the **medial striate artery,** penetrates the anterior perforated substance and irrigates the anterior region of the globus pallidus, the head of the caudate, and the anterior limb and genu of the internal capsule. It also gives

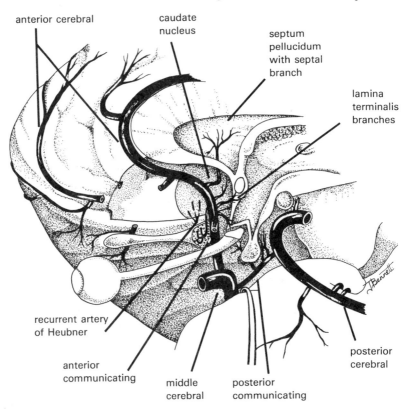

Fig. 22-20. Vascular supply. Regional details.

off fine nutrient vessels to the corpus callosum.

Cortical Branches

Branches from the main trunk of the anterior cerebral artery (Fig. 22-14) spread along the medial surface of the frontal and parietal lobes. The terminals of these branches reach the superior and medial borders of the hemispheres and end in a watershed area (confluence line) with corresponding terminal branches of the middle cerebral artery (Fig. 22-16).

Significant functional features of the region supplied by the anterior cerebral artery are described below.

Cortical branches—primary motor and sensory area of the leg region (lesion: paralysis and sensory deficits of the contralateral limb); medial frontal cortex (lesion: mental confusion).

Core branches—genu and anterior limb of the internal capsule with the corticospinal pathway for head and arm; anterior region of corpus striatum, corpus callosum (lesion: motor deficits, apraxias); region of the lamina terminalis (lesion: prolonged state of unconsciousness).

The two anterior cerebral arteries are connected by the anterior communicating artery.

Middle Cerebral Artery

The **middle cerebral artery** (Figs. 22-11, 22-19, and 22-21) courses laterally below the anterior perforated substance to reach the lateral fissure, where it runs covered by the frontal parietal and temporal lobes, emerging at the posterior end of the fissure as several branches. Through its course the middle cerebral artery gives off **central branches** and **cortical branches.**

Central Branches

The **central branches** (Fig. 22-21) consist of two groups of **medial** and **lateral striate arteries,** which originate from the first portion of the artery, perforate the anterior perforated substance and irrigate the corpus striatum, and anterior limb, genu, and posterior limb of the internal capsule.

Cortical Branches

The **cortical branches** (Fig. 22-19) fan out covering most of the lateral surface of the hemisphere and most of the orbital surface of the frontal lobe (Fig. 22-16). Their terminal branches form a nearly circular watershed area with the anterior and posterior cerebral arteries.

Many important cortical functional areas are irrigated by the middle cerebral artery (Fig. 22-22). The syndrome of **middle cerebral artery occlusion** includes contralateral hemiplegia and hemianesthesia, homonymous hemianopia (geniculocalcarine radiation), and aphasias (which are more pronounced if the lesion is in the left hemisphere). A unilateral lesion causes no obvious impairment of hearing, because of

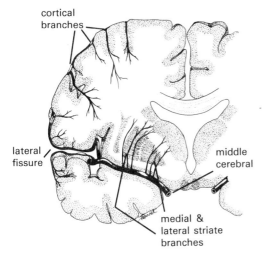

cortical branches

lateral fissure

middle cerebral

medial & lateral striate branches

Fig. 22-21. Middle cerebral artery.

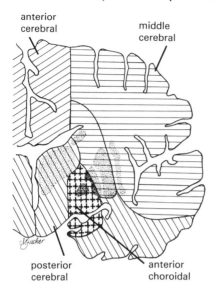

Fig. 22-22. Cerebrum. Regional vascular supply.

the bilateral cortical projection from the organ of Corti.

Note: The student must recognize that all the described vessels and corresponding areas of infarct do not match with the site of occlusion. Most commonly, the occlusion occurs in another vessel which compromises the circulation in one or a number of its branches (Fig. 22-23).

Cerebral Veins

Internal Cerebral Veins

The **internal cerebral veins** are illustrated in Figure 22-24. They receive the **thalamostriate vein (vena terminalis)** and **choroidal veins.** The internal cerebral veins unite beneath the splenium of the corpus callosum to form the **great cerebral vein of Galen,** which empties into the straight sinus in the midline of the tentorium cerebelli.

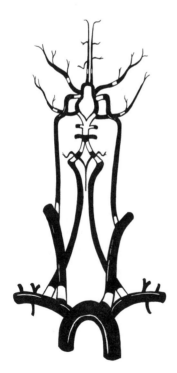

Fig. 22-23. Common regions of vascular occlusions.

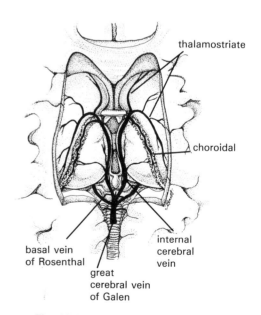

Fig. 22-24. Internal cerebral veins.

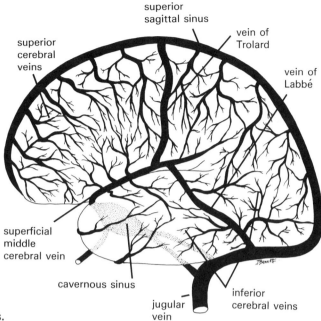

Fig. 22-25. External cerebral veins.

External Cerebral Veins

The **external cerebral veins** are shown in Figures 22-25 and 22-26. The veins empty their blood as follows:

superior cerebral veins—superior sagittal sinus;

superficial middle cerebral vein—cavernous sinus;

deep middle cerebral and anterior cerebral veins—basal vein of Rosenthal; and

basal vein of Rosenthal—great cerebral vein of Galen.

Collateral Circulation Through Venous Anastomosis

The veins of Trolard and Labbé are anastomotic veins between the external cerebral veins (Fig. 22-25).

Other venous collateral circulation between extracranial and intracranial veins (emissary veins) is depicted in Figure 22-27.

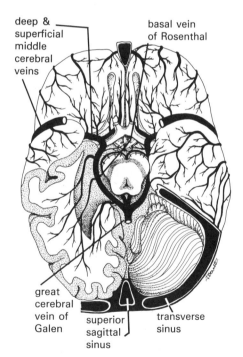

Fig. 22-26. Base of the brain. Venous circulation.

Tearing and bleeding of emissary vessels crossing the meningeal layers may occur even with a small trauma, causing accumu-

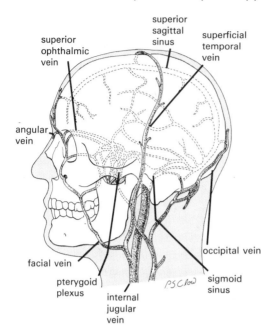

superior sagittal sinus

superior ophthalmic vein

superficial temporal vein

angular vein

facial vein

occipital vein

pterygoid plexus

internal jugular vein

PSClow

sigmoid sinus

Fig. 22-27. Venous collateral circulation.

lation of blood between the meningeal spaces.

Cerebrovascular Disease—Strokes

Abrupt deficiencies in neurological function due to impairment of the cerebral circulation are called **cerebrovascular (CV) strokes** or, less accurately, **cerebral apoplexy.**

The impairment of the cerebral circulation may be due to **occlusion** or **hemorrhage.** Occlusions are most commonly due to a thrombus, an embolus (embolism), or vasoconstriction caused by systemic or local hypertension.

Common regions of vascular occlusion are illustrated in Figure 22-23.

Hemorrhages are most frequently due to rupture of an aneurysm (which is an abnormal localized dilatation of the arterial lumen), hypertension, arteriovenous malformations, or trauma.

The region deprived of circulating blood, i.e., a region suffering an infarct, produces ischemic cell changes with neuronal death. Some strokes are of short duration (lasting from a minute to hours) with subsequent full recovery of functions, like **transient ischemic attacks (TIA),** which are due to focal ischemic events. A transient ischemic event generalized to the brain produces loss of consciousness (fainting or **syncope**).

There are many causes for these episodic attacks; for instance, just standing up from a sitting position may produce systemic hypotension and pronounced reduction in cerebral blood flow, triggering weakness, dizziness, and fainting.

The episodic attacks are important as warning signs and clues to the diagnosis of potential strokes that could cause permanent neurological deficiencies or death. Such a drastic outcome may be possible to prevent, if proper prophylactic therapy is implemented as soon as such attacks are recognized for what they may lead to.

Cerebral Vascular Innervation

The superior cervical sympathetic ganglion innervates the internal carotid artery and its branches, arteries, arterioles, and small veins but not the capillaries. The three cervical sympathetic ganglia innervate the vertebrobasilar system.

The existence not only of noradrenergic terminals but also of cholinergic terminals (vasodilators) has been proven.

The nucleus locus ceruleus may be a source of noradrenergic innervation.

Table 22-1. Autoregulation of Brain Blood Flow

Constants	Capillaries	Blood
↑ $PaCO_2$	↑ Dilation	↑ Circulation
↓ PaO_2	↑ Dilation	↑ Circulation
↓ pH (↑ acid)	↑ Dilation	↑ Circulation
↑ Lactic acid	↑ Dilation	↑ Circulation

The capillaries may change their caliber independently of the arteries and arterioles.

Most important in determining dilatation or constriction of the capillaries are the CO_2, O_2, and pH constants as summarized in Table 22-1 in normal conditions.

Autoregulation or Brain Blood Flow

Autoregulation of brain flow is the change in arterial diameter following changes in systemic blood pressure to maintain flow at a constant rate.

This is realized by the aforementioned autoregulatory mechanisms (blood constants, CO_2, pH, and vascular innervation). If the arterial blood pressure goes out of the range of 60 to 150 mm Hg, these mechanisms become inefficient.

The brain also regulates its blood flow as functionally required. It increases or diminishes it in each region of the brain in accordance with the degree of its functional activity.

The coupling mechanisms between the cerebral metabolism and cerebral blood flow are considered to play an important role in brain function.

A Major Potential Obstacle in Cerebral Circulation

The increase in the difference between the arterial pressure and cerebral venous sinuses pressure is a major factor in increasing cerebral circulation.

A critical or fatal situation occurs when the increase of intracranial pressure (which is transmitted to the venous sinuses with stagnation of venous blood circulation) reduces the pressure difference between arterial cerebral circulation and venous sinus circulation beyond the powers of autoregulation. It is critical because either reduction or increment of arterial pressure offers a health risk. Increase of arterial pressure increases even more the intracranial pressure; reduction of arterial pressure reduces blood circulation.

If no action is taken in cases of patients suffering from increased intracranial pressure, the lack of proper blood circulation produces brain edema. This further increases the intracranial pressure and impairs blood circulation, which results in brain anoxia and ends in death.

Patients with traumatic head injuries should be placed under observation for 12 hours for signs of an increase in intracranial pressure, because the development of edema or hemorrhage may cause such an increase.

Collateral Circulation Through Arterial Anastomoses

A list of **arterial anastomoses** is presented in Table 22-2. These play an important role in circulating the blood, if the on-

Table 22-2. Arterial Anastomoses

Extracranial anastomoses
Vertebral artery ⟷ Muscular branches ⟶ Occipital artery
Extra-intracranial anastomoses
External carotid (facial, maxillary, temporal) ↔ Internal carotid (ophthalmic artery)
Intracranial anastomoses
Vertebrobasilar vessels ↔ Posterior communicating artery ↔ Internal carotid vessels
Confluence of branches of anterior, middle, and posterior cerebral arteries (i.e., confluence line or watershed area)

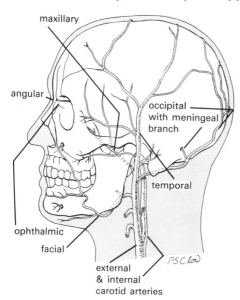

maxillary

angular

occipital
with meningeal
branch

temporal

ophthalmic

facial

external
& internal
carotid arteries

PSClow

Fig. 22-28. Arterial collateral circulation.

set of circulatory demands is slow and progressive. Sudden demands may not permit sufficient development of anastomoses as required (Fig. 22-28).

The possibility of collateral circulation in the watershed areas (confluence lines) (Fig. 22-16) has been established.

Cerebral Angiography

The cerebrovascular system can be visualized by injecting a contrast into the carotid or vertebral arteries. The roentgenographic images obtained are called **angiograms.**

Suggested Readings

Bergland RM, Page RB: Pituitary-brain vascular relations: A new paradigm, Science (Washington DC) 204:18–24, 1979.

Burrows EH, Leeds NE: Neuroradiology, Churchill Livingstone, New York, 1981.

Carpenter MB: Human Neuroanatomy. Seventh Edition. Williams and Wilkins, Baltimore, pp. 600–630, 1976.

Duvernay HM: Human Brain Stem Vessels, Springer-Verlag, New York, 1978.

Fisher CM: The anatomy and pathology of the cerebral vasculature. In Meyer JS, Ed.: Modern Concepts of Cerebrovascular Disease, Spectrum Publications, New York, pp. 1–41, 1975.

Go KG, Baethmann AO, Eds.: Recent Progress in the Study and Therapy of Brain Edema, Plenum Press, New York, 1983.

Heistad DD, Marcus ML, Eds.: Cerebral Blood Flow. Developments in Neuroscience, 14, Elsevier Excerpta Medica, Elsevier Science Publishers, New York, 1982.

Ingvar DH, Lassen NA, Eds.: Brain Work. The Coupling of Function, Metabolism and Blood Flow in the Brain, Munksgaard, 1975.

Lassen NA, Ingvar DH, Skinhöj E: Brain function and blood flow, Sci Am 239(4):62–71, 1978.

Osborn AG: Introduction to Cerebral Angiography, Harper and Row, Hagerstown, 1980.

Raichle ME, Eichling JO, Grubb RL, Hartmann BK: Central noradrenergic regulation of the brain microcirculation. In Pappius HM, Feindel W, Eds.: Dynamics of Brain Edema, pp. 11–17, Springer-Verlag, Berlin, 1976.

Rennels ML, Nelson E: Capillary innervation in the mammalian central nervous system: An electron microscopic demonstration, Anat Rec 144:233–241, 1975.

Smith CG: Basic Neuroanatomy. Second Edition. University of Toronto Press, Toronto, pp. 222–246, 1971.

Thomas DJ, Bannister R: Preservation of autoregulation of cerebral blood flow in autonomic failure, J Neurol Sci 44:205–212, 1980.

23

Neurotransmitters

A **neurotransmitter** or **transmitter substance** is defined as a substance that is released synaptically by one neuron and that subsequently affects another neuron or effector organ in a specific manner.

Acetylcholine (ACh) was, in the mid 1920's, the first substance to be identified as a neurotransmitter.

Generally, each nerve cell releases only one type of transmitter substance (Dale's hypothesis), although evidence supporting the concept of cotransmitters (one or more transmitters released together from the same neuron) has recently been described.

Transmitters produce their effect by interacting with receptors located on the surface of the receiving nerve cell. Each neurotransmitter fits with a specific receptor whose chemical configuration forms the basis of its specificity.

Each transmitter has its own characteristic action, which may be excitatory or inhibitory, quick or slow, of short or lasting effect.

Neurotransmitters may have either presynaptic or postsynaptic effects or both (Fig. 23-1).

Once the neurotransmitter action is effected, the action of the transmitter substance is normally terminated by one of a number of mechanisms.

A single neuron may possess a variety of different transmitter receptors and may therefore be the target for several neurotransmitters.

Not every neuron in a given nucleus is necessarily the target for the same transmitter substances. A nucleus may be composed of intrinsic neurons involved in local circuits and producing one type of neurotransmitter, terminals of afferent neurons that originate from distant regions and that release another transmitter substance, and efferent projection neurons releasing yet another neurotransmitter in another structure.

These elements may be components in a chain in which the neurotransmitters are interdependent.

Metabolic abnormalities are known to occur in which the transmitter substance is reduced in quantity or not produced at all (synthesis), overproduced, produced but not released, not producing its effects, or not removed from its site of action.

Knowledge of the production, distribution, and effects of neurotransmitters is important for the understanding of neuro-

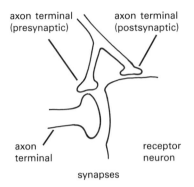

Fig. 23-1. Synaptic complex.

breaks down ACh is acetylcholinesterase (AChE). ACh is the major transmitter in the peripheral nervous system (PNS).

ACh is produced in anterior horn motor neurons, lateral horn (autonomic) neurons, and motor nuclei of cranial nerves. It is released at the neuromuscular junction of all striated muscles and in autonomic ganglia. Nearly all parasympathetic cells are cholinergic. The postganglionic sympathetic fibers to sweat glands are also cholinergic.

ACh has a powerful inhibitory effect on heart muscle.

Five regions of the brain are hitherto identified as having high densities of cholinergic (ACh-containing) nerve cells (Fig. 23-2):

logical diseases that affect the availability of neurotransmitters, the development of drug treatments for such disorders, and possible side effects of many drugs on neurotransmitter activity.

The diversity of neurotransmitter systems in the nervous system is impressive. It is possible that there may be more than 100 different transmitters, although presently only a little more than 20 have been well characterized. In Table 23-1 five distinct groups of transmitters are listed.

1. The **basal nucleus of Meynert** and its surrounding substantia innominata contain neurons rich in ACh that project broadly to frontal and parietal cortex. A recent hypothesis is that Alzheimer's type of presenile dementia may be due, or at least correlated with, the massive degeneration of this cholinergic basal nucleus-cortex system.

Acetylcholine

Acetylcholine (ACh) is synthesized from choline by the enzyme choline acetyltransferase (ChAc). The enzyme that

2. The **septohippocampal cholinergic system** is composed of cholinergic septal neurons which send their axons through the fornix to the hippocampal

Table 23-1. Classification of Neurotransmitters

Cholinergic	Aminergic	Amino Acids	Neuropeptides	Purines
Acetylcholine	Norepinephrine Dopamine Serotonin (5-hydroxytryptamine)	γ aminobutyric acid (GABA) Glycine Glutamate Aspartate	Substance P Enkephalin Endorphin Somatostatin VIP Cholecystokinin ACTH Thyrotropin releasing hormone (TRH) Vasopressin Oxytocin Neurotensin	Adenosine Adenosinetriphosphate (ATP)

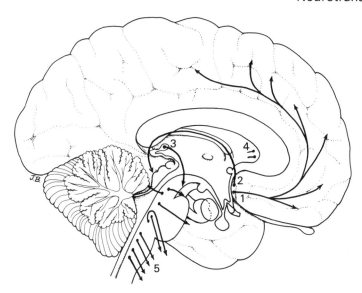

Fig. 23-2. Cholinergic system. (1) Basal nucleus of Meynert → frontal and parietal cortex; (2) septohippocampal system; (3) habenulointerpeduncular system; (4) intrinsic striatal neurons; (5) motor nuclei of cranial nerves.

formation.

3. The **habenulointerpeduncular cholinergic system** consists of neurons of the medial habenular nuclei which send their axons to the interpeduncular nucleus in the midbrain. The habenula and the interpeduncular nucleus have the highest concentrations of ChAc in the brain.

4. Many intrinsic neurons which form local circuits within the **striatum** (caudate and putamen) release ACh. Huntington's chorea has been correlated with the loss of these striatal cholinergic interneurons.

5. Motor nuclei of cranial nerves (see Chs. 13 and 14).

Aminergic Transmitters

Aminergic (monoamine) transmitters, known as biogenic amines, can be classified as **catecholamines** (norepinephrine and dopamine), and **indoleamine** (serotonin).

Norepinephrine

Norepinephrine (NE) (noradrenaline) is found in the peripheral nervous system as the transmitter between the sympathetic postganglionic terminals and effector cells or neurons of the enteric plexus. An exception is the sympathetic cholinergic neurons which innervate the sweat glands.

The number of neurons in the central nervous system (CNS) synthesizing NE is unimpressive. Nevertheless, such neurons have remarkable axonal branching which together reach every region of the CNS. NE is always inhibitory in its action, slow, and of lasting effect.

There are two principal NE systems in the CNS:

1. The **lateral tegmental NE system** (Fig. 23-3), also called the **brain stem NE system,** originates in neurons of the lateral tegmentum of the medulla and pons as well as in cells of the dorsal vagal nucleus and the solitary nucleus. They reach the spinal cord, brain stem, hypothalamus, and basal telencephalon.

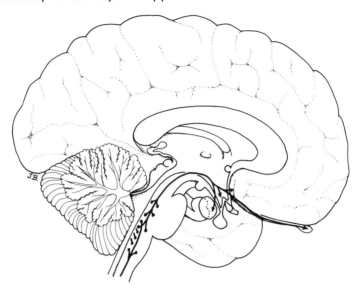

Fig. 23-3. Lateral tegmental noradrenergic system.

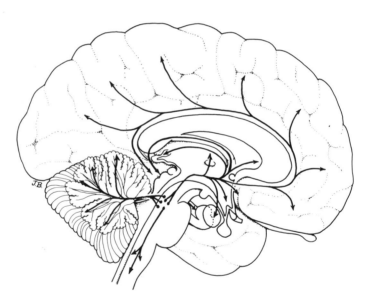

Fig. 23-4. Locus ceruleus noradrenergic system.

2. The NE neurons of the **locus ceruleus NE system** (Fig. 23-4) are located in the nucleus locus ceruleus. They send their axons to the spinal cord, brain stem, cerebellum, hypothalamus, thalamus, basal telencephalon, and the entire isocortex. The axon fibers of the NE neurons that course toward the cerebrum form part of the central tegmental tract, dorsal longitudinal fasciculus, and medial forebrain bundle.

These NE systems have been implicated in many functions such as learning and memory, sleep-wake cycle regulation, anxiety, and pain perception. Furthermore, because of their endings around vessels and capillaries, their possible role in regu-

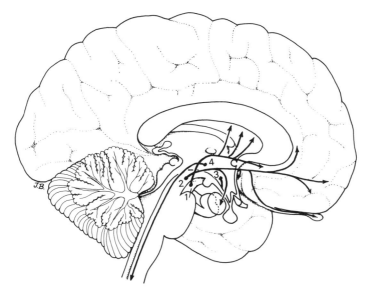

Fig. 23-5. Dopaminergic system. (1) Nigrostriatal system; (2) mesolimbic system; (3) tuberoinfundibular system; (4) hypothalamospinal system.

lating the cerebral blood flow has been suggested.

Most NE neurons appear to be part of the reticular formation. This system of neurons is thought to be involved in selectively reducing irrelevant stimuli and allowing the activity of the relevant ones to predominate. Different models that attempt to correlate NE overproduction with mania and NE deficiency with depression have been proposed.

Dopamine

In **dopamine (DA)** neurons, the amino acid tyrosin is converted to L-dihydroxyphenylalanine (L-DOPA) by the enzyme tyrosine hydroxylase. L-DOPA is in turn converted to the active transmitter substance DA by a decarboxylating enzyme.

At least seven distinct DA-containing systems have been identified. In two of the four major DA systems the neuron cell bodies are contained in the midbrain. The other two originate in the hypothalamus.

Midbrain

The two systems originating in the midbrain are known as the **mesotelencephalic (dopaminergic) system.** Its two subsystems (Fig. 23-5) are described below.

The Nigrostriatal System

DA neurons of the substantia nigra project their axons mainly to the dorsal part of the striatum through the nigrostriatal tract, which courses lateral to the hypothalamus.

In patients suffering from parkinsonism, a reduction in the number of nigrostriatal dopaminergic neurons has frequently been found.

Decrease of DA also appears to occur during the aging process in association with irregular and slow movements.

The nigrostriatal DA neurons normally innervate cholinergic nerve cells in the striatum. Thus, the loss of DA neurons in Parkinson's disease causes an imbalance of normal DA/ACh function in the striatum. Also, drugs that similarly upset the striatal

DA/ACh balance may also produce symptoms that mimic parkinsonism.

Such cases of DA/ACh imbalance and DA decrease support the view that the nigrostriatal system plays a role in motor coordination.

The Mesocortical Dopaminergic System

This system originates in the ventral tegmental area of Tsai and substantia nigra. Its fibers project through the medial forebrain bundle to the medial frontal, anterior cingulate, and entorhinal regions of the cortex, as well as the olfactory bulb and related olfactory areas. Deeper projections reach the septal area, nucleus accumbens, and amygdala.

It has been suggested that hyperactivity of the mesolimbic DA system may have some correlation with schizophrenia.

Hypothalamus

The other two major DA systems, which originate in the hypothalamus, are described below.

The Tuberoinfundibular DA System

Neurons of the arcuate nucleus, abundant with DA, project their axons to the nearby median eminence and neurohypophysis. Hyperactivity or hypoactivity of this DA system appears to have an inhibitory effect on the release of prolactin and melanocyte stimulating hormones, respectively.

The Hypothalamospinal DA system.

Neurons from the posterior hypothalamic region project to posterior and intermediate gray columns of the spinal cord.

Serotonin (5-Hydroxytryptamine)

More than 95 percent of the body's **serotonin** is found outside the nervous system (gastrointestinal tract and blood platelets). The number of neurons releasing serotonin is sparse. Their cell bodies are concentrated principally within the raphe nuclei. In spite of the restricted cell

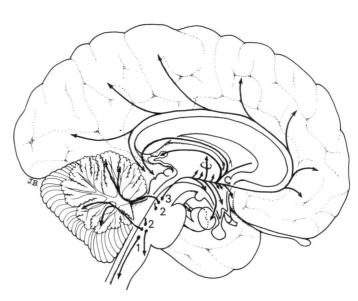

Fig. 23-6. Serotonergic system. (1) Raphespinal system; (2) raphecerebellar and raphe brain stem system; (3) raphecerebral system.

population, the role of serotonin as a neurotransmitter and its impact on brain function is of major importance.

The origin and termination of the three serotonin systems are mentioned on page 339 and illustrated in Figure 23-6. The raphe magnus projection to the substantia gelatinosa is described on page 297. Electrical stimulation of the nucleus raphe magnus produces strong and lasting analgesia. The serotonin system has a number of similarities as well as differences with the norepinephrine system. Some of the similarities are listed below.

1. Both systems consist of small clusters of neurons in the brain stem reticular formation.
2. Both diffuse through the nervous system with overlapping projections.
3. The locus ceruleus NE path is like a mirror image of the serotonergic path.
4. Both have a powerful effect on brain functions, e.g., mood states (mania and depression), behavior, and thermoregulation.

Some of the differences between the two systems are that serotonin is more selective (i.e., less diffuse) in its targets; serotonin fibers innervate the ependyma and circumventricular organs and release 5-hydroxytryptamine into the ventricle; and their receptors and mechanisms of action are different.

Amino Acids

The four **amino acids** that have been established as neurotransmitters are γ **aminobutyric acid (GABA), glycine, glutamate,** and **aspartate.**

Others, e.g., **taurine, proline,** and **histamine,** are suggested to be transmitter substances as well.

γ Aminobutyric Acid

γ **aminobutyric acid (GABA)** is produced from glutamate by the enzyme glutamic acid decarboxylase (GAD). This enzyme is found only in GABA neurons. GABA is the most common inhibitory transmitter in the brain, involved in 30 percent of all brain synapses.

Some of the GABAergic systems (Fig. 23-7) are described below.

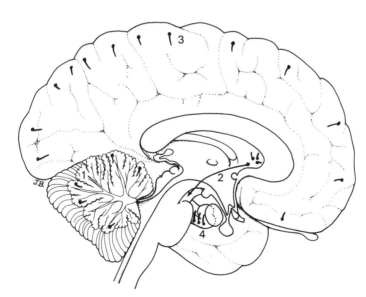

Fig. 23-7. GABAergic system. (1) Cerebellar system; (2) striatonigral system; (3) cerebrocortical system; (4) hippocampal system.

Cerebellar

Purkinje cells, the only output of the cerebellar cortex, release GABA at their axon terminals and inhibit the activity of the receiving neurons, e.g., the cerebellar and vestibular nuclei and basket cells. The basket cells also release GABA.

Striatonigral

Cells from the striatum reach the substantia nigra and release GABA, which inhibits the release of DA. There are also many intrinsic GABA neurons within the striatum which influence local circuits.

In patients suffering from Huntington's chorea, there is a loss of GABA neurons in the striatum, an increase of DA/ACh in the striatum, and widespread atrophy of the frontal cortex.

Intrinsic Cerebrocortical

The stellate neurons of the cerebral cortex produce and release GABA, influencing their local circuits.

Hippocampal

Hippocampal basket cells also produce GABA and inhibit the hippocampal local circuits.

Glycine

Glycine is an inhibitory transmitter found mainly in the spinal cord. Many of the interneurons found in the intermediate and anterior horn use glycine as their transmitter in local circuits.

Glutamate and Aspartate

Glutamate and **aspartate** occur in all body tissues. The role as neurotransmitters of these two amino acids is accepted. They are considered to be excitatory transmitters. Some of the neuronal sites of production (Fig. 23-8) are (1) cerebral cortex

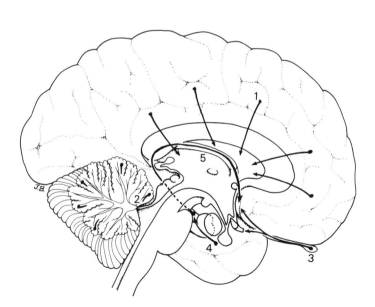

Fig. 23-8. Glutamate system. (1) Corticospinal system; (2) cerebellar system; (3) olfactory system; (4) entorhinohippocampal system; (5) hippocamposeptal system.

neurons projecting fibers to the caudate (corticostriatal path); (2) the cerebellar granule cells giving rise to parallel fibers that stimulate Purkinje cells; (3) the olfactory bulb neurons stimulating the pyriform lobe through the lateral olfactory stria; (4) the entorhinal cortex stimulating the hippocampus through the perforant path; and (5) the hippocampus connecting with the septal area.

algesia gave new impetus and perspective to the study of neuropeptides as neurotransmitters. These substances appear to have many other effects related to brain function yet to be explored.

Some of the neuropeptides are substance P (SP), endorphins, enkephalins, somatostatin, vasoactive intestinal polypeptide (VIP), cholecystokinin (CCK), and adenocorticotrophic hormone (ACTH).

Neuropeptides

Peptides are chains of amino acids. The first peptide to be established as a transmitter in the nervous system, i.e., **neuropeptide,** was **substance P,** which was discovered in 1931. It was followed by a number of hypothalamic and pituitary hormones. The interest in neuropeptides intensified with the identification of **endorphins** (endogenous morphines) in 1975. The conceptualization of the nervous system as having its own device capable of generating opiate substances and releasing them at specific opiate receptors to produce an-

Substance P

Substance P was first isolated from horse brain and intestine as a precipitate. It is slow acting but produces a lasting inhibitory effect on neuron firing and an ACh-like influence on smooth muscle. However, this effect is mediated by specific SP receptors.

Some of the SP systems (Fig. 23-9) are described below.

1. Small neurons of the spinal and cranial ganglia release SP at their primary afferent terminals (substantia gelatinosa

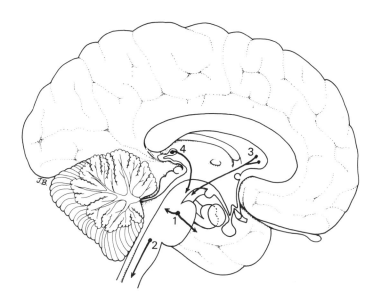

Fig. 23-9. Substance P system. (1) Cranial ganglia; (2) medullospinal system; (3) striatonigral system; (4) habenulointerpeduncular system.

and cranial nerve sensory nuclei), modulating somatic sensation.

2. SP neurons from the medulla oblongata also project to the substantia gelatinosa.

3. SP neurons from the striatum appear to reach the substantia nigra through the striatonigral path (together with GABA fibers). In patients with Huntington's chorea, SP and GABA are reduced in the substantia nigra due to the degeneration of the striatonigral path.

4. The medial habenular nucleus sends fibers to the interpeduncular nucleus and releases SP through the interpeduncular tract. Also, fibers of the hypothalamus, amygdala, and anterior frontal cortex carry SP.

Endorphins

Three of the **endorphins** commonly found in the body are known as **alpha, beta,** and **gamma endorphins.** Of the three, the beta endorphin has the largest representation in the brain. The majority of beta endorphin neurons are found in the hypothalamus (arcuate nucleus, mammillary body, and periventricular gray) and some in the amygdala (Fig. 23-10). These endorphin neurons reach mainly other hypothalamic regions (e.g., the pituitary gland) as well as structures of the midbrain and upper pons. Endorphins are considered to play a major role in the neuroendocrine system.

Enkephalins

Enkephalins are a subgroup of two types of endorphins, i.e., **methionin enkephalin (met-enkephalin)** and **leucine enkephalin (leu-enkephalin).** The enkephalins are widely distributed throughout the central and peripheral nervous systems. Apart from the broad distribution of enkephalinergic neurons, other characteristics of this neurotransmitter system (Fig. 23-11) are described.

Principally it forms part of local circuits.
A high concentration of enkephalin arriving from striatal neurons is located in the pallidum.

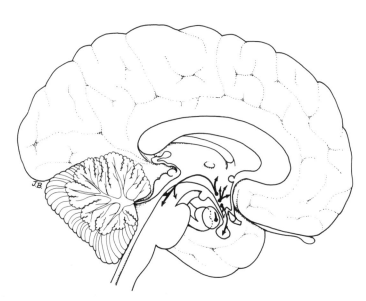

Fig. 23-10. Beta endorphin system.

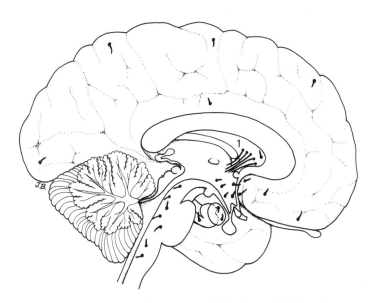

Fig. 23-11. Enkephalin system. (1) Striatopallidal system.

The role of enkephalins has been attributed to endocrine and analgesic functions. However, many other functions are presently being hypothesized and investigated.

Somatostatin

Somatostatin was first identified as one of the releasing (RF) and inhibiting (IF) factors of the hypothalamus regulating the production of growth or somatotrophic hormone (STH) of the adenohypophysis. Somatostatin neurons are found in the hypothalamus mainly in the periventricular gray with different fiber projections, e.g., to the median eminence and infundibular region entering the pituitary portal system. They have also been found in other regions, e.g., among the spinal and cranial ganglia neurons and their fibers, ending in the substantia gelatinosa and cranial nerve nuclei; in the cerebral cortex; in the intesti-

nal wall as well as other non-neuronal cells of the body, such as in the pancreas.

Vasoactive Intestinal Polypeptide

A peptide identified as a VIP was first characterized as a gut hormone. Later it was found in different neural regions, for example, in the cerebral cortex, forming part of local circuits, and the median eminence of the hypothalamus. Its function is being researched.

Cholecystokinin

Cholecystokinin is another peptide first classified as a gut hormone, which was later found to be the most common peptide in the brain. Its function as a neurotransmitter is being debated. Its role is associated with cerebral blood flow as well as neuroendocrine and cortical activities.

Adenocorticotrophic Hormone

Although **ACTH** is a substance primarily found in the pituitary gland, there are other brain regions producing it, e.g., the arcuate nucleus and region as well as other areas of the hypothalamus with fibers reaching other regions of the hypothalamus, thalamus, periaqueductal gray, and reticular formation. The destruction of the pituitary gland is not followed by a reduction of ACTH in the brain. Its potential function and role as a neurotransmitter are being debated. It is known that ACTH plays a part in motivational mechanisms, stress, learning, and memory processes.

Many other peptides are the subject of recent studies which intend to find out whether they are true neurotransmitters or modulators. Most of these peptides are found in the hypothalamus and are related to neuroendocrine activities of the nervous system.

Purines

The presence of a population of neurons in the walls of the alimentary tract that are neither adrenergic nor cholinergic is now well-established. These gastrointestinal neurons of the PNS are stimulated by cholinergic terminals and produce an inhibitory effect on the smooth muscle by the release of **adenosinetriphosphate (ATP)**.

ATP is a purine nucleotide and ATP neurons are therefore known as purinergic. ATP released by purinergic neurons behaves at the smooth muscle

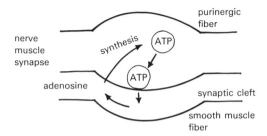

Fig. 23-12. Neurotransmitter ATP cycle.

junction as a true neurotransmitter (Fig. 23-12).

ATP is inactivated at the neuromuscular junction by enzymes. Its product, **adenosine,** returns to the presynaptic nerve terminal to resynthesize ATP. It appears that the excitatory action of cholinergic fibers in the alimentary tract, combined with the transient inhibitory action of purinergic fibers and followed by a powerful rebound contraction, forms the basis of peristaltic propagation.

Two Types of Acetylcholine Receptors

Some ACh receptors can also be activated by the alkaloid **nicotine.** These **nicotinic receptors** can be blocked by curare.

Other ACh receptors can also be activated by the alkaloid **muscarine.** These **muscarinic receptors** can be blocked by atropine.

Two Types of Norepinephrine Receptors

Some NE receptors can be activated by **phenylephrine** although not as powerfully as by NE. These so-called **alpha adrenergic receptors** can be blocked by phenoxybenzamine.

Other NE receptors are more powerfully activated by **isoproterenol** than by NE. These so-called **beta adrenergic receptors** can be blocked by dichloroisoproterenol (DCl).

General Comments

The continuous development of new neurochemical tracing methods and metabolic imaging techniques has greatly increased our knowledge in all areas of the neurosciences. The exponential growth of data related to neurotransmitters is refining our understanding of the nervous system in health and disease. Neurology, psychiatry, nutrition sciences, and drug therapy are just a few examples of areas where the impact of such new knowledge is operant.

A subsequent major conceptual change worthy of mention involves the autonomic nervous system. The discovery of other neurotransmitters besides the cholinergic and adrenergic substances in the autonomic nervous system has made the complexity of this system obvious. Scientists now conceive it as one in its own right, a system with a great many intrinsic operant mechanisms. Although coordination with the nervous system as a whole is secured through neural links, neuroendocrine mechanisms are now seen to play a very important role.

Note: In reference to neurotransmitter cell groups, the student may find them listed in the literature from A1 to A15 and from B1 to B9 instead of the conventional nomenclature.

A1 to A15 refer to 15 specific regional groups of catecholaminergic neurons (dopamine and norepinephrine) and B1 to B9 to 9 specific regional groups of indoleaminergic neurons (serotonin).

Effects of Drug Therapy

The administration of the drug L-DOPA (a precursor in the synthesis of DA

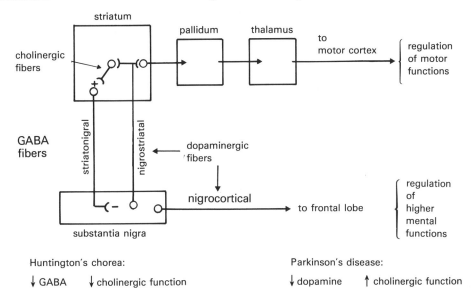

Fig. 23-13. Interactions of neurotransmitters.

to ameliorate the signs of parkinsonism) over a period of time may end up producing schizophrenic states.

The administration of some antischizophrenic drugs may among other things block DA receptors and end up causing signs of parkinsonism to appear (Fig. 23-13).

Suggested Readings

Andrew RD, Dudek FE: Analysis of intracellularly recorded phasic bursting by mammalian neuroendocrine cells, J Neurophysiol 51:552–566, 1984.

Bloom FE: Neurohumoral transmission and the central nervous system. In Goodman LS, Gilman A, Eds.: The Pharmacological Basis of Therapeutics, Macmillan, New York, pp. 235–257, 1980.

Burnstock G, Bell C: Peripheral autonomic transmission. In Hubbard JI, Ed.: The Peripheral Nervous System, Plenum Press, New York, 1974.

Burnstock G, Costa M: Adrenergic Neurons, Their Organisation, Function and Development in the Peripheral Nervous System, Chapman and Hall, London, 1975.

Cooper JR, Bloom FE, Roth RH: The Biochemical Basis of Neuropharmacology, Oxford University Press, New York, 1982.

Emson PC, Ed.: Chemical Neuroanatomy, Raven Press, New York, 1983.

Fuxe P, Roberts K, Schwarcz R, Eds.: Exitotoxins, Macmillan, New York, 1983.

Moore RY: Catecholamine neuron systems in brain, Ann Neurol 12:321–327, 1982.

Saunders SL, Reifel CW, Shin SH: Desmosomes between mammotrophs suggest the existence of a functional syncytium, Acta Anat 114:74–80, 1982.

Siegel GJ, Albers RW, Katzman R, Agranoff BW, Eds.: Basic Neurochemistry. Second Edition. Little, Brown and Co., Boston, 1976.

Zimmerman AE, Milligan JV, Joneja MG: Scanning electron microscopy of rat neurointermediate (NI) lobe cells in culture, Acta Anat 110:259–269, 1981.

Appendix I

Brain Atlas

Nuclear Magnetic Resonance Imaging

Imaging techniques for diagnostic procedures, like conventional x-rays, angiography, ultrasonic imaging, and x-ray computed tomography (CT) scans, are well-established in clinical practice. Recently, **positron emission tomography (PET)** and **nuclear magnetic resonance (NMR)** techniques are progressing from their experimental phases to become accepted in diagnostic procedures.

An NMR device uses radiowaves and a strong magnetic field to produce an image of the analyzed structure. The magnetic field causes some of the hydrogen nuclei within the structure to line up. The device subsequently emits a pulsed radiowave that causes some of the nuclei to flip out of alignment. When the pulse is switched off, these nuclei return to their original position, releasing characteristic electromagnetic signals that are received by the imaging system. A computer then converts these signals into two-dimensional images on the video screen of the system's console.

Health care professionals can store, recall, and manipulate the images in many ways to allow detailed study of a patient's internal structure.

NMR devices do not use ionizing radiation.

The potentials of NMR techniques for the investigation of cellular metabolism appear to be very promising. The NMR images shown here are presented through the courtesy of General Electric.

Note: The term nuclear resonance imaging is being replaced with the newer term **magnetic resonance imaging (MRI)**.

Serial Sections of the Brain in Coronal, Horizontal, and Sagittal Planes

The keys of the coordinates are represented in Figures A-6 and A-7. They are defined by the midsagittal 0 plane, the horizontal 0 plane of the anterior commissure–posterior pommissure (AC–PC) line, and the coronal 0 plane of the midsagittal point of the AC–PC line.

Following this system of coordinates with their 0 planes (1) successive coronal planes increase and decrease their values in the anterior and posterior direction, respectively; (2) successive horizontal planes increase and decrease their values in the upward and downward direction, respectively; and (3) successive sagittal planes increase their values in the lateral direction.

Note: To facilitate an overview of all the planes, no labels have been included for these maps. The numbers in the scales indicate centimeters. In Chapters 8 and 9 the student will find labels to identify the structures shown in each plane.

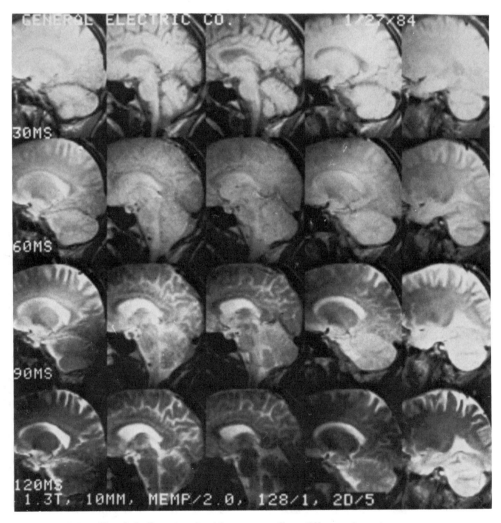

Fig. A-1. Four sagittal images at five different locations.

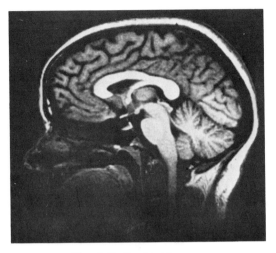

Fig. A-2. Sagittal image.

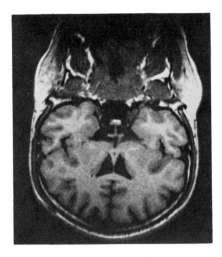

Fig. A-3. Coronal image.

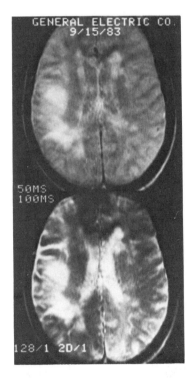

Fig. A-4. Image showing unusually severe
and asymmetric demyelination.

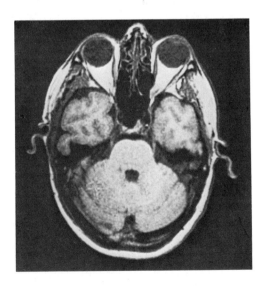

Fig. A-5. Horizontal image.

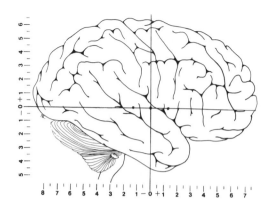

Fig. A-6. Coordinate system and scale (numbers indicate centimeters).

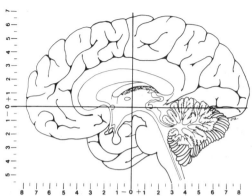

Fig. A-7. Coordinate system and scale (numbers indicate centimeters).

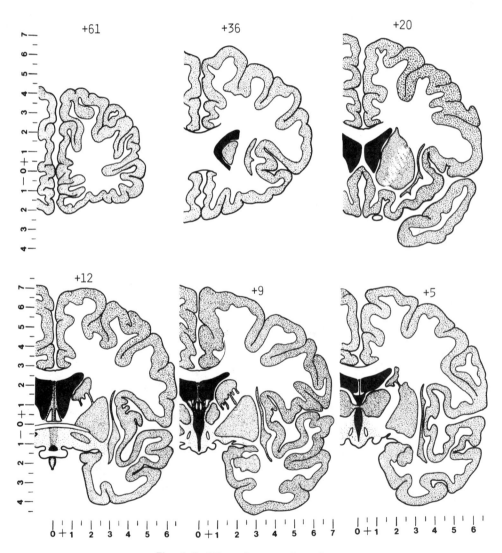

+61   +36   +20

+12   +9   +5

Fig. A-8. Atlas of coronal sections.

404

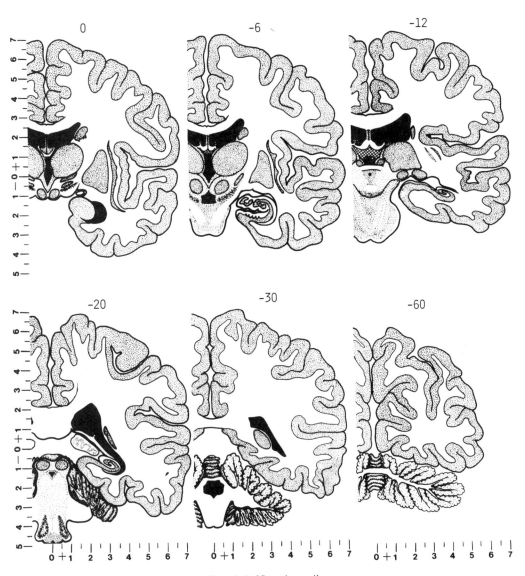

Fig. A-8 (Continued).

405

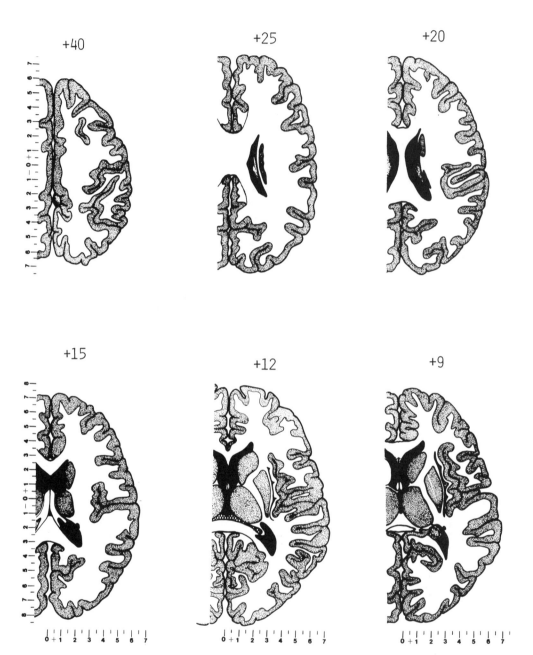

Fig. A-9. Atlas of horizontal sections.

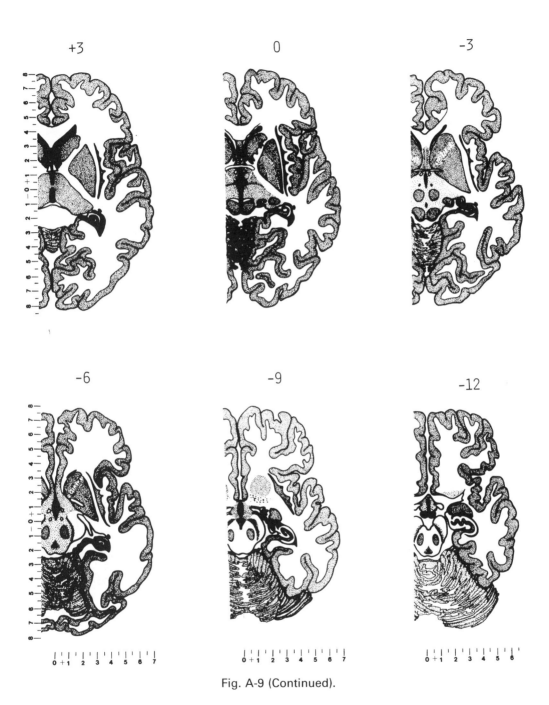

Fig. A-9 (Continued).

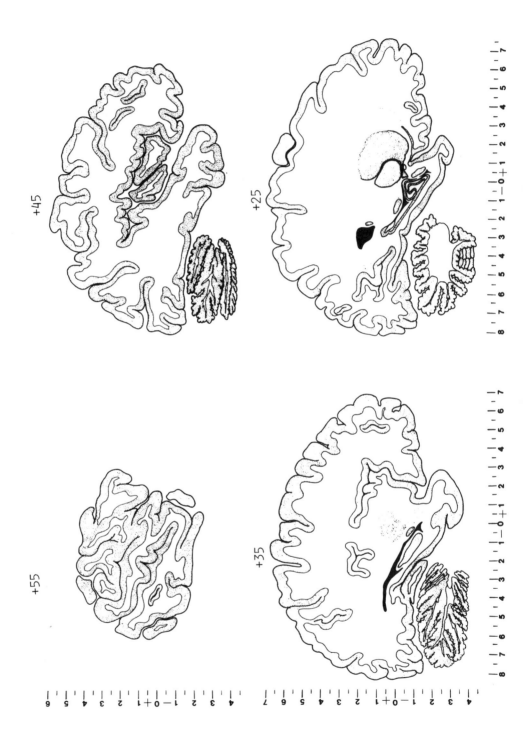

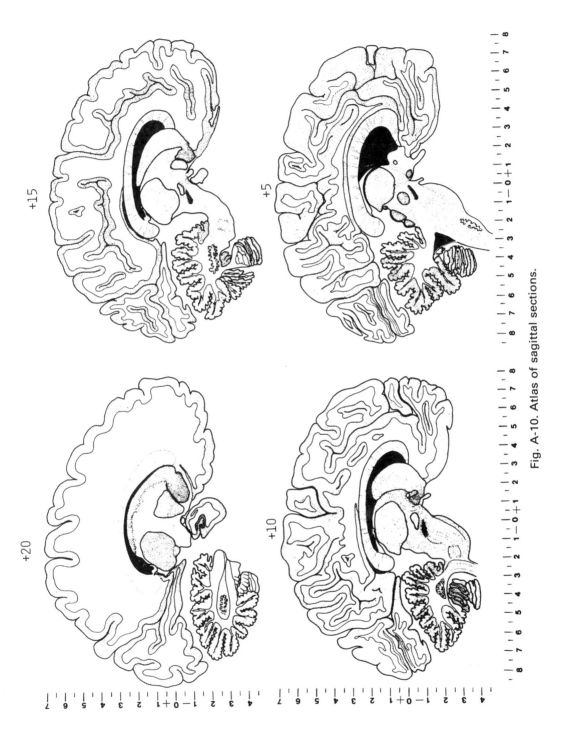

+20

+15

+10

+5

Fig. A-10. Atlas of sagittal sections.

409

Appendix II

Glossary of Neuroanatomical Terms

Acalculia (*a* neg.; L. *calculare* to compute.) Aphasia characterized by inability to work even simple arithmetic problems.

Adhesio (L. *adhaerere* to stick to.)

Adiadochokinesis (*a* neg.; Gr. *diadochos* succeeding; *kinesis* movement.) Inability to perform rapidly alternating movements.

Agnosia (*a* neg.; Gr. *gnosis* knowledge.) Loss of ability to recognize familiar sensory stimuli.

Agraphia (*a* neg.; Gr. *graphein* to write.) Aphasia characterized by loss of ability to write.

Ala (L. wing.)

Ala cinerea (L. *ala* wing; *cinereus* ashy.) Vagal triangle in floor of fourth ventricle.

Alba (L. *albus* white.)

Alexia (*a* neg.; Gr. *lexis* word.) Aphasia characterized by loss of ability to understand written symbols.

Allocortex (Gr. *allos* other; L. *cortex* bark.) The partly laminated cortex.

Alveus (L. trough.) Layer of myelinated fibers on the ventricular surface of the hippocampus.

Amaurosis (Gr. darkening.) Partial or total blindness.

Ammon. Egyptian god, represented with a ram's horns.

Ammon's horn. Synonym of hippocampus.

Amygdala (Gr. *amygdale* almond.)

Anisocoria (Gr. *anisos* unequal; Gr. *kore* pupil.) Inequality of the diameter of the pupils.

Ansa (L. handle.)

Antidromic (Gr. *antidromein* to run in a contrary direction.) Conducting impulses in the direction opposite to the usual direction.

Aphasia (*a* neg.; Gr. *phasis* speech.) Impairment of language due to lesion of associative and/or integrative cortical language areas.

Apraxia (*a* neg.; Gr. *praxis* action.) Inability to perform complex learned movements despite the presence of normal muscle power, coordination, and sensation.

Arachnoid (Gr. *arachne* spider.) Outer layer of the leptomeninges.

Arbor vitae (L. tree of life.)

Archi (Gr. beginning.)

Area postrema. Narrow ridge of glial and vascular tissue along the lateral edge of the caudal portion of the fourth ventricle.

Astereognosis (*a* neg.; Gr. *stereos* solid, having three dimensions; *gnosis* knowledge.) Inability to recognize objects by touching or grasping them.

Astrocyte (Gr. *astros* star; *kytos* cell.) A type of glial cell.

Asynergia (*a* neg.; Gr. *synergia* cooperation.) Faulty coordination of groups of muscles.

Ataxia (*a* neg.; Gr. *taxis* order.) Loss of power of muscle coordination.

Athetosis (Gr. *athetos* without position; *osis* condition.) An affection of the nervous system.

Autonomic (Gr. *autos* self; *nomos* law.) Self-governing.

Axolemma (Gr. *axon* axis; *lemma* husk.) Axon membrane.

Axon hillock (Gr. *axon* axis; *hillock* diminuitive of As. *hyll* small elevation.) Region of the neuronal body devoid of Nissl granules from which the axon arises.

Axon reaction. Changes in the neuronal body following damage to its axon.

Axoplasm (Gr. *axon* axis; *plasma* from *plassein* to form.) Axonal cytoplasm.

Baroreceptor (Gr. *baros* weight.) Receptor, sensor stimulated by changes in pressure.

Basis (Gr. base; **basilar** adjective.)

Basis pedunculi. Ventral portion of the cerebral peduncle composed of the pes pedunculi and substantia nigra.

Brachium (L. arm.)

Bradykinesia (Gr. *bradys* slow; *kinesis* movement.) Abnormally slow movements.

Bulb (L. *bulbus* a rounded mass.) Old term for the medulla oblongata. In the context of corticobulbar tracts, bulbar refers to the brain stem.

Calamus (L. a reed.)

Calamus scriptorius. Floor of the tapered caudal portion of the fourth ventricle; shaped like a pen point.

Calcar avis (L. *calcar* spur; *avis* bird.) Eminence of the medial wall of the posterior horn of the lateral ventricle, overlapping part of the calcarine fissure.

Cauda equina (L. *cauda* tail; *equus* horse; horsetail.) Lumbosacral nerve roots.

Caudate (L. having a tail.)

Cerebellum (L. little brain; diminuitive of *cerebrum* brain.)

Cerebrum (L. brain.) The part of the brain composed of diencephalon and cerebral hemispheres.

Chorda (L. from Gr. *chorde* string, cord.)

Choroid (Gr. *chorion* skin; *eidos* form.)

Chromaffin (Gr. *chroma* color; L. *affinis* affinity.)

Chromatolysis (Gr. *chromato* bearing relation to chromatin (*chroma* color); *lysis* dissolution.) Disintegration of Nissl bodies.

Cingulum (L. girdle.) Association bundle of fibers within the cingulate gyrus.

Claustrum (L. barrier.) A thin sheet of gray matter between the insula and lentiform nucleus.

Clava (L. club.)

Clivus (L. slope or hill.)

Colliculus (L. mound.) A small eminence.

Commissure (L. *commissura* a joining together.)

Convolution (L. *convolutus* rolled together.) Synonymous to gyrus.

Corona (L. from Gr. *korone* crown.)

Corpus (L. body.)

Corpus callosum (L. *corpus* body; *callosus* hard.) The largest commissure of the cerebral hemispheres.

Corpus striatum (L. *corpus* body; *striatus* striped.) A mass of gray matter made of caudate, putamen, and pallidum.

Cortex (L. bark.) The surface layer of an organ, e.g., of the cerebral hemispheres; of the cerebellum.

Crus (L. leg.)

Crus cerebri. Cerebral peduncle.

Culmen (L. summit.)

Cuneus (L. wedge.)

Decussation (L. *decussatio,* from *decussare* to cross in the form of an X.) Place where nerve fibers cross the midline, or the fibers which cross.

Dendrite (Gr. *dendron* tree.) Process of a neuron which conducts impulses toward the cell body.

Dentate (L. *dentatus* toothed.) E.g., **dentate gyrus** of the hippocampal formation; **dentate ligament** of the spinal cord; **dentate nucleus** of the cerebellum.

Diencephalon (Gr. *dia* through; *enkephalos* brain.) Part of the cerebrum consisting of the thalamus, hypothalamus, subthalamus, and epithalamus.

Diplopia (Gr. *diplous* double; *ope* sight.) Double vision.

Dura (L. *durus* hard.)

Dura mater (L. *durus* hard; *mater* mother.) The outer, heavy layer of the meninges.

Dys (Gr. combining form signifying difficult, painful, bad, disordered, etc.; the opposite of **eu-**.)

Dysarthria (Gr. *dys* difficult, bad; *arthroun* to articulate.) Disturbance of articulation due to paralysis, lacking coordination, or spasticity of the muscles used for speaking.

Dysmetria (Gr. *dys* difficult, bad; *metron* measure.) Disorder in the control of the range of movements.

Dysphagia (Gr. *dys* difficult, bad; *phagein* to eat.) Difficulty in swallowing.

Ectoderm (Gr. *ektos* outside; *derma* skin.) Outer layer of the embryo from which the nervous system develops.

Emboliform (Gr. *embolos* plug; L. *forma* form.) E.g., **emboliform nucleus** of the cerebellum.

Endo (Gr. *endon* within.) Prefix indicating within.

Engram (Gr. *en* in; *gramma* mark.) Trace left in the psyche by experience (psychology) or in the protoplasm by stimuli (biology). Term used in the context of some hypotheses on memory.

Entorhinal (Gr. *entos* inside; *rhis* nose.) Within the rhinencephalon.

Ependyma (Gr. *epi* upon; *endyma* garment.) Lining of the brain ventricles and central canal.

Epithalamus (Gr. *epi* upon; *thalamus* inner chamber.) Region of the diencephalon posterior and dorsal to the thalamus.

Falx (L. sickle).

Falx cerebri. Sickle-shaped dural fold located between the two cerebral hemispheres.

Fascia (L. ribbon, sheet, band, bundle.) E.g., **dentate fascia.**

Fasciculus (L. diminuitive of *fascia.*) A bundle of fibers.

Fastigium (L. the top of a gabled roof.) Summit of the roof of the fourth ventricle, e.g., **fastigial nucleus** of the cerebellum.

Fenestra (L. window.)

Fimbria (L. fringe.) Any fringe-like structure. **Fimbria hippocampi:** band of fibers on the medial edge of the hippocampus.

Foramen (L. opening.)

Forceps (L. a pair of tongues.) **Forceps major** and **minor** of corpus callosum: frontal and occipital fibers of the corpus callosum.

Fornix (L. arch.) One of the two fiber tracts beneath the corpus callosum extending from the fimbria of the hippocampus to the mammillary body.

Fossa (L. ditch.) E.g., **rhomboid fossa:** floor of the fourth ventricle.

Fovea (L. a small pit or depression.) E.g., **fovea centralis:** slight depression in the center of the macula lutea of the retina.

Funiculus (L. diminuitive of *funis* cord.) E.g., **anterior funiculus:** the anterior white matter division of the spinal cord.

Ganglion (Gr. swelling.) A group of nerve cell bodies located outside the central nervous system.

Geniculate (L. *geniculare* to bend the knee.) E.g., **geniculate nucleus.**

Genu (L. knee.) E.g., **genu** of corpus callosum.

Glia (Gr. glue.) E.g., **glial cells.**

Glioblast (Gr. *glia* glue; *blastos* germ.) An embryonic glial cell.

Globus pallidus (L. *globus* ball; *pallidus* pale.) Medial portion of the lentiform nucleus.

Glomerulus (L. diminuitive of *glomus* ball of yarn.)

Glomus choroideum. Expanded portion of the choroid plexus in the atrium of the lateral ventricle.

Gracilis (L. slender.) E.g., **fasciculus gracilis** of the spinal cord.

Granule (L. *granulum,* diminuitive of *granum* grain.) E.g., **granule cells:** small neurons.

Gyrus (L. from Gr. *gyros* circle.) E.g., **cerebral gyrus:** cerebral convolution.

Habenula (L. diminuitive of *habena* bridle, rein, or strap.) A small swelling in the epithalamus.

Hemi- (Gr. half.) E.g., **hemiplegia:** paralysis of one side of the body.

Hippocampus (Gr. sea horse.) A gyrus of the hippocampal formation that produces an elevation on the floor of the inferior horn of the lateral ventricle.

Homeostasis (Gr. *homoios* like; *stasis* position.) The maintenance of the internal stability of the organism.

Hydrocephalus (Gr. *hydro* water; *kephale* head.) Excessive accumulation of cerebrospinal fluid.

Hyper- (Gr. beyond, above, over.) Used as a prefix. E.g., **hyperacusis:** abnormal acuteness of the sense of hearing.

Hypo- (Gr. under.) Also a prefix denoting deficiency.

Hypesthesia (Gr. hypo; *aesthesis* sensation.) Impairment of sensation.

Hypothalamus. A region under the thalamus.

Incisure (L. *incisura* a slit or notch.)

Indusium (L. a garment.) **Indusium griseum:** thin layer of gray matter on the upper surface of the corpus callosum.

Infundibulum (L. funnel.) Ventral evagination of the third ventricle from which the neurohypophysis is derived.

Insula (L. island.) The cerebral cortex forming the floor of the lateral fissure.

Internuncial (L. *inter* between; *nuncius* messenger.) E.g., **internuncial neuron:** neuron serving as a link between other neurons.

Interoceptor (L. *internus* internal; *recipere* to receive.) Sensory end organ within viscera.

Intra (L. within.) E.g., **intrathecal:** within the subarachnoid space.

Iso- (Gr. *isos* equal.) E.g., **isocortex.**

Kine- (Gr. *kinein* to move; *kinesis* motion.)

Kinesiology (Gr. *kinesis* motion; *logos* word.) The science of movement.

Kinesthesia (Gr. *kinesis* motion; *aisthesis* sensation.) The sense of perception of movement.

Koniocortex (Gr. *konios* dust; *cortex* bark.) Cortex with predominant granular layers typical of sensory areas.

Lamina (L. plate, layer.) E.g., **lamina terminalis:** anterior wall of the third ventricle.

Lemniscus (L. from Gr. *lemniskos* fillet.) E.g., **medial lemniscus:** bundle of nerve fibers in the central nervous system.

Lentiform (L. *lens* lentil; *forma* form.) **Lentiform nucleus:** lentil-shaped nucleus which with the caudate constitutes the corpus striatum.

Leptomeninges (Gr. *leptos* slender; *meninx* membrane.) The arachnoid and pia mater. **Leptomeninx:** one layer of the leptomeninges.

Limbus (L. border.) **Limbic lobe:** cortical region consisting of cingulate and parahippocampal gyri and septal area.

Limen (L. threshold.) **Limen insulae:** the ventral part of the insula.

Locus ceruleus (L. *locus* place; *coeruleus*

bluish.) A bluish tinted eminence of the floor of the fourth ventricle.

Macro- (Gr. *makros* large.) E.g., **macroglia.**

Macula (L. spot.) E.g., **macula lutea** of the eye.

Mammillary (L. *mammilla,* diminuitive of *mamma* breast.) **Mammillary bodies:** small swellings on the ventral surface of the hypothalamus.

Massa interthalamica. Midline nuclear mass interconnecting the thalami across the third ventricle.

Mater (L. mother.) E.g., **pia mater.**

Matter (L. *materia* substance.) E.g., **white matter.**

Medulla (L. marrow.) When used alone in neuroanatomy it usually means medulla oblongata or the caudal portion of the brain stem. **Medulla spinalis:** the spinal cord.

Meninx (Gr. membrane; pl. *meninges.*)

Mesencephalon (Gr. *mesos* middle; *enkephalos* brain.) The midbrain.

Meta (Gr. after.) E.g., **metathalamus:** the medial and lateral geniculate bodies. **Metencephalon:** the pons or the pons and cerebellum.

Mimetic (Gr. *mimetikos* imitative.)

Miosis (Gr. *meiosis* diminution.) E.g., constriction of the pupils.

Mnemonic (Gr. *mnemonikos* pertaining to memory.)

Myelencephalon (Gr. *myelos* marrow; *enkephalos* brain.)

Medulla oblongata. The caudal portion of the rhombencephalon.

Myelin (Gr. *myelos* marrow.) White lipidoproteic substance forming sheaths around axons.

Neo- (Gr. new.) E.g., **neocerebellum:** the phylogenetically newest part of the cerebellum; **neostriatum:** the phylogenetically newest part of the corpus striatum.

Neurite. Old term for the axis cylinder meaning the axon of a neuron.

Neurobiotaxis (Gr. *neuron* nerve; *bios* life; *taxis* arrangement.) The tendency of the nerve cells to migrate during development toward the principal source of stimuli.

Neuroblast (Gr. *neuron* nerve; *blastos* germ.) An embryonic nerve cell.

Neuropil (Gr. *neuron* nerve; *pilos* felt.) Mesh of cell processes, found between cell bodies in the gray matter.

Node (L. *nodus* knot.) E.g., **node of Ranvier.**

Nucleus (L. nut.)

Nystagmus (Gr. *nystagmos* nodding.) An involuntary oscillation of the eyes.

Obex (L. bolt, barrier.) Point on the mid-dorsal surface of the medulla covering the caudal tip of the fourth ventricle.

Oligodendroglia (Gr. *oligos* little, scanty; *dendron* tree; *glia* glue.) Glial cells with few cytoplasmic processes.

Operculum (L. lid.) E.g., **frontal, parietal,** and **temporal lobes opercula** covering the insula.

Paleo- (Gr. *palaios* ancient.) E.g., **paleostriatum:** the phylogenetically older part of the corpus striatum, i.e., the pallidum or globus pallidus.

Pallidum (L. *pallidus* pale.)

Palsy. Synonym for paralysis.

Para- (Gr. *para* beyond, beside, near.) E.g., **paravertebral ganglion:** sympathetic ganglion beside the vertebra.

Paralysis (Gr. *paralyein* to weaken.) Loss of voluntary muscle movement.

Peri- (Gr. *peri* around.) E.g., **perineurium:** the two or more connective tissue sheaths surrounding each fascicle of fibers.

Pes (L. foot.) E.g., **pes hippocampi:** the anterior part of the hippocampus, which is shaped like a paw; **pes pedunculi:** the ventral white matter region of the midbrain composed of pyramidal and corticopontine tracts.

Pia (L. *pius* tender, soft.) E.g., **pia mater:** the innermost meningeal layer.

Pineal (L. *pinea* pine cone.) **Pineal body.**

Piriform. See pyriform.

Plexus (L. a twining.) Interwoven fibers or vessels.

Pneumoencephalography (Gr. *pneuma* air; *enkephalos* brain; *graphein* to write.) A method of visualizing the ventricular system by roentgen ray after replacement of cerebrospinal fluid by air.

Pons (L. bridge.) Portion of brain stem between medulla oblongata and midbrain.

Pre- (L. *prae* before.) E.g., **preoptic region:** region anterior to the optic chiasm.

Proprioceptor (L. *proprius* one's own; *receptor* receiver.) One of the sensory endings within muscles, tendons, joints, and the vestibular portion of the internal ear.

Prosencephalon (Gr. *pros* before; *enkephalos* brain.) The cerebrum, consisting of diencephalon and telencephalon.

Ptosis (Gr. a falling.) Drooping of the upper eyelid.

Pulvinar (L. *pulvinus* pillow.) The posterior portion of the thalamus.

Putamen (L. shell.) Lateral portion of the lentiform nucleus.

Pyriform (L. *pirum* pear; *forma* form.) Pear-shaped. Also piriform. **Pyriform area:** pear-shaped area consisting of uncus, limen insulae, and entorhinal area.

Quadrigeminal (L. *quadrigeminus* fourfold, forming a group of four.) E.g., **quadrigeminal bodies** of the tectum of the midbrain.

Quadriplegia (L. *quattuor* four; *plege* a stroke; blow.) Paralysis of the four limbs.

Raphe (Gr. *rhaphe* seam.) Term used for some structures placed in the midline. E.g., **raphe nuclei** of the reticular formation.

Restiform (L. *restis* cord; *forma* form.) Shaped like a rope. E.g., **restiform body** or inferior cerebellar peduncle.

Reticular (L. *reticularis* pertaining to or resembling a net.) E.g., **reticular formation.**

Rhinal (Gr. *rhis* nose.) Pertaining to the nose.

Rhizotomy (Gr. *rhiza* root; *tome* a cutting.) Surgical division of any root.

Rhombencephalon (Gr. *rhombos* magic wheel; *enkephalos* brain.) Portion of the brain stem consisting of the pons and medulla.

Rostrum (L. beak.) E.g., **rostrum** of the corpus callosum.

Ruber (L. red.) E.g., **nucleus ruber:** red nucleus.

Saccadic (Fr. *saccader* to jerk.) E.g., **saccadic eye movements.**

Sella turcica (L. *sella* saddle; *turcicus* Turkish.) Saddle shaped depression in the sphenoid bone containing the pituitary gland.

Septum (L. *saeptum* fence.)

Septum pellucidum (L. *saeptum* fence; *pellucidus* from *per* through; *lucere* to shine.) Membrane between the corpus callosum and the fornix forming most of the medial wall of the anterior horn of the lateral ventricle.

Somesthetic (Gr. *soma* body; *aisthesis* perception.) Perception of the body involving the general body senses exclusive of the visceral and special senses.

Splanchnic (Gr. *splanchna* viscera.) E.g., **splanchnic nerves.**

Splenium (Gr. *splenion* bandage.) E.g., **splenium** of the corpus callosum.

Strabismus (Gr. *strabismos* a squinting.)

Stratum (L. layer, blanket; pl. *strata.*) E.g., **strata** of the superior colliculus.

Stria (L. furrow, limit, stripe.) E.g., **olfactory stria.**

Subiculum (L. diminuitive of *subex* a layer.) Transitional cortex between the parahippocampal gyrus and the hippocampus.

Sub- (L. *sub* under.) E.g., **subdural:** beneath the dura.

Sulcus (L. groove, furrow.)

Sympathetic (Gr. *syn* with; *pathos* suffering.)

Synapse (Gr. *synapsis* a conjunction, connection.)

Syringomyelia (Gr. *syrinx* a tube; *myelos* marrow.) A condition in which there is central cavitation of the spinal cord.

Tanycyte (Gr. *tanyein* to stretch; *kytos* cell.) A specialized ependymal cell.

Tapetum (L. *tapeta* carpet.) Fibers of the corpus callosum as they spread over the lateral ventricle forming a cover on the lateral wall of the inferior horn.

Tectum (L. roof.) E.g., **tectum** of the midbrain.

Tegmentum (L. covering.) E.g., **tegmentum** of the brain stem.

Tela (L. web.) E.g., **tela choroidea.**

Telencephalon (Gr. *telos* end; *enkephalos* brain.) Cerebral hemispheres.

Telodendria (Gr. *telos* end; *dendron* tree.) The terminal branches of axons.

Tenia (L. from Gr. *tainia* band, tape.) E.g., **tenia thalami:** line of attachment of the choroid plexus of the third ventricle along the stria medullaris of the thalamus.

Tentorium (L. tent.) E.g., **tentorium cerebelli:** dural fold interposed between the cerebrum and cerebellum.

Tetraplegia (Gr. *tetra* four; *plege* a stroke, blow.) Paralysis of the four limbs.

Thalamus (Gr. *thalamos* inner chamber.) Region of the diencephalon.

Theca (L. a case, sheath.) E.g., **intrathecal:** within the subarachnoid space.

Tomography (Gr. *tome* a cutting; *graphein* to write.) Sectional radiography.

Torcular (L. wine-press.) **Torcular Herophili:** the confluence of dural sinuses in the occipital region.

Tuber (L. knot, swelling.) E.g., **tuber cinereum:** elevation on the ventral surface of the diencephalon between the mammillary bodies and the optic chiasm.

Uncus (L. hook.) The hooked back portion of the rostral end of the parahippocampal gyrus.

Uncinate fasciculus. Fibers connecting the frontal and temporal lobes.

Utricle (L. little womb.) Region of the membraneous labyrinth.

Uvula (L. little grape.)

Velum (L. veil, curtain.) E.g., **superior medullary velum.**

Ventricle (L. *ventriculus* little belly.) E.g., **brain ventricles.**

Vermis (L. worm.) The median portion of the cerebellum.

Vertigo (L. movement.) Sensation of turning.

Appendix III

Bibliography

Adams RD, Victor M: Principles of Neurology. Second Edition. McGraw-Hill, New York, 1979.

Adams RD, Victor M: Principles of Neurology, McGraw-Hill, New York, pp. 52–59, 1977.

Afifi AK, Bergman RA: Basic Neuroscience, Urban and Schwarzenberg, Baltimore-Munich, 1980.

Angevine JB Jr, Cotman CW: Principles of Neuroanatomy, Oxford University Press, New York, 1981.

Bannister R: Brain's Clinical Neurology. Sixth Edition. Oxford University Press, Oxford, 1984.

Barr ML: The Human Nervous System, An Anatomical Viewpoint. Third Edition. Harper and Row, Hagerstown, 1979.

Bickerstaff ER: Neurological Examination in Clinical Practice. Third Edition. Blackwell Scientific Publications, Oxford, 1975.

Bourne GH, Ed.: Structure and Function of Nervous Tissue, Academic Press, New York, Vol. 1, 1968; Vol. 2, 1969; Vol. 3, 1969; Vol. 4, 1972; Vol. 5, 1972; Vol. 6, 1972.

Brodal A: Neurological Anatomy in Relation to Clinical Medicine. Third Edition. Oxford University Press, New York, 1981.

Bullock TH, Orkand R, Grinnell A: Introduction to Nervous Systems, WH Freeman, San Francisco, 1977.

Burrows EH, Leeds NE: Neuroradiology, Churchill Livingstone, New York, 1981.

Carpenter MB: Human Neuroanatomy. Seventh Edition. Williams and Wilkins, Baltimore, 1976.

Carpenter MB, Sutin J: Human Neuroanatomy. Eighth Edition. Williams and Wilkins, Baltimore, 1983.

Chusid JG: Correlative Neuroanatomy and Functional Neurology. Seventeenth Edition. Lange Medical Publications, Los Altos, 1979.

Cotman CW, McGaugh JL: Behavioral Neuroscience: An Introduction, Academic Press, New York, 1980.

Crosby EC, Humphrey T, Lauer EW: Correlative Anatomy of the Nervous System, Macmillan Co., New York, 1962.

Curtis BA, Jacobson S, Marcus EM: An Introduction to the Neurosciences, WB Saunders, Philadelphia, 1972.

Daube JR, Sandok BA, Regan TJ, Westmoreland BF: Medical Neurosciences: An Approach to Anatomy, Pathology and Physiology by Systems and Levels, Little, Brown and Co., Boston, 1978.

Edelman G, Mountcastle V: The Mindful Brain, MIT Press, Cambridge, 1978.

Everett NB: Functional Neuroanatomy. Sixth Edition. Lea and Febiger, Philadelphia, 1971.

Gardner E: Fundamentals of Neurology—A Psychophysiological Approach. Sixth Edition. WB Saunders, Philadelphia, 1975.

Gazzaniga MS, Ed.: Handbook of Cognitive Neuroscience, Plenum Press, New York, 1984.

Golden CJ, Vicente PJ, Eds.: Foundations of Clinical Neuropsychology, Plenum Press, New York, 1983.

Granit R: The Purpositive Brain, MIT Press, Cambridge, 1977.

Haughton VM, Ed.: Computer Tomography of the Spine. Contemporary Issues in Computed Tomography, Vol. 2. Churchill Livingstone, New York, 1983.

Heilman KM, Valenstein E: Clinical Neurophysiology. Second Edition. Oxford University Press, New York, 1984.

Heimer L: The Human Brain and Spinal Cord: Functional Neuroanatomy and Dissection Guide, Springer-Verlag, New York, 1983.

Herrick CJ: Neurological Foundations of Animal Behavior, Hafner, New York, 1962.

Herrick CJ: Brains of Rats and Men, Hafner, New York, 1963.

House EL, Pansky P, Siegel A: A Systematic Approach to Neuroscience. Third Edition. McGraw-Hill, New York, 1979.

Hubbard JI, Ed.: The Peripheral Nervous System, Plenum Press, New York, 1974.

Ingram WR: A Review of Anatomical Neurology, University Park Press, Baltimore, 1976.

Isaacson RL: The Limbic System, Plenum Press, New York, 1974.

Jacobson M: Developmental Neurobiology. Second Edition. Brain Books, Evanston, 1978.

Kandel ER, Schwatz JH, Eds.: Principles of Neural Science, Elsevier, New York, 1981.

Kuffler SW, Nicholls JC: A Cellular Approach to the Function of the Nervous System, Sinauer Associates, Sunderland, 1976.

Larsell O, Janssen J: The Comparative Anatomy and Histology of the Cerebellum, the Human Cerebellum, Cerebellar Connections and Cerebellar Cortex, University of Minnesota Press, Minneapolis, 1972.

Lewis AJ: Mechanisms of Neurological Disease, Little, Brown and Co., Boston, 1976.

Liebman M: Neuroanatomy Made Easy and Understandable, University Park Press, Baltimore, 1979.

Lockhart I: Desk Reference for Neuroanatomy: A Guide to Essential Terms, Springer-Verlag, New York, 1977.

Lorenz K: The Foundations of Ethology, Springer-Verlag, New York, 1981.

Lund RD: Development and Plasticity of the Brain: An Introduction, Oxford University Press, New York, 1978.

Martinez Martinez PFA: Neuroanatomy: Development and Structure of the Central Nervous System, WB Saunders, Philadelphia, 1982.

McGeer P, Eccles JC, McGeer E: Molecular Neurobiology of the Mammalian Brain, Plenum Press, New York, 1978.

Merrit H: A Textbook of Neurology. Sixth Edition. Lea and Febiger, Philadelphia, 1979.

Minckler J, Ed.: Introduction to Neuroscience, CV Mosby Co., St. Louis, 1972.

Moore KL: The Developing Human: Clinically Oriented Embryology. Second Edition. WB Saunders, Philadelphia, 1977.

Mountcastle VB, Ed.: Medical Physiology. Thirteenth Edition. Vol. 1. CV Mosby, St. Louis, 1974.

Noback CR, Demarest RJ: The Human Nervous System: Basic Principles of Neurobiology. Second Edition. McGraw-Hill, New York, 1975.

Noback CR, Demarest RJ: The Nervous System: Introduction and Review. Second Edition. McGraw-Hill, New York, 1977.

Nolte J: The Human Brain: An Introduction to Its Functional Anatomy, CV Mosby Co., St. Louis, 1981.

Palay SL, Chan-Palay V, Eds.: The Cerebellum—New Vistas, Experimental Brain Research, Supplementum 6, Springer-Verlag, New York, 1982.

Palm G: Neural Assemblies: An Alternative Approach to Artificial Intelligence, Studies of Brain Function, Vol. 7, Springer-Verlag, New York, 1982.

Pansky B, Allen DJ: Review of Neuroscience, Macmillan Co., New York, 1980.

Papez JW: Comparative Neurology, Crowell, New York, 1929.

Patten J: Neurological Differential Diagnosis, Springer-Verlag, New York, 1977.

Patton HD, Sundsten JW, Crill WE, Swanson PD: Introduction to Basic Neurology, WB Saunders, Philadelphia, 1976.

Pearlman AL, Collins RC, Eds.: Neurological Pathophysiology. Third Edition. Oxford University Press, New York, 1984.

Peele TL: The Neuroanatomic Basis for Clinical Neurology. Third Edition. McGraw-Hill, New York, 1977.

Peters A, Palay SL, Webster HdeF: The Fine Structure of the Nervous System: The Neurons and Supporting Cells, WB Saunders, Philadelphia, 1976.

Pfaff DW, Ed.: Ethical Questions in Brain and Behavior: Problems and Opportunities, Springer-Verlag, New York, 1983.

Pfeiffer SE, Ed.: Neuroscience Approached Through Cell Culture, Vol. 1, CPR Press, Inc., Boca Raton, 1982.

Pfeiffer SE, Ed.: Neuroscience Approached Through Cell Culture, Vol. 2, CPR Press, Inc., Boca Raton, 1983.

Popper KR, Eccles JC: The Self and Its Brain, Springer-Verlag, Heidelberg, 1977.

Poritsky R: Neuroanatomical Pathways, WB Saunders, Philadelphia, 1984.

Robertson DM, Dinsdale HB: The Nervous System, Structure and Function in Disease. Monograph Series, Williams and Wilkins Co., Baltimore, 1972.

Rosenberg RN, Ed.: The Clinical Neurosciences, Churchill Livingstone, New York, 1983.

Sarnat HB, Netsky MG: Evolution of the Nervous System, Oxford University Press, New York, 1974.

Shepherd GM: The Synaptic Organization of the Brain: An Introduction, Oxford University Press, New York, 1974.

Shepherd GM: Neurobiology, Oxford University Press, New York, 1983.

Sidman RL, Sidman M: Neuroanatomy: A Programmed Text, Vol. 1, Little, Brown and Co., Boston, 1965.

Snell RS: Clinical Neuroanatomy for Medical Students, Little, Brown and Co., Boston, 1980.

Tyrer JH, Sutherland JM, Eadie MJ: Exercises in Neurological Diagnosis, Churchill Livingstone, New York, 1981.

Watts GO: Dynamic Neuroscience: Its Application to Brain Disorders, Harper and Row, Publishers, Inc., Hagerstown, 1975.

Weiss PA: The Science of Life: The Living System—A System for Living, Futura, Mt. Kisco, 1973.

Williams PL, Warwick R: Functional Neuroanatomy of Man, WB Saunders, Philadelphia, 1975.

Willis WD, Grossman RG: Medical Neurobiology: Neuroanatomical and Neurophysiological Principles Basic to Clinical Neuroscience. Third Edition. CV Mosby Co., St. Louis, 1981.

Young JZ: Programs of the Brain, Oxford University Press, Oxford, 1978.

Atlases

Angevine JB Jr, Mancall EL, Yakovlev PI: The Human Cerebellum, An Atlas of Gross Topography in Serial Sections, Little, Brown and Co., Boston, 1961.

Babel J, Bischoff A, Spoendlin H: Ultrastructure of the Peripheral Nervous System and Sense Organs: Atlas of Normal and Pathologic Anatomy, CV Mosby Co., St. Louis, 1970.

Bertram EGM, Moore KL: An Atlas of the Human Brain and Spinal Cord, Williams and Wilkins, Baltimore, 1982.

Bossy J: Atlas of Neuroanatomy and Special Sense Organs, WB Saunders, Philadelphia, 1970.

Clemente CD: Anatomy: A Regional Atlas of the Human Body. Second Edition. Urban and Schwarzenberg, Baltimore, 1981.

Collins RD: Illustrated Manual of Neurologic Diagnosis, JB Lippincott Co., Philadelphia, 1962.

DeArmond SJ, Fusco MM, Dewey MM: Structure of the Human Brain: A Photographic Atlas. Second Edition. Oxford University Press, New York, 1976.

Dunkerley GB: A Basic Atlas of the Human Nervous System, FA Davis, Philadelphia, 1975.

Fix JD, Punte CS: Atlas of the Human Brain Stem and Spinal Cord, University Park Press, Baltimore, 1981.

Ford DH, Illari J, Schadé JP: Atlas of the Human Brain. Third Edition. Elsevier/North-Holland, Amsterdam and New York, 1978.

Gawler J, Bull JWD, Du Bourlay GH, Marshall

J: Computerized Axial Tomography: The Normal EMI Scan, J Neurol Neurosurg Psychiatry 38:935–947, 1975.

Gluhbegovic N, Williams TH: The Human Brain: A Photographic Guide, Harper and Row, Publishers, Inc., Hagerstown, 1980.

Haines DE: Neuroanatomy: An Atlas of Structures, Sections, and Systems, Urban and Schwarzenberg, Baltimore, 1983.

Heiss W-D, Phelps ME, Eds.: Positron Emission Tomography of the Brain, Springer-Verlag, New York, 1983.

Igarashi S, Kamiya T: Atlas of the Vertebrate Brain, University Park Press, Tokyo, 1972.

Ludwig E, Klingler J: Atlas Cerebri Humani, Little, Brown and Co., Boston, 1956.

Miller RA, Burack E: Atlas of the Central Nervous System in Man. Third Edition. Williams and Wilkins, Baltimore, 1982.

Montemurro DG, Bruni JE: The Human Brain in Dissection, WB Saunders, Philadelphia, 1981.

Netter FH: Nervous System, Part I, Anatomy and Physiology, CIBA Collection of Medical Illustrations, CIBA Pharmaceutical Co., Newark, 1958.

Nieuwenhuys R, Voogd J, van Huijzen C: The Human Central Nervous System: A Synopsis and Atlas. Second Edition. Springer-Verlag, Berlin-Heidelberg, 1981.

Peters A, Palay S, Webster HdeF: The Fine Structure of the Nervous System, WB Saunders, Philadelphia, 1976.

Rasmussen AT: Atlas of Cross Section Anatomy of the Brain: Guide to the Study of the Morphology and Fiber Tracts of the Human Brain, Blakiston Division, McGraw-Hill, New York, 1951.

Riley HA: An Atlas of the Basal Ganglia, Brain Stem and Spinal Cord, Hafner, New York, 1960.

Roberts M, Hanaway K: Atlas of the Human Brain in Section, Lea and Febiger, Philadelphia, 1970.

Salamon G: Atlas of the Arteries of the Human Brain, Sandoz Editions, Paris, 1973.

Schnitzlein HN, Hartley EW, Murtagh FR, Grundy L, Fargher JT: Computed Tomography of the Head and Spine: A Photographic Color Atlas of CT, Gross, and Microscopic Anatomy, Urban and Schwarzenberg, Baltimore, 1983.

Singer M, Yakovlev PI: The Human Brain in Sagittal Section, Charles C Thomas, Springfield, 1964.

Smith CG: Serial Dissections of the Human Brain, Gage Publishing Limited, Toronto, 1981.

Walmsley R, Murphy TR: Jamieson's Illustrations of Regional Anatomy. Ninth Edition. Section I. Central Nervous System, Churchill Livingstone, Edinburgh, 1971.

Watson C: Basic Human Neuroanatomy: An Introductory Atlas. Second Edition. Little, Brown and Co., Boston, 1977.

Wicke L: Atlas of Radiologic Anatomy. Third Edition. Urban and Schwarzenberg, Baltimore, 1982.

Zuleger S, Staubesand J: Atlas of the Central Nervous System in Sectional Planes, Urban and Schwarzenberg, Baltimore-Munich, 1977.

Index

Page numbers followed by f represent figures; numbers followed by t represent tables.